T0348628

Endocrine Hypertension

Editor

AMIR H. HAMRAHIAN

ENDOCRINOLOGY AND METABOLISM CLINICS OF NORTH AMERICA

www.endo.theclinics.com

Consulting Editor
ADRIANA G. IOACHIMESCU

December 2019 • Volume 48 • Number 4

ELSEVIER

1600 John F. Kennedy Boulevard • Suite 1800 • Philadelphia, Pennsylvania, 19103-2899

http://www.theclinics.com

ENDOCRINOLOGY AND METABOLISM CLINICS OF NORTH AMERICA Volume 48, Number 4
December 2019 ISSN 0889-8529, ISBN 13: 978-0-323-68323-4

Editor: Katerina Heidhausen
Developmental Editor: Casey Potter

Endocrinology and Metabolism Clinics of North America (ISSN 0889-8529) is published quarterly by Elsevier Inc., 360 Park Avenue South, New York, NY 10010-1710. Months of issue are March, June, September, and December. Periodicals postage paid at New York, NY and additional mailing offices. Subscription prices are USD 371.00 per year for US individuals, USD 761.00 per year for US institutions, USD 100.00 per year for US students and residents, USD 454.00 per year for Canadian individuals, USD 941.00 per year for Canadian institutions, USD 497.00 per year for international individuals, USD 941.00 per year for international institutions, and USD 245.00 per year for international and Canadian and foreign students/residents. To receive student/resident rate, orders must be accompanied by name of affiliated institution, date of term, and the signature of program/residency coordinator on institution letterhead. Orders will be billed at individual rate until proof of status is received. Foreign air speed delivery is included in all *Clinics* subscription prices. All prices are subject to change without notice. **POSTMASTER:** Send address changes to *Endocrinology and Metabolism Clinics of North America*, Elsevier Health Sciences Division, Subscription Customer Service, 3251 Riverport Lane, Maryland Heights, MO 63043. **Customer Service: Telephone: 1-800-654-2452** (U.S. and Canada); **1-314-447-8871** (outside U.S. and Canada). **Fax: 1-314-447-8029. E-mail: journalscustomerservice-usa@elsevier.com (for print support); journalsonlinesupport-usa@elsevier.com (for online support).**

Reprints. For copies of 100 or more, of articles in this publication, please contact the Commercial Rights Department, Elsevier Inc., 360 Park Avenue South, New York, NY 10010-1710; phone: +1-212-633-3874; fax: +1-212-633-3820; E-mail: reprints@elsevier.com.

Endocrinology and Metabolism Clinics of North America is covered in *MEDLINE/PubMed (Index Medicus), EMBASE/Excerpta Medica, Current Contents/Clinical Medicine, Current Contents/Life Sciences, Science Citation Index, ISI/BIOMED, BIOSIS,* and *Chemical Abstracts.*

Contributors

CONSULTING EDITOR

ADRIANA G. IOACHIMESCU, MD, PhD, FACE
Professor of Medicine (Endocrinology) and Neurosurgery, Emory University School of Medicine, Atlanta, Georgia, USA

EDITOR

AMIR H. HAMRAHIAN, MD
Associate Professor of Medicine, Division of Endocrinology, Diabetes and Metabolism, Johns Hopkins University, Baltimore, Maryland, USA

AUTHORS

SHOBANA ATHIMULAM, MBBS
Clinical Fellow, Division of Endocrinology, Diabetes, Metabolism and Nutrition, Mayo Clinic, Rochester, Minnesota, USA

IRINA BANCOS, MD
Consultant, Division of Endocrinology, Diabetes, Metabolism and Nutrition, Mayo Clinic, Rochester, Minnesota, USA

FILIPPO CECCATO, MD, PhD
Endocrinology Unit, Department of Medicine DIMED, University-Hospital of Padova, Padova, Italy

OSCAR H. CINGOLANI, MD
Associate Professor of Medicine, Division of Cardiology, Director, Hypertension Program, Johns Hopkins University Hospital, Baltimore, Maryland, USA

SALVATORE M. CORSELLO, MD
Professor, Endocrinology, Fondazione Policlinico Universitario Agostino Gemelli, IRCCS - Università Cattolica del Sacro Cuore, Rome, Italy

DANAE A. DELIVANIS, MD, PhD
Department of Endocrinology, Diabetes and Metabolism, Evangelismos Hospital, Athens, Greece; Division of Endocrinology, Diabetes, Metabolism, and Nutrition, Mayo Clinic, Rochester, Minnesota, USA

MURRAY D. ESLER, MB, PhD
Baker IDI Heart and Diabetes Institute, Melbourne, Australia; Dobney Hypertension Centre, Royal Perth Hospital Campus-University of Western Australia, Perth, Australia

MATTHEW C. FOY, MD
Division of Nephrology, Louisiana State University Health Science Center, Baton Rouge, Louisiana, USA

HANS K. GHAYEE, DO
Department of Medicine, Division of Endocrinology, University of Florida, Malcom Randall VA Medical Center, Gainesville, Florida, USA

MELISSA K. GONZALES, BS
Section on Medical Neuroendocrinology, *Eunice Kennedy Shriver* National Institute of Child Health and Human Development, National Institutes of Health, Bethesda, Maryland, USA

SRIRAM GUBBI, MD
Diabetes, Endocrinology, and Obesity Branch, National Institute of Diabetes and Digestive and Kidney Diseases, National Institutes of Health, Bethesda, Maryland, USA

FADY HANNAH-SHMOUNI, MD, FRCPC
Internal Medicine-Endocrinology, Hypertension, and Metabolic Genetics, Section on Endocrinology and Genetics, *Eunice Kennedy Shriver* National Institute of Child Health and Human Development, National Institutes of Health, Bethesda, Maryland, USA

SANDRA M. HERRMANN, MD
Associate Professor of Medicine, Division of Nephrology and Hypertension, Mayo Clinic, Rochester, Minnesota, USA

GREGORY L. HUNDEMER, MD, MPH
Division of Nephrology, Ottawa Hospital Research Institute, University of Ottawa, Ottawa, Ontario, Canada

CHRISTIAN A. KOCH, MD, PhD
Professor, The University of Tennessee Health Science Center, Memphis, Tennessee, USA

NATALIA LAZIK, MD, PhD
Senior Associate Consultant, Department of Internal Medicine, Mayo Clinic, Rochester, Minnesota, USA

GIUSEPPE MAIOLINO, MD, PhD
Clinica dell'Ipertensione Arteriosa, Department of Medicine, DIMED, University of Padova, Padova, Italy

DIVYA MAMILLA, MBBS
Section on Medical Neuroendocrinology, *Eunice Kennedy Shriver* National Institute of Child Health and Human Development, National Institutes of Health, Bethesda, Maryland, USA

FRANCO MANTERO, MD
Endocrinology Unit, Department of Medicine DIMED, University-Hospital of Padova, Padova, Italy

AARTI MATHUR, MD, FACS
Assistant Professor, Department of Surgery, Johns Hopkins University School of Medicine, Baltimore, Maryland, USA

LYNNETTE K. NIEMAN, MD
Senior Investigator, Diabetes, Endocrinology and Obesity Branch, The National Institute of Diabetes and Digestive and Kidney Diseases, National Institutes of Health, Bethesda, Maryland, USA

KAREL PACAK, MD, PhD, DSc, FACE
Chief, Section on Medical Neuroendocrinology, Professor of Medicine, *Eunice Kennedy Shriver* National Institute of Child Health and Human Development, National Institutes of Health, Bethesda, Maryland, USA

ROSA MARIA PARAGLIOLA, MD, PhD
Endocrinology, Fondazione Policlinico Universitario Agostino Gemelli, IRCCS - Università Cattolica del Sacro Cuore, Rome, Italy

JASON D. PRESCOTT, MD, PhD, FACS
Assistant Professor, Department of Surgery, Johns Hopkins University School of Medicine, Baltimore, Maryland, USA

SORAYA PUGLISI, MD
Internal Medicine 1, Department of Clinical and Biological Sciences, University of Turin, San Luigi Gonzaga Hospital, Orbassano, Italy

GIAN PAOLO ROSSI, MD, FAHA, FACC
Arterial Hypertension Unit, Clinica dell'Ipertensione Arteriosa, Department of Medicine, DIMED University Hospital, University of Padova, Padova, Italy

TERESA M. SECCIA, MD, PhD
Clinica dell'Ipertensione Arteriosa, Department of Medicine, DIMED, University of Padova, Padova, Italy

JESSICA SHANK, MD
Department of Surgery, Johns Hopkins University School of Medicine, Baltimore, Maryland, USA

J. DAVID SPENCE, MD, FRCPC, FAHA
Professor of Neurology and Clinical Pharmacology, Stroke Prevention & Atherosclerosis Research Centre, Robarts Research Institute, Western University, London, Ontario, Canada

CHRISTOPHER JOHN SPERATI, MD, MHS
Division of Nephrology, Johns Hopkins University School of Medicine, Baltimore, Maryland, USA

CONSTANTINE A. STRATAKIS, MD, D(Med)Sci
Scientific Director, *Eunice Kennedy Shriver* National Institute of Child Health and Human Development, National Institutes of Health, Bethesda, Maryland, USA

MASSIMO TERZOLO, MD
Internal Medicine 1, Department of Clinical and Biological Sciences, University of Turin, San Luigi Gonzaga Hospital, Orbassano, Italy

SERGEI G. TEVOSIAN, PhD
Department of Physiological Sciences, College of Veterinary Medicine, University of Florida, Gainesville, Florida, USA

STEPHEN C. TEXTOR, MD
Professor of Medicine, Division of Nephrology and Hypertension, Mayo Clinic, Rochester, Minnesota, USA

STYLIANOS TSAGARAKIS, MD, PhD, FRCP
Department of Endocrinology, Diabetes and Metabolism, Evangelismos Hospital, Athens, Greece

ANAND VAIDYA, MD, MMSc
Director, Center for Adrenal Disorders, Brigham and Women's Hospital, Harvard Medical School, Boston, Massachusetts, USA

JOBAN VAISHNAV, MD
Division of Cardiology, Johns Hopkins University School of Medicine, Baltimore, Maryland, USA

DIMITRA-ARGYRO VASSILIADI, MD, PhD
Department of Endocrinology, Diabetes and Metabolism, Evangelismos Hospital, Athens, Greece

Contents

Secondary hypertension is associated with increased cardiovascular risk and exaggerated target organ damage, not only due to the higher and more sustained blood pressure values often observed in these patients but also because certain forms of hypertension can increase cardiovascular risk and organ damage by the neurohormonal and/or molecular pathways activation they exert. Early identification of secondary forms of hypertension can help mitigate organ damage and prevent cardiovascular complications. Signs and symptoms distinction among types of secondary hypertension is essential in order to prevent complications.

Hypertension is one of the commonest chronic diseases contributing to cardiovascular disease. Idiopathic (primary) hypertension accounts for approximately 85% of the diagnosed cases, and 15% of hypertensive patients have other contributing conditions leading to elevated blood pressure (secondary hypertension). Endocrine hypertension is a common secondary cause of hypertension. The most common causes of endocrine hypertension are excess production of mineralocorticoids (ie, primary hyperaldosteronism), glucocorticoids (Cushing syndrome), and catecholamines (pheochromocytoma). After biochemical confirmation of hormonal excess, appropriate use of imaging modalities, both functional and anatomic, should occur for the diagnostic workup of these patients and for location of the source of hormonal excess.

Primary aldosteronism used to be considered a rare cause of secondary hypertension. However, accruing evidence indicates that primary aldosteronism is more common than previously recognized. The implications of this increased prevalence are important to public health because autonomous aldosterone production contributes to cardiovascular disease and can be treated in a targeted manner. This article focuses on clinical approaches for diagnosing primary aldosteronism more frequently and earlier in its course, as well as practical treatment objectives to reduce the risk for incident cardiovascular disease.

The clinical manifestations are similar but not identical to those in excess circulating catecholamines. The underlying symptomatic mechanism includes augmented cardiovascular responsiveness to catecholamines alongside heightened sympathetic nervous stimulation. The psychological characteristics are probably attributed to the component of repressed emotions related to a past traumatic episode or repressive coping style. Successful management can be achieved by strong collaboration between a hypertension specialist and a psychiatrist or psychologist with expertise in cognitive-behavioral panic management.

Renovascular disease (RVD) is a major cause of secondary hypertension. Atherosclerotic renal artery stenosis is the most common type of RVD followed by fibromuscular dysplasia. It has long been recognized as the prototype of angiotensin-dependent hypertension. However, the mechanisms underlying the physiopathology of hypertensive occlusive vascular renal disease are complex and distinction between the different causes of RVD should be made. Recognition of these distinct types of RVD with different degrees of renal occlusive disease is important for management. The greatest challenge is to individualize and implement the best approach for each patient in the setting of widely different comorbidities.

Hypertension is one of the most frequent complications in acromegaly, with a median frequency of 33.6% (range, 11%–54.7%). Although the pathogenesis has not been fully elucidated, it probably results from concomitant factors leading to expansion of extracellular fluid volume, increase of peripheral vascular resistance, and development of sleep apnea syndrome. Because the effect of normalization of growth hormone and insulinlike growth factor 1 excess on blood pressure levels is unclear, an early diagnosis of hypertension and prompt antihypertensive treatment are eagerly recommended, regardless of the specific treatment of the acromegalic disease and the level of biochemical control attained.

Essential hypertension is a highly prevalent disease in the general population. Secondary hypertension is characterized by a specific and potentially reversible cause of increased blood pressure levels. Some secondary endocrine forms of hypertension are common (caused by uncontrolled cortisol, aldosterone, or catecholamines production). This article describes rare monogenic forms of hypertension, characterized by electrolyte disorders and suppressed renin-aldosterone axis. They represent simple models for the physiology of renal control of sodium levels and plasma volume, thus reaching a high scientific interest. Furthermore, they could explain some features closer to the essential phenotype of hypertension, suggesting a mechanistically driven personalized treatment.

Jessica Shank, Jason D. Prescott, and Aarti Mathur

Increased hormonal secretion of aldosterone, cortisol, or catecholamines from an adrenal gland can produce a variety of undesirable symptoms, including hypertension, which may be the initial presenting symptom. Consequences of secondary hypertension can result in potential cardiovascular and cerebrovascular complications at higher rates than in those with essential hypertension. Once a biochemical diagnosis is confirmed, targeted pharmacotherapy can be initiated to improve hypertension and may be corrected with surgical intervention. Adrenalectomy can be curative and can reverse the risk of cardiovascular sequelae once blood pressure control is achieved. This article discusses perioperative and operative considerations of adrenal causes of hypertension.

ENDOCRINOLOGY AND METABOLISM CLINICS OF NORTH AMERICA

SERIES OF RELATED INTEREST

Medical Clinics
https://www.medical.theclinics.com

VISIT THE CLINICS ONLINE!
Access your subscription at:
www.theclinics.com

Foreword

Updates in Endocrine Hypertension

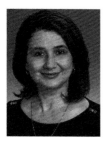

Adriana G. Ioachimescu, MD, PhD, FACE
Consulting Editor

The "Endocrine Hypertension" issue of the *Endocrinology and Metabolism Clinics of North America* is a collection of articles that provides an update on secondary causes of hypertension, with emphasis on hormonal factors. The guest editor is Dr Amir H. Hamrahian, Associate Professor of Medicine at Johns Hopkins University, a well-known expert in the field of adrenal and pituitary diseases who authored several American Association of Endocrinologists disease state reviews on adrenal nodules, Cushing disease, and acromegaly.

Systemic arterial hypertension is the most common modifiable risk factor for cardio-vascular morbidity and mortality. While primary hypertension affects approximately 90% patients, those with secondary hypertension are at risk of late diagnosis, delayed treatment, and detrimental health consequences. Case selection and appropriate choice of biochemical and radiological testing are of paramount importance. In this issue, the authors emphasize the diagnostic steps required for the diagnosis of primary aldosteronism, pheochromocytoma, paraganglioma, hypercortisolism, and acromegaly, as well as renovascular, drug-induced, and monogenic hypertension. In addition, the authors tackle new biochemical assays and update the readers on pertinent genetic testing. A separate article is dedicated to the adrenal venous sampling and its caveats.

Management of endocrine hypertension is multifaceted and requires a thorough understanding of disease pathogenesis and multidisciplinary approach. Our issue apprises the readers on surgical methods for removal of adrenal tumors causing endocrine hypertension as well as medical treatment options. In addition, refractory hypertension and hypertension during pregnancy are thoroughly reviewed in dedicated articles.

I hope you will find this issue of the *Endocrinology and Metabolism Clinics of North America* informative and helpful in your practice. This issue is a great resource for

Endocrinol Metab Clin N Am 48 (2019) xiii–xiv
https://doi.org/10.1016/j.ecl.2019.09.002
0889-8529/19/© 2019 Published by Elsevier Inc.

endo.theclinics.com

primary care physicians and internists who usually first evaluate the patients with hypertension as well as endocrinologists and other specialists. I thank Dr Hamrahian for guest editing this important issue and the authors for their excellent contributions. As always, I am grateful to the Elsevier editorial staff for their support.

Adriana G. Ioachimescu, MD, PhD, FACE
Emory University School of Medicine
1365 B Clifton Road, Northeast, B6209
Atlanta, GA 30322, USA

E-mail address:
aioachi@emory.edu

Preface

More Needs to Be Done for Patients with Endocrine Hypertension

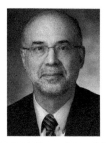

Amir H. Hamrahian, MD
Editor

Hypertension is one of the most common health disorders contributing to significant morbidity and mortality. By a conservative estimate, about 5% to 10% of patients with hypertension have a secondary identifiable endocrine cause in the general primary care office setting. This number increases up to 20% in patients with a more severe hypertension. The ability to come up with an identifiable cause is of great importance since in many instances effective medical and surgical treatment is available, with the potential for a cure. Understanding the underlying pathophysiology has improved our strategies of tackling these challenging cases by improving our case selection, and through biochemical as well as radiologic approaches in the past couple of decades.

Endocrine hypertension is an area that requires continued education. Many clinicians may be less familiar with the scope of the disease compared with some of the other disciplines, such as diabetes, thyroid, and bone disorders, which make up the bulk of their practice. The proper identification of patients to be screened for endocrine hypertension is crucial. A relaxed screening approach will overwhelm clinicians by having them deal with many false positive results, and a restrictive approach will decrease the chance of identifying causes that are potentially curable in many instances.

Among the important barriers in proper evaluation of patients with endocrine hypertension is the lack of significant experience with rarer disorders, a shortage of resources, and adequate time necessary for proper evaluation of such patients in busy clinical practices. The lack of expertise to handle such patients may lead to proper evaluation and treatment in only a fraction of the patients.

An important update in the current issue is a significant change in our understanding of primary aldosteronism and the scope of the disease from an uncommon disease to a common condition. This may extend to even normotensive patients with an impact on

Endocrinol Metab Clin N Am 48 (2019) xv–xvi
https://doi.org/10.1016/j.ecl.2019.09.001
0889-8529/19/© 2019 Published by Elsevier Inc.

their cardiovascular morbidity and mortality. Treatment of patients with subtle forms of autonomous hyperaldosteronism may have an impact on reducing their long-term complications.

The general trend toward measuring several endocrine hormones by liquid chromatography with tandem mass spectrometry provides us with an opportunity for better diagnosis and monitoring, and the challenge of revisiting the previously established diagnostic cutoffs. There will be a learning curve in our implementation of new assays in the evaluation of patients with suspected endocrine hypertension with more studies to come.

The current issue is primarily designed for clinicians with practical information on biochemical evaluation, imaging studies, differential diagnosis, and clinically relevant updates on genetic testing by some of the experts in the field. This is another step toward the management of a complex and frequently challenging disorder for which many of us do not receive enough training.

Amir H. Hamrahian, MD
Division of Endocrinology, Diabetes and Metabolism
Johns Hopkins University
1830 East Monument Street, Suite 333
Baltimore, MD 21287, USA

E-mail address:
ahamrah1@jhmi.edu

Cardiovascular Risks and Organ Damage in Secondary Hypertension

Oscar H. Cingolani, MD

KEYWORDS

- Target organ damage • Secondary hypertension • Cardiovascular risk • Assessment
- Risk factors

KEY POINTS

- Secondary hypertension is associated with increased cardiovascular risk and exaggerated target organ damage.
- Early identification of secondary forms of hypertension can help mitigate organ damage and prevent cardiovascular complications.
- Signs and symptoms distinction among types of secondary hypertension is essential in order to prevent complications.

Worldwide, approximately 3.5 billion adults have blood pressure (BP) levels that are suboptimal and roughly 900 million adults have a systolic BP of greater than or equal to 140 mm Hg. Between 1990 and 2015, there was a 43% increase in the total global number of healthy life years lost to suboptimal BP control. The Global Burden of Disease study has shown that uncontrolled hypertension continues to be the most important single-risk factor contributing to all-cause mortality, leading to 9.4 million deaths and more than 200 million lost in healthy life years each year.[1] Hypertension is the number one preventable risk factor for cardiovascular disease, chronic kidney disease, and cognitive impairment and is the leading single cause for disability.[1] High BP should not be seen as a binary problem. The relationship between BP and risk is continuous, starting at BPs as low as 115/75 mm Hg.[1,2] Successful prevention and treatment of hypertension (even lowering BP by a few mm Hg) is key to reducing disease burden and promoting longevity in the world's population.[2]

Patients with secondary hypertension carry an increased cardiovascular risk and greater impact on target organs, not only due to the higher and more sustained BP values often observed in these patients but also because certain forms of

Disclosures: The author has nothing to disclose.
Division of Cardiology, Hypertension Program, Johns Hopkins University Hospital, 601 North Caroline Street, Outpatient Center, 7th Floor, Suite 7263, Baltimore, MD 21287, USA
E-mail address: ocingol1@jhmi.edu

Endocrinol Metab Clin N Am 48 (2019) 657–666
https://doi.org/10.1016/j.ecl.2019.08.015
0889-8529/19/© 2019 Elsevier Inc. All rights reserved.

endo.theclinics.com

hypertension, as described later, can increase cardiovascular risk and organ damage by the neurohormonal and/or molecular pathways activation they exert. For example, angiotensin-II and aldosterone play a crucial part in hypertension as well as in target organ damage and cardiovascular risk (relative risk). Catecholamines can activate platelets and increase the risk of stroke and acute coronary events. Those hypertension animal models characterized by elevated levels of these hormones have revealed more renal and cardiac fibrosis as well as worsening hypertensive heart disease.[3] The author as well as other investigators have described the molecular machinery activated in high renin-angiotensin-aldosterone system models of hypertension, as well as its impact on cardiac structure and function.[4]

In this section, the author review those identifiable sources of hypertension that have been shown to carry an increased cardiovascular risk and briefly describe the mechanisms involved (**Table 1**), but before going through each specific scenario, it is important to understand that regardless of the secondary cause, BP can be in most instances controlled with antihypertensive drugs early in the course. A high degree of suspicion should alert the clinician to consider secondary forms when the impact on target organs (left ventricular hypertrophy, proteinuria, hypertensive retinopathy on fundoscopic eye examination) are often disproportionate for the degree of BP observed.

PRIMARY ALDOSTERONISM

Primary aldosteronism (PA) refers to inappropriately high aldosterone synthesis that is independent of the renin-angiotensin system and is not suppressed by sodium loading. If renal parenchymal disease is excluded, PA is now thought to be among the most common identifiable forms of hypertension. In the first 262 cases of PA diagnosed at the Mayo Clinic (1957–1986), the highest BP was 260/155 mm Hg and mean ($\pm$SD) was 184/112 $\pm$ 28/16 mm Hg.[5] Patients with aldosterone-producing adenomas tend to have higher BPs than those with idiopathic hyperaldosteronism. Hypokalemia led to muscle weakness and cramping, headaches, palpitations, polydipsia, polyuria, and nocturia. Periodic paralysis is a very rare presentation in whites, but it is not an infrequent in patients of Asian descent. Another rare presentation can be tetany associated with a decrease in ionized calcium and marked hypokalemic alkalosis.[5]

By binding to the mineralocorticoid receptor, aldosterone induces nongenomic effects (that is, without directly modifying gene expression) that include activation of the amiloride sensitive sodium channel, commonly known as the epithelial sodium channel, and results in the stimulation of renal sodium reabsorption in the cortical collecting duct.[6] Aldosterone also has many other effects that contribute to endothelial dysfunction, vasoconstriction, and hypertension.[6] These include vascular smooth muscle cell proliferation, fibroblast activation and vascular extracellular matrix deposition, vascular remodeling, fibrosis, and increased oxidative stress,[6] all of which are responsible for causing diastolic dysfunction, stiffness of the arteries, and renal failure.

Different studies suggest that patients with PA have more pronounced target organ damage (TOD) and experience more cardiovascular events. Those with persistent hypokalemia are at increased risk of developing medullary renal cysts, with progressive renal failure. This feature can also help clinicians to suspect PA when these typical findings are seen on renal imaging studies.[7] When matched for BP levels and duration of hypertension, PA patients have exaggerated cardiac hypertrophy and worsening diastolic function when compared with other forms of hypertension.[8] This is because of the known trophic effect of aldosterone on myocytes and other cells.[9] In patients with aldosterone-producing adenomas, adrenalectomy has been shown to reverse

Table 1
Secondary hypertension forms associated with increased cardiovascular risk and target organ damage

Condition	Prevalence	Impact on Target Organ and Cardiovascular Risk
Primary aldosteronism	5%–11%	Disproportionate cardiac hypertrophy; diastolic dysfunction; renal cysts with progressive renal failure. 2.5-fold increase in stroke, 1.7-fold increase in CAD, 3.5-fold increase in atrial fibrillation, and 2-fold increase in HF when compared with patients with primary hypertension.[11]
Renal artery stenosis	1%–5%	Associated with a 2-fold increase in CAD. Cardiovascular events and death is 16% per year, 6 times more frequent than end-stage renal disease.[12] If FMD present, suspect other vessels involved (carotids, cerebral, coronary arteries) with risk of dissection.
Obstructive sleep apnea	4%–6%	Augmented sympathetic tone leads to increased platelet reactivity, with enhanced risk for arrhythmias and acute coronary syndromes.[20–22] Increased aldosterone activity.
Cushing syndrome	0.1%	High prevalence (>60%) of glucose intolerance with metabolic syndrome (high LDL cholesterol, low HDL cholesterol), increased response to vasoconstrictors can complicate surgical procedures.[32] Similar risks as in PA due to the mineralocorticoid effects of steroids.
Pheochromocytoma	0.1%	Enhanced sympathetic tone increases the risk of arrhythmias, ACS, and HF. Suspect PHEO in acute HF syndromes mimicking myocarditis or stress cardiomyopathy.[36–38]
Hyperthyroidism	1%–2%	Systolic hypertension. Increased risk of arrhythmias (AF), tachycardia-induced cardiomyopathy.[43,44] Cardiac hypertrophy.[45]
Hypothyroidism	1%–10%	Diastolic hypertension. Hypercholesterolemia, heart failure (in severe cases). Increased risk of atrial fibrillation.
Coarctation of the aorta	4 in 10,000 live birth. 4%–6% of congenital heart defects.	Hypertension in upper extremities. Increased interstitial fibrosis in heart, kidneys, and arteries (secondary Aldo). Often associated with other congenital cardiac abnormalities.[49,50] Cardiac abnormalities can be reversed if treated early.

Abbreviations: ACS, acute coronary syndromes; AF, atrial fibrillation; CAD, coronary artery disease; FMD, fibromuscular dysplasia; HDL, high-density lipoprotein; HF, heart failure; LDL, low-density lipoprotein; PA, primary aldosteronism; PHEO, pheochromocytomas.

hypertrophy.[9] Milliez et al. showed that in patients with either aldosterone-producing adenoma or adrenal hyperplasia, the risk of stroke, atrial fibrillation, or myocardial infarction was elevated when compared with matched primary hypertensive controls without PA.[10] Finally, a large meta-analysis identified 31 studies including 3838 patients with PA and 9284 patients with primary hypertension. After a median of 8·8 years from the diagnosis of hypertension, and compared with patients with essential hypertension, those individuals with PA had an increased risk of stroke (odds ratio [OR] 2.58, 95% confidence interval [CI] 1.93–3.45), coronary artery disease (1.77, 1.10–2.83), atrial fibrillation (3.52, 2.06–5.99), and heart failure (2.05, 1.11–3.78).[11] These results were consistent for patients with both aldosterone-producing adenoma and bilateral adrenal hyperplasia, with no difference between these subgroups. Similarly, PA increased the risk of diabetes (OR 1.33, 95% CI 1.01–1.74), metabolic syndrome (1.53, 1.22–1.91), and left ventricular hypertrophy (2.29, 1.65–3.17).[11] Taking all this together, it is clear that suspecting PA with prompt diagnosis and treatment is essential to prevent morbidity and mortality in these patients.

RENAL ARTERY STENOSIS

As mentioned in the specific section, renal artery stenosis (RAS) is the most common form of secondary hypertension in certain countries, head to head with PA. RAS can be roughly divided into atherosclerotic disease and fibromuscular dysplasia (FMD). Early recognition of the latter is key, because these patients are often young, and interventional treatment is highly successful in curing the disease.

The risk of cardiovascular events increases exponentially with ascending levels of BP as in other conditions, yet the progression of renal failure is more pronounced than in primary hypertension. In a series involving 220 patients with atherosclerotic disease, followed by ultrasound, progression of renal stenosis was seen in 31% over 3 years, including in those without significant initial stenosis.[12] Of those with initial stenosis of less than 60%, 28% progressed, as opposed to 49% with renal arterial stenosis greater than 60%. RAS was associated with an almost 2-fold increased risk of coronary artery disease in the Cardiovascular Health Study.[13] In another study involving patients older than 65 years with new diagnosis of RAS, the risk of cardiovascular events and death was 16% per year, 6 times more than end-stage renal disease.[12]

If FMD is detected, other vascular beds (ie, cerebrovascular, coronary arteries) should be screened due to the prevalent association with other organs.[14] These patients can present with coronary artery or cerebrovascular arteries dissections, presenting with myocardial infarction or stroke, respectively.[15] Findings from the US registry for FMD showed that from 912 patients with this condition, aneurysm occurred in 200 patients (21.7%) and dissection in 237 patients (25.7%); in total, 384 patients (41.7%) had an aneurysm and/or a dissection by the time of FMD diagnosis. The extracranial carotid, renal, and intracranial arteries were the most common sites of aneurysm; dissection most often occurred in the extracranial carotid, vertebral, renal, and coronary arteries. Patients with FMD with dissection were younger at presentation (48.4 vs 53.5 years of age, respectively; $P<.0001$) and experienced more neurologic symptoms and other end-organ ischemic events than those without dissection. One-third of the patients with aneurysm (63 of 200) underwent therapeutic intervention for aneurysm repair.[15]

OBSTRUCTIVE SLEEP APNEA

Obstructive sleep apnea (OSA) has been associated with hypertension, and although some controversy exists, it is accepted by most as an identifiable cause of hypertension.[16,17] It is characterized by recurrent obstructive apneas and hypopneas caused by partial collapse of the upper airways during sleep. Both nocturnal (nondipping) and daytime BP are increased. Mechanism proposed to explain the BP elevation in OSA is increased sympathetic nerve activity.[18,19] As a result, these patients have more persistent BP elevations with the consequent increased cardiovascular risk. The augmented sympathetic tone has been linked to increased platelet aggregation and also risk for arrhythmias.[20–22] The hypoxemia observed in these patients plays a critical role in the risk, possibly due, at least in part, to activation of hypoxia-inducible factors.[23] Also, an overactive renin-angiotensin-aldosterone system has been described in this syndrome.[24] In fact, in patients with resistant hypertension and OSA, there seems to be an association between aldosterone levels and apnea-hypopnea episodes, whereas mineralocorticoid receptor blockers have been shown to improve apnea episodes and also lower BP in these patients.[25,26] In a study by Møller and colleagues,[27] patients with OSA had significantly increased BP and heart rate and a reduced nocturnal BP drop. Both angiotensin II and aldosterone were significantly higher in OSA than in control subjects. Positive correlations were found between angiotensin II and daytime BP. Continuous positive airway pressure (CPAP) therapy resulted in a decrease in BP, and this CPAP-induced reduction in BP was correlated with a decrease in both plasma renin and plasma angiotensin II concentration. Another study also found elevated levels of endothelin-1 (ET-1) in patients with OSA. ET-1 is a known vasoconstrictor, and elevated levels are associated with increased vascular and cardiac hypertrophy, inflammation, and cardiovascular disease.[28]

CUSHING SYNDROME

Cushing syndrome is a rare syndrome affecting 0.1% of the general population and resulting from prolonged exposure to excess glucocorticoids. Patients with this syndrome display a typical body habitus with obesity, facial plethora, buffalo hump, hirsutism, and purple striae.[29] Cardiovascular complications in patients with Cushing syndrome cause a mortality rate higher than that observed in a normal population. The latter is mainly due to metabolic alterations but also due to increased atherosclerosis and changes in cardiovascular structure and function.[30] In these patients, it is crucial to assess global cardiovascular risk and control not only hypertension but also other correlated risk factors, such as obesity, insulin resistance, dyslipidemia, and endothelial dysfunction. Increased low-density lipoprotein, decreased high-density lipoprotein, and glucose intolerance occur in 45% to 70% of patients with this condition,[31] yet this percentage could be an underestimate, because many patients with normal fasting glucose have underlying glucose intolerance, and not all patients with Cushing syndrome undergo glucose-tolerance testing. Cortisol-mediated vascular reactivity to vasoconstrictors and also the mineralocorticoid effects of cortisol are often seen in patients with Cushing syndrome, with a prevalence of approximately 80%.[32]

Complete normalization of hypercortisolism is often difficult in these patients, so close follow-up is warranted with aggressive risk factors modification. As an example, hypercortisolism carries a higher risk of myocardial rupture in patients suffering from myocardial infarction; therefore, special attention in this scenario is important.

PHEOCHROMOCYTOMA AND CATECHOLAMINE-INDUCED HYPERTENSION

Pheochromocytomas (PHEO) are tumors composed of chromafin cells that secrete cetecholamines, mainly adrenaline and noradrenaline. These tumors can be localized to the adrenal glands most of the time, yet extra adrenal PHEOs are also often found in roughly 10% of the cases. In half of the patients, PHEO produce a sustained and severe elevation of BP, as opposed to the classic "catecholamine crisis" described in the other half. Patients with this condition are sometimes quite difficult to diagnose, because they do not present with the classic symptoms. Adrenaline causes an increase in heart rate and contractility, whereas noradrenaline increases systemic vascular resistance. Zielen and colleagues[33] showed that patients with PHEO had more pronounced early TOD as compared with age- and gender-matched individuals with primary hypertension. In another study, only patients with PHEO with reverse nocturnal dipping in BP (paradoxic nocturnal elevation in BP) were the ones having more pronounced TOD.[34] These results can be confounded by the fact that night-time BP recording is not often measured in patients with PHEO. The levels of catecholamines have been shown to correlate to the impact on TOD in these patients.[35]

Patients with catecholamine excess do not always have PHEO. In fact, pseudo-pheochromocytoma is a condition that can be indistinguishable from PHEO. They present with episodic hypertension, and although some have mildly elevated levels of serum and/or urinary metanephrines, the final evaluation is negative for any cathecholamine-secreting tumor. In this setting, it is important to exclude other causes of catecholamine excess, such as stress, autonomic dysfunction/baroreflex failure, or medications/drugs. Patients with pseudopheochromocytoma seem to have an exaggerated cardiovascular response to catecholamines, with enhanced sympathetic nervous stimulation, therefore placing them at elevated cardiovascular risk. The exact mechanism is not totally understood, but elevated levels of dopamine, epinephrine, and norepinephrine have been identified as detrimental to the cardiovascular system.[36,37] Increasing number of reports suggest that PHEO should be suspected in cases of unexplained acute heart failure presentation.[38] Catecholamines are known to activate platelets, so these patients are also at increased risk of presenting with acute coronary syndromes and arrhythmias.[39–41] Occasionally, patients can present with primary adrenal hyperplasia, a condition mimicking PHEO but challenging to diagnose.[42]

THYROID DISEASE

Although not always suspected, and still neglected by some investigators, both hypo- and hyperthyroidism can be a cause of hypertension, and these patients can be at increased risk of developing TOD, independently of the levels of BP. Hypothyroidism often presents as diastolic hypertension, whereas hyperthyroidism as isolated systolic hypertension. Hypertension is caused by hypothyroidism in 3% of patients with high BP. Hypercholesterolemia is also associated with this scenario, thus increasing the risk of cardiovascular disease.[43]

Both hyperthyroidism and hypothyroidism produce changes in cardiac contractility, myocardial oxygen consumption, cardiac output, and systemic vascular resistance.[43] Although it is well known that hyperthyroidism can produce atrial fibrillation, it is less well recognized that hypothyroidism also predisposes to ventricular arrhythmias. In most cases, these cardiovascular changes are reversible when the underlying thyroid disorder is recognized and treated, therefore mandating early recognition.[43,44]

Thyroid hormone is an important regulator of cardiac gene expression. Hyperthyroidism in both humans and animal models leads to cardiac hypertrophy.[45] Cardiac genes that are modulated by thyroid hormones include sarcoplasmic reticulum Ca^{2+} adenosine triphosphatase (ATPase), phospholamban (both responsible for sarcoplasmic reticulum calcium handling), α-myosin and β-myosin heavy chains, sodium potassium ATPase (Na^+,K^+-ATPase), the voltage-gated potassium channels (Kv1.5, Kv4.2, Kv4.3), and the sodium calcium exchanger.[46,47] The β1 adrenergic receptor and thyroid hormone receptor α1 are positively and negatively regulated by thyroid hormone, respectively.[43]

COARCTATION OF THE AORTA

Coarctation of the aorta (CoA) is a recognized congenital heart disease, responsible for hypertension in the upper libs with decreased flow distal to the narrowed aorta. As a result, the heart and brain are exposed to markedly elevated BP, with secondary aldosteronism caused by renal hypoperfusion.[48,49] This leads to structural changes in the heart and vessels, leading to cardiac hypertrophy and extensive interstitial fibrosis that can result in dilated cardiomyopathy if not diagnosed and treated early.[50] It is associated with several other cardiac and vascular anomalies, such as bicuspid aortic valve, ventricular septal defect, patent ductus arteriosus, and aortic arch hypoplasia. Without treatment, the outcome for patients with CoA is poor. Historical data on the natural history of patients with CoA who survived beyond infancy showed a mean age of death of 34 years and 75% mortality by age 43 years. Death was from congestive heart failure, aortic dissection or rupture, endocarditis, and intracranial bleeding.[49] The most important noncardiac associated lesion is cerebral aneurysm present in up to 10% of patients. This is 5 times higher than that in the general population.[51] CoA can also be acquired: Takayasu disease and more rarely giant cell arteritis can present with narrowing of the aorta, producing similar TOD.[52] These patients have invariably high erythrocyte sedimentation rate on routine laboratory testing.

SUMMARY

Secondary forms of hypertension typically carry an increased cardiovascular risk and exaggerated TOD. These findings are due to the more sustain and often higher levels of BP seen in these patients, but also due to the secondary effect of hormones and the molecular machinery activated by these specific subtypes, leading to worsening interstitial fibrosis, cardiac hypertrophy and elevated incidence of stroke, renal failure, and coronary events. Clinicians should always think of secondary hypertension when evaluating these patients, and if criteria are met, then proceed with indicated testing for early recognition and treatment in order to mitigate damage and prevent cardiovascular events.

ACKNOWLEDGMENTS

This work was supported by the PJ Schafer memmorial award, The Dunk Hypertension Fund and The Magic that Matters Award.

REFERENCES

1. GBD 2015 Risk Factors Collaborators, Forouzanfar MH, Afshin A, Alexander LT, et al. Global, regional, and national comparative risk assessment of 79 behavioral, environmental and occupational, and metabolic risks or clusters of risks, 1990–2015: a systematic analysis for the Global Burden of Disease Study 2015. Lancet 2016;388:1659–724.
2. Blood Pressure Lowering Treatment Trialists' Collaboration. Blood pressure-lowering treatment based on cardiovascular risk: a meta-analysis of individual patient data. Lancet 2014;384:591–8.
3. Grassi G, Ram VS. Evidence for a critical role of the sympathetic nervous system in hypertension. J Am Soc Hypertens 2016;10(5):457–66.
4. Cingolani OH, Pérez NG, Ennis IL, et al. In vivo key role of reactive oxygen species and NHE-1 activation in determining excessive cardiac hypertrophy. Pflugers Arch 2011;462(5):733–43.

5. Young WF Jr, Klee GG. Primary aldosteronism. Diagnostic evaluation. Endocrinol Metab Clin North Am 1988;17:367–95.

6. Funder JW. Primary aldosteronism. Hypertension 2019;74(3):458–66.

7. Torres VE, Young WF Jr, Offord KP, et al. Association of hypokalemia, aldosteronism and renal cysts. N Engl J Med 1990;322:345–51.

8. Stowasser M, Sharman J, Leano R, et al. Evidence for abnormal left ventricular structure and function in normotensive individuals with familial hyperaldosteronism type I. J Clin Endocrinol Metab 2005;90(9):5070–6.

9. Rossi GP, Saccheto A, Visentin P, et al. Changes in left ventricular anatomy and function in patients with primary aldosteronism. Hypertension 1996;27:1039–45.

10. Milliez P, Girerd X, Plouin PF, et al. Evidence for an increased rate of cardiovascular events in patients with primary aldosteronism. J Am Coll Cardiol 2005;45(8):1243–8.

11. Monticoni S, D'Ascenzo F, Moretti C, et al. Cardiovascular events and target organ damage in primary aldosteronism compared with essential hypertension: a systematic review and meta-analysis. LancetDiabetes Endocrinol 2018;6(1):41–50.

12. Kalra PA, Guo H, Kausz AT, et al. Atherosclerotic renovascular disease in United States patients aged 67 years or older: risk factors, revascularization, and prognosis. Kidney Int 2005;68:293–301.

13. Edwards MS, Craven TE, Burke GL, et al. Renovascular disease and the risk of adverse coronary events in the elderly: a prospective, population-based study. Arch Intern Med 2005;165(2):207–13.

14. Slovut DP, Olin JW. Fibromuscular dysplasia. N Engl J Med 2004;350:1862–71.

15. Kadian-Dodov D, Gornik HL, Gu X, et al. Dissection and aneurysm in patients with fibromuscular dysplasia: findings from the U.S. registry for FMD. J Am Coll Cardiol 2016;68(2):176–85.

16. Pedrosa RP, Drager LF, Gonzaga CC, et al. Obstructive sleep apnea: the most common secondary cause of hypertension associated with resistant hypertension. Hypertension 2011;58:811–7.

17. Logan AG, Perlikowski SM, Mente A, et al. High prevalence of unrecognized sleep apnoea in drug-resistant hypertension. J Hypertens 2001;19:2271–7.

18. Fletcher EC. Sympathetic over activity in the etiology of hypertension of obstructive sleep apnea. Sleep 2003;26:15–9.

19. Leuenberger UA, Brubaker D, Quraishi S, et al. Effects of intermittent hypoxia on sympathetic activity and blood pressure in humans. Auton Neurosci 2005;121:87–93.

20. Alonso-Fernandez A, Garcia-Rio F, Racionero MA, et al. Cardiac rhythm disturbances and ST-segment depression episodes in patients with obstructive sleep apnea-hypopnea syndrome and its mechanisms. Chest 2005;127:15–22.

21. Ludka O, Konecny T, Somers V. Sleep apnea, cardiac arrhythmias, and sudden death. Tex Heart Inst J 2011;38(4):340–3.

22. Gong W, Wang X, Fan J, et al. Impact of obstructive sleep apnea on platelet function profiles in patients with acute coronary syndrome taking dual antiplatelet therapy. J Am Heart Assoc 2018;7(15):e008808.

23. Martinez CA, Kerr B, Jin C, et al. Obstructive sleep apnea activates HIF-1 in a hypoxia dose-dependent manner in HCT116 colorectal carcinoma cells. Int J Mol Sci 2019;20(2).

24. Goodfriend TL, Calhoun DA. Resistant hypertension, obesity, sleep apnea, and aldosterone: theory and therapy. Hypertension 2004;43:518–24.

25. Ke X, Guo W, Peng H, et al. Association of aldosterone excess and apnea-hypopnea index in patients with resistant hypertension. Sci Rep 2017;7:45241.
26. Yang L, Zhang H, Cai M, et al. Effect of spironolactone on patients with resistant hypertension and obstructive sleep apnea. Clin Exp Hypertens 2016;38(5):464–8.
27. Møller DS, Lind P, Strunge B, et al. Abnormal vasoactive hormones and 24-hour blood pressure in obstructive sleep apnea. Am J Hypertens 2003;16(4):274–80.
28. Gjørup PH, Sadauskiene L, Wessels J, et al. Abnormally increased endothelin-1 in plasma during the night in obstructive sleep apnea: relation to blood pressure and severity of disease. Am J Hypertens 2007;20(1):44–52.
29. Raff H, Carroll T. Cushing's syndrome: from physiological principles to diagnosis and clinical care. J Physiol 2015;593(3):493–506.
30. Marchand L, Segrestin B, Lapoirie M, et al. Dilated cardiomyopathy revealing cushing disease: a case report and literature review. Medicine (Baltimore) 2015;94(46):e2011.
31. Pivonello R, De Leo M, Vitale P, et al. Pathophysiology of diabetes mellitus in Cushing's syndrome. Neuroendocrinology 2010;92(Suppl 1):77–81.
32. Torpy DJ, Mullen N, Ilias I, et al. Association of hypertension and hypokalemia with Cushing's syndrome caused by ectopic ACTH secretion: a series of 58 cases. Ann N Y Acad Sci 2002;970:134–44.
33. Zielen P, Peczkowska M, Prejbisz A, et al. Early target organ damage in patients with pheochromocytoma, obstructive sleep apnea and essential hypertension. J Hypertens 2010;28:e307–8.
34. Petrák O, Rosa J, Holaj R, et al. Blood pressure profile, catecholamine phenotype and target organ damage in pheochromocytoma/paraganglioma. J Clin Endocrinol Metab 2019. https://doi.org/10.1210/jc.2018-02644.
35. Noshiro T, Watanabe T, Akama H, et al. Changes in clinical features and long-term prognosis in patients with pheochromocytoma. Am J Hypertens 2000;13(1 Pt 1):35–43.
36. Garcha AS, Cohen DL. Catecholamine excess: pseudopheochromocytoma and beyond. Adv ChronicKidney Dis 2015;22(3):218–23.
37. Brener MI, Keramati AR, Mirski MA, et al. A sudden change of heart: a case of rapidly reversed stress cardiomyopathy in a critically ill patient. Cardiol Res 2016;7(3):119–21.
38. Afana M, Panchal RJ, Simon RM, et al. Pheochromocytoma-induced Takotsubo cardiomyopathy. Tex Heart Inst J 2019;46(2):124–7.
39. Tafreshi S, Naqvi SY, Thomas S. Extra-adrenal pheochromocytoma presenting as inverse takotsubo-pattern cardiomyopathy treated with surgical resection. BMJCase Rep 2018;11(1).
40. Anderson EJ, Efird JT, Kiser AC, et al. Plasma catecholamine levels on the morning of surgery predict post-operative atrial fibrillation. JACC Clin Electrophysiol 2017;3(12):1456–65.
41. Chen S, Du C, Shen M, et al. Sympathetic stimulation facilitates thrombopoiesis by promoting megakaryocyte adhesion, migration, and proplatelet formation. Blood 2016;127(8):1024–35.
42. Cingolani OH, Heath J, McDonald M. A Nervous Heart. Circulation 2014;129(9):e358–9.
43. Klein I, Danzi S. Thyroid disease and the heart. Circulation 2007;116(15):1725–35 [Review].
44. Kahaly GJ, Dillmann WH. Thyroid hormone action in the heart. Endocr Rev 2005;26:704–28.

45. Biondi B, Palmieri EA, Fazio S, et al. Endogenous subclinical hyperthyroidism affects quality of life and cardiac morphology and function in young and middle-aged patients. J Clin Endocrinol Metab 2000;85:4701–5.
46. Ladenson PW, Sherman SI, Baughman KL, et al. Reversible alterations in myocardial gene expression in a young man with dilated cardiomyopathy and hypothyroidism. Proc Natl Acad Sci US A 1992;89:5251–5.
47. Klein I, Ojamaa K. Thyroid hormone and the cardiovascular system. N Engl J Med 2001;344:501–9.
48. Torok RD, Campbell MJ, Fleming GA, et al. Coarctation of the aorta: management from infancy to adulthood. World J Cardiol 2015;7(11):765–75.
49. Campbell M. Natural history of coarctation of the aorta. Br Heart J 1970;32(5): 633–40.
50. Cangussu LR, Lopes MR, Barbosa RHA. The importance of the early diagnosis of aorta coarctation. Rev Assoc Med Bras(1992) 2019;65(2):240–5.
51. Alkashkari W, Albugami S, Hijazi ZM. Management of coarctation of the aorta in adult patients: state of the art. Korean Circ J 2019;49(4):298–313.
52. Lande A. Takayasu's arteritis and congenital coarctation of the descending thoracic and abdominal aorta: a critical review. AJR Am J Roentgenol 1976; 127(2):227–33.

Adrenal Imaging in Patients with Endocrine Hypertension

Danae A. Delivanis, MD, PhD[a,b,1],
Dimitra-Argyro Vassiliadi, MD, PhD[a],
Stylianos Tsagarakis, MD, PhD, FRCP[a,*]

KEYWORDS

- Computed tomography • Endocrine hypertension • Magnetic resonance imaging
- Radionuclide imaging • Cushing syndrome • Pheochromocytoma
- Primary aldosteronism

KEY POINTS

- Endocrine adrenal hypertension is a common cause of secondary hypertension. Biochemical confirmation of the disease should occur before using imaging modalities.
- Primary aldosteronism is a common cause of secondary hypertension. Once biochemically confirmed, abdominal computed tomographic (CT) imaging followed by adrenal venous sampling is the most commonly used diagnostic test to identify the source of hormonal excess (unilateral vs bilateral disease).
- In adrenocorticotropic hormone–independent Cushing syndrome, abdominal CT and MRI are the main imaging modalities used, whereas adrenal venous sampling may be considered in selected cases.
- Catecholamine-secreting tumors are located in adrenal and extraadrenal, predominantly abdominal, sites.
- Anatomic imaging is useful to locate these tumors. Various functional imaging modalities are available for tumor localization and for identification of patients who may benefit from radiopharmaceutical therapy.

INTRODUCTION

Hypertension is one of the commonest health burdens contributing to cardiovascular morbidity and mortality. In the vast majority hypertension is idiopathic. In a substantial proportion of patients, particularly in children and young adults, hypertension is

The authors have nothing to disclose.
[a] Department of Endocrinology, Diabetes and Metabolism, Evangelismos Hospital, 45 Ipsilantou Street, Athens 106 76, Greece; [b] Division of Endocrinology, Diabetes, Metabolism, and Nutrition, Mayo Clinic, Rochester, MN, USA
[1] Present address: Riga Feraiou 48-50, Patras 26221, Greece.
* Corresponding author.
E-mail address: stsagara@otenet.gr

Endocrinol Metab Clin N Am 48 (2019) 667–680
https://doi.org/10.1016/j.ecl.2019.08.001
0889-8529/19/© 2019 Elsevier Inc. All rights reserved.

endo.theclinics.com

secondary to a distinct cause that can be diagnostically detected and therapeutically cured. Among the secondary causes, endocrine hypertension is common, and among the endocrine hypertension cases adrenal causes are the most prevalent. Adrenal endocrine hypertension is diagnosed in patients with excess production of mineralocorticoids (primary aldosteronism), glucocorticoids (Cushing syndrome [CS]), and catecholamines (pheochromocytoma).[1] Because hormones are not "visualized," adrenal imaging cannot be used to establish the diagnosis of these conditions. Nevertheless, following a biochemical diagnosis, adrenal imaging plays a pivotal role in the diagnostic workup of these disorders. In this article, structural and functional adrenal imaging modalities in current use are presented and reviewed.

ADRENAL IMAGING IN PRIMARY HYPERALDOSTERONISM

Primary aldosteronism (PA) is responsible for 5% to 13% of cases of hypertension.[2,3] The most frequent causes of PA are bilateral idiopathic hyperaldosteronism (or idiopathic hyperplasia [IHA], 60%–70%) and unilateral aldosterone-producing adenomas (APAs) (30%–40%).[1] Less common forms include unilateral adrenal hyperplasia (caused by micronodular or macronodular hyperplasia of the zona glomerulosa), pure aldosterone producing adrenocortical carcinomas, different types of familial hyperaldosteronism, and ectopic aldosterone-secreting tumors.

It has long been appreciated that radiology plays no role in the initial diagnosis of PA. The diagnosis of PA is solely biochemical. Once the diagnosis of PA has been established, it is crucial to distinguish between the principal causes of PA, namely between unilateral and bilateral disease, as treatment options are different. Differentiating between these 2 entities on clinical and biochemical grounds is imprecise.

Cross-sectional Imaging—Abdominal Computed Tomography and MRI

Once the diagnosis of PA has been confirmed, the patient should undergo abdominal computed tomography (CT) with 2- to 3-mm thick slices of the adrenal glands. APAs usually present as solitary, low (<10) Hounsfield units (HU) density in unenhanced CT imaging; diffuse hyperplasia is characterized by diffuse uniform thickening of adrenal cortex, which maintains the normal adrenal architecture (**Fig. 1**A). Nodules may be microscopic (micronodular) or visible (macronodular). When a unilateral, large (>4 cm) heterogeneous adrenal mass with internal calcifications and hemorrhages is found on CT in a patient with PA, then adrenocortical carcinoma should be suspected.[4] Several studies have compared diagnostic performance of CT with MRI.[5,6] Although there are no significant differences in the diagnostic performance between these 2 imaging procedures, adrenal CT has been more widely used thanks to its superior spatial resolution, lower cost, and more widespread experience and availability.

The limitations of adrenal CT imaging (**Table 1**) are that (1) APAs can be as small as 3 mm in size and therefore easily missed on CT imaging; (2) patients with hyperplasia may have almost normal-appearing adrenal glands on CT, making it hard to differentiate between small APAs and adrenal hyperplasia[7]; and (3) the prevalence of nonfunctioning adrenal adenomas is high especially in the elderly population and therefore many patients with biochemical evidence of PA and a unilateral adrenal mass turn out to have bilateral hyperplasia, and patients with bilateral lesions may end up having aldosteronoma in one adrenal gland and a nonfunctioning adrenal nodule in the other.[8,9]

Based on current guidelines adrenal venous sampling (AVS) is the gold-standard examination to differentiate between unilateral versus bilateral disease.[10] In a systematic

A

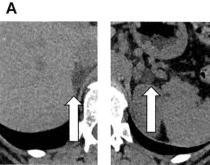

Vein	Aldosterone pg/ml	Cortisol µg/dl	Aldosterone/ Cortisol	Lateralization Ratio
R adrenal vein	39,000	1,100	36	1.4
Peripheral vein	382	25		
L adrenal vein	9,100	350	26	
Peripheral vein	461	23		

B

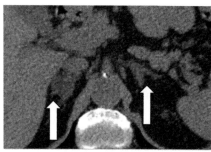

Vein	Aldosterone pg/ml	Cortisol µg/dl	Aldosterone/ Cortisol	Lateralization Ratio
L adrenal vein	>20,000	646	31	23.1
R adrenal vein	1,660	1,230	1.3	
Peripheral vein	366	37.4		

Fig. 1. (*A*) Axial images of unenhanced adrenal CT in a 56-year-old woman with resistant hypertension and PA showing bilateral adrenal nodules (*left* 1.3 cm, *right* 1.4 cm) (*arrows*). Sequential adrenal venous sampling with ACTH stimulation demonstrated bilateral aldosterone secretion (lateralization index<4). (*B*) Axial image from unenhanced adrenal CT in a 62-year-old man with resistant hypertension and PA shows a right adrenal nodule 2.5 cm in diameter and a normal-appearing left adrenal (*arrows*). Simultaneous bilateral adrenal venous sampling with ACTH stimulation lateralized cortisol to the left adrenal gland leading to successful laparoscopic left adrenalectomy. ACTH, adrenocorticotropic hormone.

Table 1
Advantages and disadvantages of adrenal imaging methods for subtyping patients with primary aldosteronism

Modalities	Advantages	Disadvantages
Computed tomography	• High spatial resolution • Concurrent evaluation of other organs • Widely available • Noninvasive • Relative cheap	• High/moderate radiation exposure • Contrast media use • Limited sensitivity • Not specific anatomic information
Nuclear imaging NP-59	• Detection of hypermetabolic adrenal tumors that may be missed on CT or MRI	• Poor spatial resolution • Less anatomic information • Time consuming, high radiation exposure • Tracer not widely available
Metomidate imaging	• Specific binding to CYP11B2 • Noninvasive	• Limited availability (cyclotron needed) • Radiation exposure moderate • Lower selectivity to CYP11B2 than CYP11B1 • Very limited data available
18F-CDP2230	• Higher selectivity to CYP11B2 than CYP11B1	• Very limited data

review of 38 studies (950 patients with PA), adrenal CT/MRI results were discordant to AVS in 37.8% of cases (using AVS as the gold standard).[11] If only imaging was considered, then 14.6% of patients with bilateral hyperplasia would have undergone inappropriate unilateral adrenalectomy, 19.1% with unilateral secretion on AVS would have been offered medical therapy instead of curative adrenalectomy, and 3.9% would have undergone adrenalectomy on the wrong side given that AVS showed unilateral secretion on the opposite side of CT/MRI abnormalities (**Fig. 1**B).[11]

In an attempt to improve specificity of adrenal CT imaging, several investigators have measured intracellular lipid content of APAs on unenhanced CT imaging[12] or chemical shift on MRI[13] and compared it with that of nonfunctioning adrenal adenomas. Results, however, were equivocal, and there was a large overlap in lipid content between APAs and nonfunctioning adenomas. Similarly, to improve diagnostic performance of CT in diagnosing IHA, several investigators have proposed measuring adrenal limb width on CT to differentiate IHA from APA.[14,15] In a retrospective study of 28 patients with PA, Lingam and colleagues[15] showed that a mean adrenal limb width of greater than 3 mm reached a sensitivity of 100% to diagnose IHA and an adrenal mean limb width greater than 5 mm achieved a specificity of 100%. Based on a proposed algorithm by Lingman and colleagues, adrenal gland width greater than 5 mm highly suggests IHA; however, in most of the cases adrenal gland width is less than 5 mm and therefore AVS is again the test of choice.

Adrenal Functional Imaging—Adrenal Scintigraphy

It is widely accepted that AVS provides the best lateralization for PA etiology.[16] However, occasionally AVS is not readily available and/or AVS results are inconclusive or contradict the CT results. Under these circumstances, several investigators in the past supported the use of functional adrenal imaging with I-131-6β-iodomethyl-19-norcholesterol (NP-59) scintigraphy as a supplementary diagnostic tool.[17]

I-131 NP-59 is a radiolabeled cholesterol analogue that circulates in the blood stream bound to low-density lipoproteins and is taken up and stored in adrenocortical cells. Preparation for this test is cumbersome and complicated. Dexamethasone (8 mg per day for >1 week) is needed to suppress the radiopharmaceutical uptake to the normal adrenal gland, and[18] scanning is usually performed in multiple occasions after intravenous injection of I-131 NP-59. Unilateral uptake on early images indicates unilateral adenoma or unilateral hyperplasia. Symmetric uptakes on early images suggest bilateral autonomous hyperplasia.[19] The reported sensitivity for detecting an APA varies widely, ranging from 47% to 100%[20–22] and depends mainly on the size of the adenoma.[22,23] A lateralizing scan can be seen in nonfunctional adrenal cortical adenomas (false positive), and uptake of the tracer is poor in small APAs (false negative). Overall, I-131 NP-59 scintigraphy has been mostly abandoned due to several major disadvantages (see **Table 1**).

Functional Adrenal Imaging Using Radiolabeled PET Tracers

In most recent years, new promising radioisotope agents specific for adrenocortical tissue coupled with PET/CT imaging are being studied in patients with PA.[24] Specifically, radioisotopes with high binding specificity to CYP11B2 (aldosterone synthase) are of critical importance in adrenal imaging of patients with PA. CYP11B2 is the key enzyme in aldosterone synthesis, and it has been reported that in smaller APAs, the expression density of CYP11B1 (11β-hydroxylase) decreases and that of CYP11B2 increases.[25] Therefore, for subtyping patients with PA, a molecular tracer specific to CYP11B2 is of critical importance.[26]

Great interest was first developed on ^{11}C-metomidate, the methyl analogue of etomidate, a potent inhibitor of CYP11B1 and CYP11B2. Burton and colleagues[27] studied 39 patients with PA and 5 with nonfunctioning adenomas. ^{11}C-metomidate when coupled with PET/CT imaging and after dexamethasone pretreatment, achieved a sensitivity of 76% and specificity of 87% to distinguish unilateral APAs from bilateral idiopathic hyperplasia when compared with AVS. However, diagnostic accuracy was not high enough for ^{11}C-metomidate PET/CT to replace AVS.

Using another etomidate derivative, ^{123}I-iodometomidate, Hahner and colleagues[28] studied 51 patients with relative large (median tumor size 5.6 cm, range 2.3–21.7 cm) adrenal tumors and found that ^{123}I-iodometomidate was successful in differentiating adrenocortical tumors from lesions of nonadrenocortical origin with a sensitivity of 89% and specificity of 85%. However, no significant association of tracer uptake with hormonal activity was observed.

Despite these promising results, ^{11}C-metomidate agents can only be used in medical centers in close proximity to a cyclotron due to their short half-life; they cannot differentiate between benign and malignant adrenocortical lesions given that both express CYP11B enzymes and show low selectivity for CYP11B2 over CYP11B1 enzymes, therefore mandating dexamethasone pretreatment in order to avoid accumulation of the agents in normal adrenal tissue.

In order to overcome some of the above limitations, promising results arise from in vitro and animal studies of the newer radioisotope ^{18}F-CDP2230. In the study of Abe and colleagues,[29] ^{18}F-CDP2230, compared with ^{11}C-metomidate, showed a 15 times higher selectivity for CYP11B2 over CYP11B1 and was accumulated in the adrenal glands with low background uptake, making it an attractive diagnostic test in patients with PA. Whether ^{18}F-CDP2230 distinguishes APA from hyperplasia remains to be investigated.

Gaining more experience with these newer radioisotopes may eventually prevail their use as an adjuvant diagnostic tool in patients with PA with inconclusive results on AVS or when AVS is not available.

ADRENAL IMAGING IN CUSHING SYNDROME

Hypertension is one of the most frequent features of CS occurring in 75% to 80% of patients.[30] CS is characterized by autonomous and excessive secretion of cortisol and should be considered when a hypertensive patient presents with central obesity, muscle weakness, supraclavicular fat pad, and easy bruising. CS is either adrenocorticotropic hormone (ACTH) dependent or ACTH independent. ACTH-dependent CS accounts for approximately 85% of cases and in 15% to 20% of the cases the cause is a primary adrenal neoplasm, most likely an adenoma or less likely adrenal carcinoma or bilateral adrenal nodular hyperplasia.

Cross-sectional Imaging with Computed Tomography and MRI

In ACTH-independent CS adrenal CT and/or MRI is the primary imaging modality for localization of the lesion and for ruling out adrenocortical cancer.[31] No differentiation can be made between cortisol-secreting adenomas and benign nonfunctioning adrenal masses based on imaging features alone. Hyperfunctioning adenomas are typically homogenous with smooth borders and with increased intracellular lipid content, conferring low attenuation on unenhanced CT imaging (**Fig. 2**A) and typical signal drop-out of 40% at chemical shift imaging.[32] On contrast-enhanced CT, performed 15 minutes after intravenous contrast administration, adenomas show both a rapid enhancement and a rapid washout loss of contrast, whereas nonadenomas

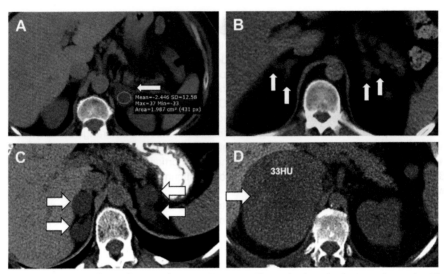

Fig. 2. (*A*) ACTH-independent CS due to a 2.8 cm unilateral adrenal adenoma (*arrow*) with low attenuation (−2.4 HU). (*B*) Bilateral micronodular adrenal hyperplasia with almost normal-appearing adrenal glands and multiple small nodules of less than 5 mm in size (*arrows*). (*C*) Primary bilateral macronodular adrenal hyperplasia, with bilateral large distinct adrenal nodules (*arrows*). (*D*) A 14 cm adrenocortical carcinoma (*arrow*) with high attenuation (>10 HU) on unenhanced CT.

typically show a slower contrast washout phase. When the 15-minute delay protocol is used, contrast-enhanced washout studies have 100% sensitivity (95%, confidence interval [CI] 75%–100%) and 92% specificity (95%, CI 62%–100%) for the diagnosis of adrenal malignancy.[33] *Adrenal wash out is measured by using the density value of the adrenal mass on unenhanced, portal venous phase and 15 minute–delayed CT scans. Absolute washout is calculated by using the formula [(HU portal venous phase)−(HU delayed)]/[(HU portal venous phase)−(HU non-enhanced)] × 100, and a value greater than 60% highly suggests adrenal adenoma, whereas relative washout is calculated by using the formula [(HU portal venous phase)−(HU delayed)]/(HU portal venous phase) × 100, and a value greater than 40% highly suggests adrenal adenoma.* With the combination of unenhanced and dynamic scans, CT represents the single most accurate modality for detection and characterization of adrenal adenomas.

On cross-sectional imaging in ACTH-independent CS, bilateral micronodular adrenal hyperplasia, also known as primary pigmented nodular adrenal dysplasia, typically shows normal-appearing adrenal glands with multiple small nodules of 2 to 5 mm size[34] (**Fig. 2**B). The adrenal nodules are macroscopically pigmented and demonstrate lower T1 and T2 signal intensity on MRI compared with the surrounded atrophic cortical tissue. Whereas, in primary bilateral macronodular adrenal hyperplasia, previously known as ACTH-independent macronodular adrenal hyperplasia, both glands are massively enlarged, with nodularity and distortion of the adrenal cortex (**Fig. 2**C). Bilateral adrenal enlargement may be seen in several forms; either as multiple large macronodules on both adrenals or more commonly as one discrete macronodule on each adrenal. Nodules vary in size from 1 to 5.5 cm and have low attenuation on unenhanced CT. On MRI, nodules are hypointense compared with liver on T1-weighted images and hyperintense or isointense compared with liver on T2-weighted images.[35,36]

Similar to aldosterone-producing ACC, cortisol-secreting ACCs are typically large (>4 cm),[37] with high attenuation (>10 HU) on unenhanced CT, and prevail a heterogeneous contrast enhancement on enhanced CT in combination with intratumoral calcifications, necrosis, and hemorrhage (**Fig. 2D**).[5,33] The sensitivity of greater than 10 HU on unenhanced CT to detect adrenal malignancy is high (100%; 95% CI: 91%, 100%); however, the specificity is poor (72%; 95% CI: 60%, 82%).[33] Additional information may be obtained by using ^{18}F-fluoro-2-deoxyglucose (FDG)-PET/CT imaging, where malignant lesions usually show a high uptake while the uptake is in the range of hepatic activity for benign lesions.[38] However, a recent systematic review and meta-analysis showed that the performance of PET/CT for detecting adrenocortical carcinoma was no better than CT.[33]

In ACTH-dependent CS, the adrenals typically appear enlarged due to chronic ACTH stimulation. The 2 types of adrenal enlargement observed on CT and MRI are either a smooth diffuse hyperplasia of both adrenal glands or nodular enlargement (micro- or macronodular).[39,40] Smooth hyperplasia is more common than nodular disease.[39] It is not uncommon in patients with ACTH-dependent CS and normal-appearing adrenals to hide micronodular disease detected only after pathologic examination of the adrenals.[35] A dominant nodule in nodular hyperplasia may easily confuse clinicians when dealing with patients with ACTH-dependent CS (**Fig. 3**).

Adrenal Venous Sampling

Treatment of adrenal CS is primarily surgical; therefore, localization of the source of excess cortisol is pivotal. In fact, an adrenal nodule usually greater than 2.5 cm in a patient with biochemical evidence of autonomous cortisol secretion correlates with the source of cortisol excess. However, particularly in the presence of bilateral lesions, several studies[41,42] have raised thoughts for the application of AVS as an additional diagnostic tool.

Specifically in a study of 34 patients with autonomous cortisol secretion who underwent successful AVS, 4 out of 14 patients with bilateral tumors were shown to have unilateral overproduction of cortisol, and 4 out of 20 patients with unilateral tumors

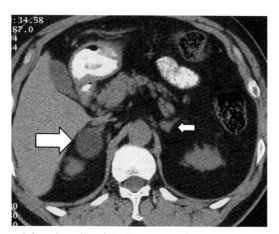

Fig. 3. A dominant right adrenal nodule (*large arrow*) in a 64-year-old man with ACTH-depending CS (cortisol post-dexamethasone, 13.2 μg/dL; increased midnight cortisol, 12.6 μg/dL; nonsupressed morning ACTH levels, 45 pg/mL). Left adrenal (*small arrow*) is slightly hyperplastic.

had bilateral cortisol secretion. This implies that CT imaging performs poorly in localizing cortisol secretion in patients with unilateral tumors (sensitivity of 73% and a specificity of 45%), if AVS is considered the gold-standard test.[41] Therefore, uncertainty exists till date on the optimal diagnostic workup and the role of AVS in patients with CS and bilateral adrenal lesions. If surgery is indicated in such patients an alternative option to AVS is removal of the largest adrenal or in case of similar size lesions removal of the easier left adrenal gland. This approach has led to clinical and biochemical improvement in most of the patients with clinical or subclinical CS.[43,44]

Adrenal Scintigraphy

I^{131}-cholesterol scintigraphy, as discussed earlier, provides an assessment of the adrenal tumor's function and has been used to evaluate cortisol secretion from the adrenal glands.[45–47] The procedure is not commonly performed anymore owing to cost and limited availability. However, several studies have shown that cholesterol scintigraphy could add valuable information about lateralization and help in selecting operation side in patients with bilateral adrenal adenomas.[45,46] In the study of Papierska and colleagues,[45] all 14 patients with subclinical hypercortisolism and bilateral adrenal tumors with unilateral predominant uptake on adrenal scintigraphy who underwent unilateral adrenalectomy showed remission of hypercortisolism in the 6-month follow-up visit. In the study of Ueland and colleagues,[41] cholesterol scintigraphy (planar and SPECT/CT images) findings were concordant with those of AVS in 13 of 18 cases (72%) and discordant in 5 (28%). No further follow-up was available in the discordant cases, and therefore, comparison of performance between these 2 modalities was not possible.

Functional adrenal imaging using radiolabeled PET tracers such as 11C-metomidate, as discussed, has been more commonly investigated in patients with PA, and only limited studies exist to date in patients with CS.[48,49]

ADRENAL IMAGING IN CATECHOLAMINE-SECRETING TUMORS

Catecholamine-secreting tumors most often arise from chromaffin cells of adrenal medulla and are referred to as pheochromocytomas (PCC), and up to 20% develop from extraadrenal chromaffin cells and are termed paragangliomas (PGL). PGL arising from the sympathetic ganglia produce catecholamines, whereas head and neck PGL arise from parasympathetic ganglia and are nonsecretory.[50] PCC and PGL (PPGL) represent a rare cause (0.2%–0.6%) of hypertension in unselected hypertensive patients.[51] Notably, up to 30% of PCC are diagnosed during the evaluation of incidentally discovered adrenal lesions.[52] Diagnosis of PPGL is crucial because if undiagnosed the patient is at high risk for cardiovascular morbidity and mortality and even life-threatening pheochromocytoma crisis. Biochemical diagnosis is based on measurement of plasma-free or 24-hour urinary fractionated metanephrines. Imaging studies are an important part of the evaluation of patients with PPGL. Imaging should follow, and not precede, the biochemical diagnosis of PPGL to locate the tumor. Imaging modalities comprise anatomic (CT and MRI) and functional imaging studies.

Anatomic Imaging—Computed Tomography and MRI

When the diagnosis of PPGL is biochemically confirmed, imaging to detect the tumor should follow. Sensitivity is high, 85% to 100%, but specificity is less than optimal with both CT and MRI.[53] PCC comprises 80% to 85% of cases, but also most of the extraadrenal tumors are located in the abdomen; therefore, imaging of the abdomen including pelvis is the first approach. In case of documented selective epinephrine secretion, adrenal imaging usually suffices because only pheochromocytoma can secrete epinephrine. Imaging of the thorax should be performed if abdomen and pelvis imaging fails to detect the tumor or in cases where metastatic disease is suspected.

The initial modality of choice, as proposed in Endocrine Society's guidelines,[50] is CT with contrast. With regard to concerns about the administration of contrast-inducing hypertensive crisis in patients with PPGL, there is evidence that administration of nonionic contrast is safe and does not necessitate adrenergic receptor blockade.[50] Although CT is the preferred modality, in special situations MRI may be used, preferentially in patients allergic to CT contrast and when radiation exposure is a concern (children, pregnant women, or patients who are expected to undergo repeated imaging).[50]

On unenhanced CT scans PCCs almost invariably appear as masses with a density of greater than 10HU and an average size of 4.5 cm. Importantly, areas of necrosis, hemorrhage, and calcifications are often present in PCC, and the region of interest for the assessment of attenuation values needs to be chosen so that it is homogenous and does not contain any of these alterations (**Fig. 4**A).[54] Another information obtained during a CT scan is the lesion's rate of contrast medium washout. High-contrast washout usually denotes a benign adrenocortical lesion; malignant lesions usually have low washout percentage. PCC do not have a constant pattern, with about 30% to 35% having high washout.[55] Thus, radiologic features of PCC overlap with those of malignant lesions and it is often difficult to differentiate between these 2 entities based on CT imaging.

MRI is more sensitive than CT for extraadrenal lesions and postoperatively for residual, recurrent or metastatic lesions[50] and also for intracardiac, juxta-cardiac, and juxta-vascular lesions, due to less cardiac and respiratory motion-induced artifacts. On MRI, PCC have a signal similar to that of liver, kidney, and muscle on T1-weighted sequences. They have a low fat content and thus there is no signal loss on chemical shift MRI, and they also characteristically display a high signal intensity on T2-weighted sequences (**Fig. 4**B), features shared with malignant lesions, lipid-poor benign adenomas, and hemorrhagic pseudocysts.[53] Medium T2 signal intensity has been reported in atypical PCC, especially those with cystic components. In addition, MRI may provide presurgery information about vessel invasion.[53]

Functional Imaging

Nuclear medicine imaging complements anatomic imaging by confirming that a lesion detected on imaging represents PPGL, especially in patients with multiple tumors. It may also help to localize PPGLs in patients with negative radiological studies or locate additional tumors at other sites or metastases.

Several radiopharmaceuticals can be used for nuclear imaging of PPGLs.[53] ^{123}I-metaiodobenzylguanidine (MIBG) scintigraphy is the traditional functional imaging modality for PPGL and is preferred over ^{131}I-MIBG due to its higher sensitivity[56] and ability to be combined with SPECT. Physiologic uptake, encountered in about 50% of normal adrenal glands, or rarely uptake by other lesions, such as adrenocortical cancer, may hinder to some degree its specificity, which ranges between 70% and 100%. Its sensitivity depends on the type of PPGL; it is best for PCC followed by PGL metastatic lesions; and it is less than 50% for SDHx-related PPGL, in particular SDHB PPGL, skull base and neck, thoracic, bladder, or recurrent PGL. ^{18}F-FDG PET scanning can better detect these latter lesions. The location, the aggressiveness, as well as the genetic background of the lesions[57] determine the localization accuracy of the tracer used. ^{18}F-FDG PET/CT is superior to anatomic imaging and ^{123}I-MIBG

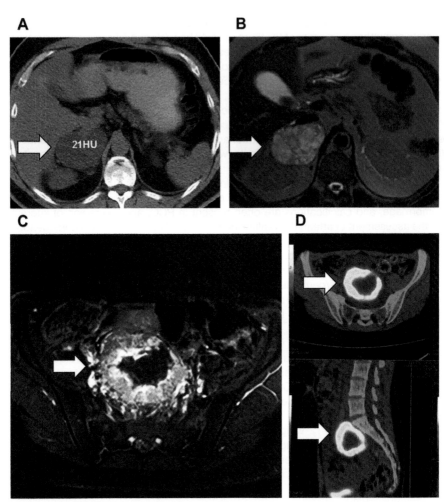

Fig. 4. (*A*) Axial image of unenhanced adrenal CT in a 46-year-old man showing a right adrenal mass of 8.9 cm in size with high attenuation (>10 HU) on unenhanced CT (*arrow*) and biochemical workup that suggest pheochromocytoma. (*B*) MRI of the same lesion displaying high signal intensity on T2-weighted sequences. (*C*) A 14-year-old girl with paroxysmal hypertension, tachycardia, and biochemical evidence of catecholamine excess with almost exclusively norepinephrine secretion (fractionated 24-hour urinary normetanephrine 15,245 μg/24 hrs, n.r. 88–444 and metanephrines <32 μg/24 hrs, n.r. 52–341). MRI of the abdomen revealed a 7.5 pelvic mass with high signal intensity on T2-weighted sequences and areas of necrosis. (*D*) The mass had increased uptake on ^{18}F-FDG PET/CT (SUVmax 12.4). Histology confirmed paraganglioma, and genetic testing revealed SDHB mutation.

for metastatic lesions[58] and for SDHx-related tumors (**Fig. 4**C, D). ^{18}F-FDOPA PET/CT is preferred for pseudohypoxic EPAS1-related PPGLs.[59]

Classic somatostatin receptor (SSTR) scintigraphy (with either [123I]Tyr3-octreotide or [111In]DTPA-octreotide) has been used in the past with suboptimal results. Newer, however, imaging modalities combining the superior spatial resolution of PET/CT with radiopharmaceuticals targeting the SSTR, such as ^{18}Ga-DOTATATE, have proved to have excellent diagnostic localization, especially for PPGLs associated with SDHx mutations.[59] Besides localization, both ^{123}I-MIBG and [18]Ga-DOTATATE imaging identify patients who would benefit from ^{123}I-MIBG therapy or peptide receptor nucleotide therapy with ^{177}Lu-DOTATE, respectively.[59]

SUMMARY

Adrenal imaging plays a pivotal role in investigating the different causes of adrenal endocrine hypertension. The diagnosis is made on clinical and biochemical grounds, and subsequent anatomic and functional adrenal imaging allows for localization of the source of hormonal excess. With the current availability of minimally invasive surgery appropriate location of the source of hormonal excess allows for optimal surgical treatment of these patients.

REFERENCES

1. Young WF Jr, Textor SC, Calhoun DA, et al. Screening for endocrine hypertension: an endocrine society scientific statement. Endocr Rev 2017;38(2):103–22.
2. Kayser SC, Dekkers T, Groenewoud HJ, et al. Study heterogeneity and estimation of prevalence of primary aldosteronism: a systematic review and meta-regression analysis. J Clin Endocrinol Metab 2016;101(7):2826–35.
3. Monticone S, Burrello J, Tizzani D, et al. Prevalence and clinical manifestations of primary aldosteronism encountered in primary care practice. J Am Coll Cardiol 2017;69(14):1811–20.
4. Seccia TM, Fassina A, Nussdorfer GG, et al. Aldosterone-producing adrenocortical carcinoma: an unusual cause of Conn's syndrome with an ominous clinical course. Endocr Relat Cancer 2005;12(1):149–59.
5. Lingam RK, Sohaib SA, Rockall AG, et al. Diagnostic performance of CT versus MR in detecting aldosterone-producing adenoma in primary hyperaldosteronism (Conn's syndrome). Eur Radiol 2004;14(10):1787–92.
6. Lumachi F, Marzola MC, Zucchetta P, et al. Non-invasive adrenal imaging in primary aldosteronism. Sensitivity and positive predictive value of radiocholesterol scintigraphy, CT scan and MRI. Nucl Med Commun 2003;24(6):683–8.
7. Gleason PE, Weinberger MH, Pratt JH, et al. Evaluation of diagnostic tests in the differential diagnosis of primary aldosteronism: unilateral adenoma versus bilateral micronodular hyperplasia. J Urol 1993;150(5 Pt 1):1365–8.
8. Magill SB, Raff H, Shaker JL, et al. Comparison of adrenal vein sampling and computed tomography in the differentiation of primary aldosteronism. J Clin Endocrinol Metab 2001;86(3):1066–71.
9. Young WF, Stanson AW, Thompson GB, et al. Role for adrenal venous sampling in primary aldosteronism. Surgery 2004;136(6):1227–35.
10. Lim V, Guo Q, Grant CS, et al. Accuracy of adrenal imaging and adrenal venous sampling in predicting surgical cure of primary aldosteronism. J Clin Endocrinol Metab 2014;99(8):2712–9.
11. Kempers MJ, Lenders JW, van Outheusden L, et al. Systematic review: diagnostic procedures to differentiate unilateral from bilateral adrenal abnormality in primary aldosteronism. Ann Intern Med 2009;151(5):329–37.
12. Yamada T, Ishibashi T, Saito H, et al. Adrenal adenomas: relationship between histologic lipid-rich cells and CT attenuation number. Eur J Radiol 2003;48(2):198–202.
13. Sohaib SA, Peppercorn PD, Allan C, et al. Primary hyperaldosteronism (Conn syndrome): MR imaging findings. Radiology 2000;214(2):527–31.

14. Vincent JM, Morrison ID, Armstrong P, et al. The size of normal adrenal glands on computed tomography. Clin Radiol 1994;49(7):453–5.

15. Lingam RK, Sohaib SA, Vlahos I, et al. CT of primary hyperaldosteronism (Conn's syndrome): the value of measuring the adrenal gland. AJR Am J Roentgenol 2003;181(3):843–9.

16. Pessina AC, Sacchetto A, Feltrin GP, et al. Identification of the etiology of primary aldosteronism with adrenal vein sampling in patients with equivocal computed tomography and magnetic resonance findings: results in 104 consecutive cases. J Clin Endocrinol Metab 2001;86(3):1083–90.

17. Yen RF, Wu VC, Liu KL, et al. 131I-6beta-iodomethyl-19-norcholesterol SPECT/CT for primary aldosteronism patients with inconclusive adrenal venous sampling and CT results. J Nucl Med 2009;50(10):1631–7.

18. Conn JW, Cohen EL, Herwig KR. The dexamethasone-modified adrenal scintiscan in hyporeninemic aldosteronism (tumor versus hyperplasia). A comparison with adrenal venography and adrenal venous aldosterone. J Lab Clin Med 1976;88(5):841–56.

19. Lombardi CP, Raffaelli M, De Crea C, et al. Noninvasive adrenal imaging in hyperaldosteronism: is it accurate for correctly identifying patients who should be selected for surgery? Langenbecks Arch Surg 2007;392(5):623–8.

20. Gross MD, Shapiro B, Shreve P. Radionuclide imaging of the adrenal cortex. Q J Nucl Med 1999;43(3):224–32.

21. Kazerooni EA, Sisson JC, Shapiro B, et al. Diagnostic accuracy and pitfalls of [iodine-131]6-beta-iodomethyl-19-norcholesterol (NP-59) imaging. J Nucl Med 1990;31(4):526–34.

22. Nomura K, Kusakabe K, Maki M, et al. Iodomethylnorcholesterol uptake in an aldosteronoma shown by dexamethasone-suppression scintigraphy: relationship to adenoma size and functional activity. J Clin Endocrinol Metab 1990;71(4):825–30.

23. Hogan MJ, McRae J, Schambelan M, et al. Location of aldosterone-producing adenomas with 131I-19-iodocholesterol. N Engl J Med 1976;294(8):410–4.

24. Powlson AS, Gurnell M, Brown MJ. Nuclear imaging in the diagnosis of primary aldosteronism. Curr Opin Endocrinol Diabetes Obes 2015;22(3):150–6.

25. Ono Y, Nakamura Y, Maekawa T, et al. Different expression of 11beta-hydroxylase and aldosterone synthase between aldosterone-producing microadenomas and macroadenomas. Hypertension 2014;64(2):438–44.

26. Lenders JWM, Eisenhofer G, Reincke M. Subtyping of patients with primary aldosteronism: an update. Horm Metab Res 2017;49(12):922–8.

27. Burton TJ, Mackenzie IS, Balan K, et al. Evaluation of the sensitivity and specificity of (11)C-metomidate positron emission tomography (PET)-CT for lateralizing aldosterone secretion by Conn's adenomas. J Clin Endocrinol Metab 2012;97(1):100–9.

28. Hahner S, Kreissl MC, Fassnacht M, et al. Functional characterization of adrenal lesions using [123I]IMTO-SPECT/CT. J Clin Endocrinol Metab 2013;98(4):1508–18.

29. Abe T, Naruse M, Young WF Jr, et al. A novel CYP11B2-specific imaging agent for detection of unilateral subtypes of primary aldosteronism. J Clin Endocrinol Metab 2016;101(3):1008–15.

30. Sacerdote A, Weiss K, Tran T, et al. Hypertension in patients with Cushing's disease: pathophysiology, diagnosis, and management. Curr Hypertens Rep 2005;7(3):212–8.

31. Park JJ, Park BK, Kim CK. Adrenal imaging for adenoma characterization: imaging features, diagnostic accuracies and differential diagnoses. Br J Radiol 2016; 89(1062):20151018.
32. Lumachi F, Marchesi P, Miotto D, et al. CT and MR imaging of the adrenal glands in cortisol-secreting tumors. Anticancer Res 2011;31(9):2923–6.
33. Dinnes J, Bancos I, Ferrante di Ruffano L, et al. Management of endocrine disease: imaging for the diagnosis of malignancy in incidentally discovered adrenal masses: a systematic review and meta-analysis. Eur J Endocrinol 2016;175(2): R51–64.
34. Peppercorn PD, Reznek RH. State-of-the-art CT and MRI of the adrenal gland. Eur Radiol 1997;7(6):822–36.
35. Sahdev A, Reznek RH, Evanson J, et al. Imaging in Cushing's syndrome. Arq Bras Endocrinol Metabol 2007;51(8):1319–28.
36. Lieberman SA, Eccleshall TR, Feldman D. ACTH-independent massive bilateral adrenal disease (AIMBAD): a subtype of Cushing's syndrome with major diagnostic and therapeutic implications. Eur J Endocrinol 1994;131(1):67–73.
37. Iniguez-Ariza NM, Kohlenberg JD, Delivanis DA, et al. Clinical, biochemical, and radiological characteristics of a single-center retrospective cohort of 705 large adrenal tumors. Mayo Clin Proc Innov Qual Outcomes 2018;2(1):30–9.
38. Delivanis DA, Bancos I, Atwell TD, et al. Diagnostic performance of unenhanced computed tomography and (18) F-fluorodeoxyglucose positron emission tomography in indeterminate adrenal tumours. Clin Endocrinol 2018;88(1):30–6.
39. Sohaib SA, Hanson JA, Newell-Price JD, et al. CT appearance of the adrenal glands in adrenocorticotrophic hormone-dependent Cushing's syndrome. AJR Am J Roentgenol 1999;172(4):997–1002.
40. Doppman JL, Miller DL, Dwyer AJ, et al. Macronodular adrenal hyperplasia in Cushing disease. Radiology 1988;166(2):347–52.
41. Ueland GA, Methlie P, Jossang DE, et al. Adrenal venous sampling for assessment of autonomous cortisol secretion. J Clin Endocrinol Metab 2018;103(12): 4553–60.
42. Young WF Jr, du Plessis H, Thompson GB, et al. The clinical conundrum of corticotropin-independent autonomous cortisol secretion in patients with bilateral adrenal masses. World J Surg 2008;32(5):856–62.
43. Perogamvros I, Vassiliadi DA, Karapanou O, et al. Biochemical and clinical benefits of unilateral adrenalectomy in patients with subclinical hypercortisolism and bilateral adrenal incidentalomas. Eur J Endocrinol 2015;173(6):719–25.
44. Debillon E, Velayoudom-Cephise F-L, Salenave S, et al. Unilateral adrenalectomy as a first-line treatment of cushing's syndrome in patients with primary bilateral macronodular adrenal hyperplasia. J Clin Endocrinol Metab 2015;100:4417–24.
45. Papierska L, Cwikla J, Rabijewski M, et al. Adrenal (131)I-6beta-iodomethylnorcholesterol scintigraphy in choosing the side for adrenalectomy in bilateral adrenal tumors with subclinical hypercortisolemia. Abdom Imaging 2015;40(7):2453–60.
46. Katabami T, Ishii S, Obi R, et al. Contralateral adrenal suppression on adrenocortical scintigraphy provides good evidence showing subclinical cortisol overproduction from unilateral adenomas. Endocr J 2016;63(12):1123–32.
47. Ricciato MP, Di Donna V, Perotti G, et al. The role of adrenal scintigraphy in the diagnosis of subclinical Cushing's syndrome and the prediction of postsurgical hypoadrenalism. World J Surg 2014;38(6):1328–35.
48. Hennings J, Lindhe O, Bergström M, et al. [11C]Metomidate positron emission tomography of adrenocortical tumors in correlation with histopathological findings. J Clin Endocrinol Metab 2006;91(4):1410–4.

49. Zettinig G, Mitterhauser M, Wadsak W, et al. Positron emission tomography imaging of adrenal masses: (18)F-fluorodeoxyglucose and the 11beta-hydroxylase tracer (11)C-metomidate. Eur J Nucl Med Mol Imaging 2004;31(9):1224–30.

50. Lenders JW, Duh QY, Eisenhofer G, et al. Pheochromocytoma and paraganglioma: an endocrine society clinical practice guideline. J Clin Endocrinol Metab 2014;99(6):1915–42.

51. Maria Ariton M, Christina S, Juan M, et al. Pheochromocytoma: clinical observations from a brooklyn tertiary hospital. Endocr Pract 2000;6(3):249–52.

52. Kopetschke R, Slisko M, Kilisli A, et al. Frequent incidental discovery of phaeochromocytoma: data from a German cohort of 201 phaeochromocytoma. Eur J Endocrinol 2009;161(2):355–61.

53. Ilias I, Pacak K. Current approaches and recommended algorithm for the diagnostic localization of pheochromocytoma. J Clin Endocrinol Metab 2004;89(2): 479–91.

54. Buitenwerf E, Korteweg T, Visser A, et al. Unenhanced CT imaging is highly sensitive to exclude pheochromocytoma: a multicenter study. Eur J Endocrinol 2018; 178(5):431–7.

55. Canu L, Van Hemert JAW, Kerstens MN, et al. CT characteristics of pheochromocytoma: relevance for the evaluation of adrenal incidentaloma. J Clin Endocrinol Metab 2019;104(2):312–8.

56. Shulkin BL, Shapiro B, Francis IR, et al. Primary extra-adrenal pheochromocytoma: positive I-123 MIBG imaging with negative I-131 MIBG imaging. Clin Nucl Med 1986;11(12):851–4.

57. Castinetti F, Kroiss A, Kumar R, et al. 15 YEARS Of PARAGANGLIOMA: imaging and imaging-based treatment of pheochromocytoma and paraganglioma. Endocr Relat Cancer 2015;22(4):T135–45.

58. Timmers HJ, Chen CC, Carrasquillo JA, et al. Staging and functional characterization of pheochromocytoma and paraganglioma by 18F-fluorodeoxyglucose (18F-FDG) positron emission tomography. J Natl Cancer Inst 2012;104(9):700–8.

59. Crona J, Taieb D, Pacak K. New perspectives on pheochromocytoma and paraganglioma: toward a molecular classification. Endocr Rev 2017;38(6):489–515.

Primary Aldosteronism Diagnosis and Management

A Clinical Approach

Gregory L. Hundemer, MD, MPH[a], Anand Vaidya, MD, MMSc[b],*

KEYWORDS

- Primary aldosteronism • Aldosterone • Cardiovascular disease • Hypertension
- Cardiovascular morbidity

KEY POINTS

- Primary aldosteronism is a relatively common yet often underdiagnosed cause of hypertension that is associated with cardiovascular disease independent of blood pressure.
- Increased screening among patients with hypertension, and more permissive criteria for acceptable aldosterone levels in the setting of a suppressed renin, may improve case detection for primary aldosteronism.
- When possible, surgical adrenalectomy is the preferred treatment to reduce cardiovascular outcomes. Mineralocorticoid receptor antagonists, along with dietary sodium restriction, can also be effective treatments when used appropriately.

INTRODUCTION

Primary aldosteronism used to be considered a rare cause of secondary hypertension. However, accruing evidence indicates that primary aldosteronism is more common than previously recognized. The implications of this increased prevalence are important to public health because autonomous aldosterone production contributes to cardiovascular disease and can be treated in a targeted manner. This article focuses on clinical approaches for diagnosing primary aldosteronism more frequently and earlier in its course, as well as practical treatment objectives to reduce the risk for incident cardiovascular disease.

PATHOPHYSIOLOGY OF PRIMARY ALDOSTERONISM

The hallmark of primary aldosteronism is autonomous secretion of aldosterone from either one or both adrenal glands, independent of angiotensin II, and often despite

Funding: This article was funded in part by grants from the National Institutes of Health R01DK115392.
[a] Division of Nephrology, Ottawa Hospital Research Institute, University of Ottawa, 501 Smyth Box 511, Ottawa, ON K1H 8L6, Canada; [b] Center for Adrenal Disorders, Brigham and Women's Hospital, Harvard Medical School, 221 Longwood Avenue, Boston, MA 02115, USA
* Corresponding author.
E-mail address: anandvaidya@bwh.harvard.edu

Endocrinol Metab Clin N Am 48 (2019) 681–700
https://doi.org/10.1016/j.ecl.2019.08.002
0889-5529/19/© 2019 Elsevier Inc. All rights reserved.

endo.theclinics.com

hypokalemia and intravascular volume expansion. Aldosterone binds to the mineralo-corticoid receptor (MR) of the principal cell in the distal nephron, inducing sodium reabsorption via the epithelial sodium channel (ENaC), and a commensurate excretion of potassium or hydrogen ions. The ENaC-mediated sodium reabsorption induces osmolar changes that drive water reabsorption, resulting in volume expansion, glomerular hyperfiltration, and suppression of renin and angiotensin II. Because angiotensin II is an important mediator of proximal nephron sodium reabsorption, suppression of angiotensin II results in greater sodium delivery to the distal nephron, thereby amplifying the aldosterone-driven sodium reabsorption and volume expansion, as well as potassium and acid excretion. These renal and hemodynamic effects explain why patients with primary aldosteronism classically present with hypertension, hypokalemia, and metabolic alkalosis.

Importantly, although the latter explains the pathophysiology mediated via the renal MR, autonomous aldosterone secretion also induces pathophysiology via activation of the extrarenal MR, particularly in the heart and cardiovascular tissues.[1–10] Specifically, the combination of a volume-expanded and/or sodium-replete state with excessive MR activation is speculated to be the mechanism for blood pressure–independent cardiovascular disease in primary aldosteronism.[1,4–7,9]

PREVALENCE

Historically considered a niche or rare cause of hypertension, recent studies suggest that primary aldosteronism is a common condition that often goes undiagnosed. The challenges in estimating prevalence are multifold. In part, true prevalence should reflect an adequate sampling of the population to provide confidence of generalizability; to date, most studies have been too small to achieve this. Second, there is no universal or international consensus on the definition of primary aldosteronism,[11,12] and there is no histopathologic or other gold standard. Thus, the flexible nature of characterizing autonomous aldosterone secretion that is sufficient to be considered "primary aldosteronism" has resulted in differing prevalence estimates from a variety of sample populations worldwide.

Regardless, primary aldosteronism is now recognized as the most common cause of endocrine hypertension. In one of the largest studies to attempt an estimate on the prevalence of primary aldosteronism, Monticone and colleagues[13] tested 1672 primary care patients with hypertension for primary aldosteronism. The investigators used strict screening and confirmatory thresholds to define primary aldosteronism and reported that 6% of their general hypertensive population had the diagnosis. Primary aldosteronism was more common in severe cases of hypertension with approximately 12% of patients with an untreated blood pressure of 160 to 179/100 to 109 mm Hg confirmed to have primary aldosteronism; however, a prevalence of 4% was observed even among patients with milder hypertension (140–159/ 80–99 mm Hg). Among the patients in this study who underwent adrenal venous sampling (AVS), approximately one-third of primary aldosteronism cases had unilateral disease (typically due to an aldosterone-producing adenoma [APA]), whereas the remaining two-thirds had bilateral disease (typically due to bilateral adrenal hyperplasia [BAH] or idiopathic hyperaldosteronism). The prevalence reported from this study was similar to that found in prior studies conducted in other countries with unique sample populations.[14–16]

It is important to note that had these investigators used slightly different criteria for their screening thresholds, or confirmatory testing cutoffs, they may have observed more modest or alarming prevalence estimates, as has been reported before,[17] thus underscoring the challenges in determining prevalence when using relatively arbitrary categorizations.

Prevalence estimates for primary aldosteronism in more severe hypertension populations, for example, resistant hypertension, are even greater at approximately 12% to 20%.[13,14,18–20] New observations suggest that even this high prevalence in resistant hypertension may be an underestimate, as it did not include milder forms of autonomous aldosterone secretion that do not meet the current (or classical) diagnostic thresholds of primary aldosteronism.[11,21]

HEALTH OUTCOMES IN PRIMARY ALDOSTERONISM BEFORE TARGETED THERAPY

The relevance of the relatively large prevalence of primary aldosteronism is best contextualized by the clinical consequences attributed to the disease, especially when it is not diagnosed early. A multitude of studies have demonstrated that before targeted therapy with MR antagonist medications or surgical adrenalectomy, patients with primary aldosteronism are at a higher risk for several adverse health outcomes compared with patients with essential hypertension, independent of blood pressure. Most of these studies have focused on cardiometabolic outcomes, including myocardial infarction,[13,22–25] heart failure,[13,24,25] stroke,[13,22–24] atrial fibrillation,[13,22–27] diabetes,[28,29] and metabolic syndrome.[29,30] A recent meta-analysis incorporated several of these studies to demonstrate that the odds ratios for nearly all clinically relevant cardiometabolic adverse outcomes was higher in patients with primary aldosteronism before targeted therapy compared with patients with essential hypertension (**Table 1**).[31] Other studies have shown that patients with primary aldosteronism before targeted therapy are also at higher risk for kidney disease,[32–37] including glomerular hyperfiltration and albuminuria, as well as death.[38]

DIAGNOSTIC APPROACH

Given the aforementioned risk for cardiometabolic disease in primary aldosteronism, it is imperative that patients with this condition be recognized early so that targeted therapy can be initiated.

Who to Screen for Primary Aldosteronism

The current Endocrine Society guidelines recommend screening for primary aldosteronism among populations in which the prevalence has been reported to be the highest (**Box 1**).[11]

Table 1
Odds ratios for outcomes in patients with primary aldosteronism when compared with similar patients with essential hypertension as reported by Monticone et al

Outcomes	Odds Ratio	95% Confidence Interval
Coronary artery disease (myocardial infarction or revascularization)	1.77	1.10–2.83
Stroke	2.58	1.93–3.45
Atrial fibrillation	3.52	2.06–5.99
Heart failure	2.05	1.11–3.78
Diabetes	1.33	1.01–1.74
Metabolic syndrome	1.53	1.22–1.91

Data from Monticone S, D'Ascenzo F, Moretti C, et al. Cardiovascular events and target organ damage in primary aldosteronism compared with essential hypertension: a systematic review and meta-analysis. Lancet Diabetes Endocrinol. 2018;6(1):41-50. Epub 2017/11/14. https://doi.org/10.1016/S2213-8587(1730319-4). PubMed PMID: 29129575.

Box 1
Indications to screen for primary aldosteronism

Blood pressure greater than 150/100 mm Hg on 3 consecutive measurements on different days

Blood pressure greater than 140/90 mm Hg resistant to 3 conventional antihypertensive medications including a diuretic

Blood pressure less than 140/90 mm Hg on 4 or more antihypertensive medications

Hypertension and hypokalemia (spontaneous or diuretic-induced)

Hypertension and adrenal incidentaloma

Hypertension and sleep apnea

Hypertension and a family history of hypertension or stroke before age 40

Hypertension and a first-degree relative with primary aldosteronism

---

It is alarming that only a small fraction of patients who meet the aforementioned indications are screened for primary aldosteronism,[39] highlighting the need for greater education of primary aldosteronism prevalence and the importance of case detection. Alternatively, it may be that screening for primary aldosteronism requires more time and resources than are available to many primary care physicians and other nonhypertension specialists. Further, although these are recommendations made by consensus and expert opinion, it should be noted that these indications are likely to identify individuals with more severe and overt forms of primary aldosteronism in whom a substantial degree of vascular injury may have already occurred. Recent studies have reported that primary aldosteronism may be prevalent in less severe forms of hypertension,[13,14,17] and even among normotensive individuals,[40–43] phenotypes that are excluded from the recommended screening guidelines.

How to Screen for Primary Aldosteronism

The most often recommended screening test for primary aldosteronism is the aldosterone-to-renin ratio (ARR).[11] ARR testing can be easily performed in the ambulatory setting typically without any additional preparation. The most widely accepted definition of a positive screen is an ARR greater than 30 ng/dL per ng/mL/h with a serum aldosterone level greater than 15 ng/dL.[11,44] Certainly, the higher the aldosterone level, and the lower the plasma renin activity (PRA), the more obvious the potential diagnosis. Rather than focusing on the ARR metric itself, we emphasize evaluating the absolute aldosterone and renin measures individually to determine whether there is inappropriate and autonomous aldosterone secretion that appears to be independent of renin. The clinical challenge is determining how low an aldosterone level can be in a patient with autonomous and inappropriate aldosterone secretion. Diagnostic cutoffs for what is considered to be a positive screen using the ARR can vary by practice and practitioner, namely because the ARR has not been calibrated or validated against a known gold standard because there exists no universal histopathologic, or other method, for the diagnosis of primary aldosteronism.

Less conservative criteria accept lower aldosterone levels (eg, >6 ng/dL or >9 ng/dL)[11,17,45] in the context of a suppressed PRA (eg, <1.0 ng/mL/h).[46] The suppression of renin, or at least a low renin, is generally a biochemical requisite to support autonomous aldosterone secretion. In this context, determination of how high an aldosterone level should be to be considered a "positive screen" is often dictated by personal style, cost-effectiveness, and other resources in specific settings. Relying on more conservative criteria (a very high aldosterone level with a low renin) may detect overt cases at the expense of missing milder ones (ie, false negatives), whereas relying on more relaxed criteria (modest or normal aldosterone levels with a low renin) may detect overt and mild cases at the expense of a greater number of false-positive screens.[12]

For decades, the main clinical measure of renin has been PRA, and this metric has been predominantly used in research studies as well. However, there is a global trend moving to replace PRA measures with renin concentrations. As this shift occurs, a recalibration of diagnostics will be needed, as will reliable comparisons to crudely convert and compare PRA with renin concentration.[11] Similarly, aldosterone assays are increasingly performed using liquid chromatography–tandem mass spectrometry (LC-MS/MS) rather than radioimmunoassay. Aldosterone measurements with LC-MS/MS have been shown to be substantially lower than other assays,[47] thus suggesting that, going forward, a new calibration of clinically relevant aldosterone levels, and arbitrary thresholds, must be considered.

A common question that arises is which, if any, antihypertensive medications must be stopped before testing to avoid false-negative results. Here again, geographic and personal stylistic practices vary. The most common culprit antihypertensive medications are those that raise renin and thus lower the ARR (ie, MR antagonists, ENaC inhibitors). If renin remains suppressed despite these medications, the renin, aldosterone, and ARR remain valid and interpretable, and therefore testing while on these medications is reasonable. However, if a patient is on one of these potentially interfering medications, and the renin is not suppressed, a washout period (that can take up to 4–6 weeks, although is usually much shorter) may be necessary before repeat testing. During this washout period, antihypertensive agents that will not affect renin measurements (eg, alpha blockers and/or hydralazine) and potassium supplementation can be used to control a patient's blood pressure and serum potassium.

Washout of angiotensin-converting enzyme (ACE) inhibitors, and angiotensin receptor blockers (ARB) is often recommended[11] because in normal physiology these medications can raise renin. However, in the pathophysiology of primary aldosteronism (reviewed earlier), renin and angiotensin II are suppressed, and therefore it is uncommon for ACE inhibitors or ARBs to impart sufficient influence to result in diagnostic misinterpretation. Beta-blockers can lower renin, and therefore increase the risk for false-positive ARR testing by decreasing the denominator[11]; however, lowering renin in normal physiology typically also lowers angiotensin II and aldosterone, and thus false-positive testing due to beta-blocker effect alone is not common. Similarly, although calcium channel blockers and diuretics can all potentially influence the ARR, for most practical purposes their influence is not sufficient to dramatically alter diagnostic testing, and measurement of the ARR while on these medications can be performed. For these reasons, many experts recommend screening when primary aldosteronism is suspected regardless of which medications are being used by the patient, and to consider an MR antagonist or ENaC inhibitor washout only if the renin is not suppressed.[48–50] When there is uncertainty in interpretation, a washout of additional medications can be considered; however, this should proceed with caution and careful monitoring because patients with primary aldosteronism can have very difficult to control hypertension and hypokalemia.

Confirmatory Testing

Confirming the screening results is often necessary. For patients with hypertension, hypokalemia, undetectable renin activity or levels, and serum aldosterone levels that are sufficiently elevated (ie, 15 or 20 ng/dL or higher), there is no need for further dynamic testing, and the diagnosis can be confirmed.[11] In a recent large prospective study, patients with very high ARR values not only had confirmed primary aldosteronism, but a high probability of having unilateral APAs.[51]

When the initial screen results are not overwhelmingly convincing, dynamic confirmatory testing can be conducted. Confirmatory tests are effectively aldosterone suppression tests; however, there is substantial variation and lack of consensus on protocols, interpretation of results, and categorical levels that indicate a "positive" or "negative" study. The 4 main recommended confirmatory tests are as follows[11,52,53]:

- Oral sodium load: Patients are instructed to consume an approximately 4000-6000mg sodium diet for 3 to 4 days with the addition of sodium chloride tablets if needed. Additional potassium supplementation is also commonly required because of an increase in kaliuresis. On the final day of the diet, a 24-hour urine specimen is collected. A 24-hour urine aldosterone excretion of more than 12 μg in the setting of 24-hour urine sodium excretion of more than 200 mEq is diagnostic of primary aldosteronism. However, values of more than 10 μg/24 hours also are strongly suggestive.
- Saline infusion test: Patients receive a 2-L infusion of isotonic saline over 4 hours. Traditionally, this test has been performed with the patient in the recumbent position; however, recent studies suggest that having the patient in a seated position increases the sensitivity without reducing the specificity in identifying primary aldosteronism.[53,54] Blood samples for renin, aldosterone, cortisol, and potassium are measured immediately before and after infusion. At the end of the infusion, a serum aldosterone level greater than 10 ng/dL is diagnostic of primary aldosteronism, a serum aldosterone level less than 5 ng/dL rules out primary aldosteronism, whereas a serum aldosterone level of 5 to 10 ng/dL is considered indeterminate. When the test is performed with the patient in a seated position, a postinfusion serum aldosterone level greater than 6 ng/dL is diagnostic of primary aldosteronism as long as the postinfusion serum cortisol level is lower than the preinfusion level to exclude an ACTH effect.
- Fludrocortisone suppression test: Patients receive fludrocortisone 0.1 mg every 6 hours for 4 days together with sodium and potassium supplementation. On day 4, serum cortisol is measured at 7 AM, and serum aldosterone, PRA, and cortisol are measured at 10 AM with the patient in a seated position. A serum aldosterone greater than 6 ng/dL with a PRA less than 1.0 ng/mL per hour and a 10 AM serum cortisol less than the 7 AM value is diagnostic of primary aldosteronism.
- Captopril challenge test: Individuals are given 25 to 50 mg of captopril after sitting or standing for at least 1 hour. Serum aldosterone and PRA are measured at time zero and at 1 and 2 hours after captopril administration, with the patient remaining seated during this period. Serum aldosterone will be suppressed in healthy individuals; however, in primary aldosteronism, aldosterone will remain elevated and PRA will remain suppressed. Many different diagnostic thresholds have bene proposed. A less than 30% suppression of aldosterone from baseline while PRA remains suppressed confirms primary aldosteronism.[11] Alternatively, an ARR greater than 20 or greater than 30 ng/dL per ng/mL per hour also can be strongly suggestive of the diagnosis.[16] Finally, a failure to suppress aldosterone to less than 11 ng/dL has also been suggested to be diagnostic.[55]

Lateralization of Disease

Once the diagnosis of primary aldosteronism has been confirmed, localization can be pursued. Cross-sectional imaging is recommended even for patients who are not interested or eligible for surgery, to exclude the rare instance of an aldosterone-producing adrenocortical carcinoma (**Fig. 1**). However, reliance on cross-sectional imaging to determine laterality is not widely recommended and can be misleading[56–59]; nonfunctional adrenal incidentalomas may exist and primary aldosteronism may be present in one or both adrenal glands without a visible abnormality on cross-sectional imaging (see **Fig. 1**). The PASO study showed that patients who underwent AVS had a substantially higher likelihood of attaining biochemical cure or biochemical improvement when compared with patients who had only computed tomography (CT)-based localization.[60] For this reason, most experts and professional societies recommend AVS for localization for most patients with primary aldosteronism who are interested and eligible for a potential adrenalectomy. In young (<35 years) patients with a clear unilateral adenoma on imaging and severe primary aldosteronism with hypokalemia, AVS may not be necessary because the visible unilateral adenoma is almost always the culprit lesion.[11,61,62]

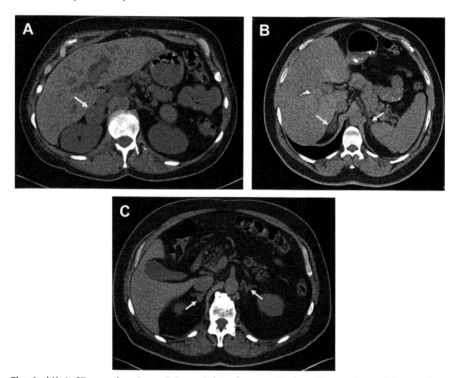

Fig. 1. (A) A CT scan showing a 3.8-cm right adrenocortical carcinoma (*arrow*) in a patient who presented with hypokalemia, hypertension, and confirmed primary aldosteronism. (B) A CT scan showing a 2.1-cm right adrenocortical adenoma (*left arrow*) and a normal-appearing left adrenal gland (*right arrow*) in a patient with confirmed primary aldosteronism. AVS confirmed bilateral aldosterone production and the patient was treated with MR antagonists. (C) A CT scan showing a 1.3-cm right adrenocortical adenoma(*left arrow*) and a normal-appearing left adrenal gland (*right arrow*) in a patient with confirmed primary aldosteronism. AVS confirmed unilateral aldosterone production from the right side, and the patient underwent a curative right adrenalectomy.

In contrast, a randomized controlled trial (the SPARTACUS trial) evaluated whether CT-based or AVS-based localization and therapy was more effective and concluded that both approaches resulted in similar blood pressure control 1 year later.[63] However, several limitations and critiques of the study design have emerged, including that the primary outcome was blood pressure control at only 1 year of follow-up, and that there may have been substantial misclassification.[64–66] Thus, although SPARTACUS was a randomized controlled trial, its results have not yet resulted in a dramatic shift in recommendations or practice.

The AVS procedure is technically challenging. and should be performed by an expert with ample experience. The optimal methodology and protocol for AVS has been the source of great debate and discussion.[67–72] The details, values, and pitfalls of AVS are discussed in a separate article in this issue.

Proposed Diagnostic Approach

Fig. 2 displays our proposed diagnostic approach for primary aldosteronism, recognizing that the condition exists across a spectrum of disease severity.

GENETICS

Genetic testing in the evaluation of primary aldosteronism is not a common part of routine clinical practice. Inheritable forms of primary aldosteronism are exceptionally rare. Recent reviews have discussed the genetics of primary aldosteronism in great detail.[12,73–77] Herein, we provide only a brief summary on the genetic aspects of primary aldosteronism that are most pertinent to clinicians in routine practice.

Glucocorticoid Remediable Aldosteronism

Glucocorticoid remediable aldosteronism (GRA), also known as familial hyperaldosteronism (FH) type I, is a rare form of primary aldosteronism due to BAH that is inherited in autosomal dominant fashion and accounts for <1% of all cases of primary aldosteronism.[78] These patients carry a mutation that results in a fusion of the promoter sequence of the CYP11B1 (11β-hydroxylase) gene and the coding sequence of the CYP11B2 (aldosterone synthase) gene resulting in ACTH-driven aldosterone secretion.[79] Patients with GRA typically present at a young age and typically carry a strong family history of primary aldosteronism, early-onset hypertension, or hemorrhagic stroke at a young age. Patients with GRA are less likely to be hypokalemic than other patients with primary aldosteronism, which may be related to the circadian nature of ACTH secretion.[80] When suspected clinically, the diagnosis should be confirmed via genetic testing[81]; however, in settings where genetic testing cannot be performed or afforded, dexamethasone suppression testing can be used as a second-line alternative. With dexamethasone suppression testing, dexamethasone can be prescribed at a dosage of 1 mg twice daily for 3 days. A serum aldosterone on day 3 of less than 4 ng/dL is considered a positive test for GRA. Once GRA is confirmed, low-dose glucocorticoids to suppress ACTH, in addition to MR antagonists, can be initiated.

Familial Hyperaldosteronism Types II to IV

Traditionally, patients with familial forms of primary aldosteronism, when GRA had been excluded, were categorized as having FH-II. FH-II is still considered to be the most common form of FH, is typically thought to be of autosomal dominant inheritance, and is clinically similar to sporadic forms of primary aldosteronism.[78,82] Until recently, the mutations responsible for FH-II have remained unknown; however, linkage analyses have mapped them to chromosome 7p22.[83,84] Two recent studies

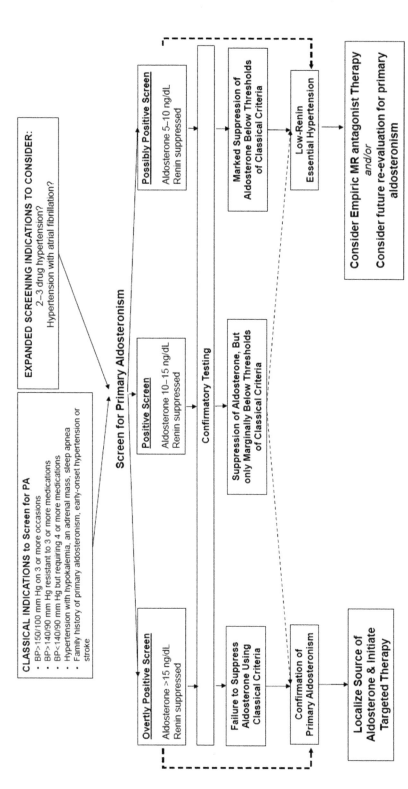

Fig. 2. Proposed diagnostic approach for diagnosis of primary aldosteronism. Biochemical screening for primary aldosteronism is generally pursued when classic indications are observed, as recommended by The Endocrine Society and others.[11] Consideration of expanded screening indications may increase the probability of detecting more cases of primary aldosteronism. A positive screen for primary aldosteronism should

demonstrated the discovery of mutations in the *CLCN2* chloride channel causing inheritable primary aldosteronism that may account for at least some cases of FH-II, thereby setting the stage for a potential reclassification of some FH-II cases.[85,86] FH-III is exceedingly rare and attributable to mutations in the *KCNJ5* potassium channel, and presents with severe childhood hypertension and primary aldosteronism.[87–89] FH-IV is also exceedingly rare and attributable to mutations in the *CACNA1H* T-type voltage-gated calcium channel.[90–93] The phenotype of FH-IV also includes neurocognitive disorders, epilepsy, and autism.[94–97] De novo mutations in the L-type voltage-gated calcium gene for *CACNA1D* can cause primary aldosteronism, and are also linked to childhood seizures and neurologic abnormalities (known as PASNA).[93,95,96]

Genetics and Pathogenesis of Aldosterone-Producing Adenomas

Although inheritable forms of primary aldosteronism remain rare, it is now becoming evident that the vast majority of APAs harbor known pathogenic mutations that result in autonomous aldosterone secretion.[98,99] For example, a recent study[98] found that 66 (88%) of 75 studied APAs had identifiable somatic mutations. The most commonly identified mutations were *KCNJ5* (43%), *CACNA1D* (21%), and *ATP1A1* (17%). *KCNJ5* mutations have been shown to be more common in women, present at a young age, associate with a more severe primary aldosteronism phenotype, and demonstrate high rates of clinical cure following adrenalectomy.[100–104] Although the voltage-gated calcium channels in zona glomerulosa cells are either directly or indirectly affected by these somatic mutations,[73–75,77] it remains unclear whether primary aldosteronism driven by these mutations is particularly susceptible to treatment with calcium channel blockers. Ultimately, testing for these mutations is not currently part of standard clinical practice and how this knowledge will practically influence routine clinical practice remains to be determined.

Aldosterone-Producing Cell Clusters

In recent years, non-neoplastic clusters of autonomous aldosterone-secreting cells, termed aldosterone-producing cell clusters (APCCs), have been identified in postmortem studies on individuals with and without primary aldosteronism.[105,106] APCCs are defined as areas of CYP11B2 expression, are known to commonly harbor pathogenic somatic mutations linked to primary aldosteronism,[107,108] can be found in normotensive and hypertensive adrenal glands, and appear to exist in greater quantities with older age.[109] APCCs have been hypothesized to represent one potential explanation for BAH (or idiopathic hyperaldosteronism),[110] age-related autonomous aldosteronism,[109,111] and a precursor lesion that may exist before neoplastic primary aldosteronism.[12]

---

suggest renin-independent aldosterone secretion, whereby aldosterone levels are relatively high in the context of a suppressed renin. In the absence of overt evidence for renin-independent aldosteronism on screening, confirmatory testing can be used to affirm the diagnosis. Failure or relative failure to suppress aldosterone on dynamic testing may confirm the diagnosis, whereas marked suppression of aldosterone may instead suggest a diagnosis of low-renin hypertension. The diagnosis of primary aldosteronism need not rely on binary thresholds, rather may exist across a continuum of severity whereby mild and nonclassic cases may be detected as well. BP, blood pressure. (*Adapted from* Vaidya A, Mulatero P, Baudrand R, et al. Expanding Spectrum of Primary Aldosteronism: Implications for Diagnosis, Pathogenesis, and Treatment. Endocr Rev 2018;39(6):1057–88; with permission.)

MANAGEMENT OF PRIMARY ALDOSTERONISM
Dietary Sodium Restriction

As with essential hypertension, dietary sodium restriction should be encouraged in patients with primary aldosteronism. Physiologically, effective reduction in dietary sodium intake can result in volume contraction leading to a rise in both renin and angiotensin II. This rise in angiotensin II leads to decreased distal sodium delivery, thereby limiting the pathologic consequences of aldosterone-MR-ENaC–mediated distal sodium reabsorption in primary aldosteronism. However, sodium restriction alone is likely inadequate to effectively mitigate the adverse long-term health outcomes in the vast majority of patients with primary aldosteronism. For instance, one prior study showed that more than half of patients with confirmed primary aldosteronism had normalization of their ARR due to substantial increases in renin after intense dietary sodium restriction to less than 50 mmol/d,[17] a degree of sodium restriction that would be extremely challenging to sustain for most individuals in North America and Europe where the mean dietary sodium intake is 150 to 200 mmol/d.[112,113]

Mineralocorticoid Receptor Antagonists

Lifelong MR antagonist therapy is recommended for patients with bilateral primary aldosteronism as well as those with unilateral primary aldosteronism who are unable to or unwilling to undergo surgical adrenalectomy.[11] The 2 most common MR antagonists are spironolactone and eplerenone, with spironolactone having approximately double the potency of eplerenone,[114] but carrying with it a risk for gynecomastia in men, which can limit adherence. MR antagonists decrease ENaC-mediated sodium reabsorption and consequent volume expansion, and decrease potassium and hydrogen ion excretion. In this regard, they are usually able to substantially reduce blood pressure (or decrease the number of antihypertensive medications) and improve potassium balance.

Despite the recommendation to use lifelong MR antagonists in primary aldosteronism, it has remained uncertain how effective these medications are in reducing long-term adverse health outcomes, when compared with comparable patients with essential hypertension, and how to dose these medications to achieve optimal clinical results. Recent cohort studies, attempting to fill this knowledge gap, have suggested that despite treatment with MR antagonists, patients with primary aldosteronism continue to have worse long-term health outcomes compared with patients with essential hypertension.[115,116] A recent large cohort study compared cardiometabolic outcomes in patients with primary aldosteronism treated with MR antagonists and age-matched patients with essential hypertension and similar blood pressure control.[117] Despite treatment with MR antagonists, patients with primary aldosteronism had a twofold higher risk for developing myocardial infarction, heart failure hospitalization, and stroke compared with patients with essential hypertension, despite similar blood pressure control. Patients with primary aldosteronism treated with MR antagonists also had substantially higher risks for developing atrial fibrillation, diabetes mellitus, chronic kidney disease,[37] and death.

Importantly, the excess risk for these adverse cardiovascular outcomes (myocardial infarction, heart failure, stroke, atrial fibrillation) and mortality was effectively limited to those patients whose renin remained suppressed (<1.0 ng/mL per hour) despite MR antagonist therapy.[117,118] Those patients with primary aldosteronism who achieved a substantial rise in renin ($\geq$1.0 ng/mL per hour), and who had also received slightly higher doses of MR antagonists, had a lower risk for incident cardiovascular events and mortality that was similar to that observed among patients with essential hypertension.[117,118] These studies, along with multiple prior studies,[22,23,31,38] highlight the fact that much of the excess risk for adverse health outcomes in primary aldosteronism occurs independent of blood pressure control; therefore, blood pressure alone may not be a sufficient marker of treatment efficacy in primary aldosteronism. In contrast, these studies suggest that a rise in renin, reflective of effective MR blockade and a subsequent volume contraction, may be a clinically useful biomarker to assess MR antagonist adequacy. To achieve a substantial rise in renin, more aggressive MR antagonist dosing is usually needed; however, this may not be always be possible, as the antiandrogenic effects of spironolactone and the risk for hyperkalemia, especially among patients with kidney disease, may be limiting factors.[37] Combining MR antagonists with sodium restriction to normalize blood pressure and potassium, and raise renin activity into the detectable range, may be the ideal treatment approach when it can be sustainably achieved.

Surgical Adrenalectomy

Surgical adrenalectomy to cure primary aldosteronism is the treatment of choice for patients with unilateral primary aldosteronism who are healthy enough to undergo the surgery.[11] This procedure is now primarily performed laparoscopically, or even retroperitoneoscopically, which has resulted in a lower complication rate and shorter hospitalizations.[119–121] Multiple studies have demonstrated high success rates in curing primary aldosteronism, as demonstrated via resolution of hypokalemia, resolution or reduced severity of hypertension, and biochemical cure.[60,122–128] Direct comparisons of surgical adrenalectomy and MR antagonist medications in the treatment of primary aldosteronism have been limited due to bias in terms of the varied demographics and clinical presentation of unilateral versus bilateral disease; however, the few studies that have attempted to control for these differences have suggested improved long-term cardiovascular outcomes, renal outcomes, and mortality with surgical adrenalectomy compared with MR antagonist therapy.[37,117,118] Therefore, in patients with unilateral primary aldosteronism who are willing and capable to safely undergo surgery, we strongly recommend this as the preferred treatment approach.

A major unanswered question in the treatment of primary aldosteronism is whether unilateral surgical adrenalectomy should be considered in specific cases of bilateral primary aldosteronism with the goal of disease attenuation, as opposed to disease cure in unilateral primary aldosteronism. As discussed previously, cohort studies suggest inferior outcomes in primary aldosteronism treated with MR antagonists as compared with both surgical adrenalectomy for unilateral disease and essential hypertension with similar blood pressure control.[37,117,118] In cases of bilateral primary aldosteronism, in which the disease is difficult to control with maximal MR antagonist dosing or in which MR antagonist dosing is limited by side effects, such as gynecomastia or hyperkalemia (eg, due to higher rates of chronic kidney disease), unilateral surgical adrenalectomy could reduce the amount of autonomous aldosterone secretion that needs to be treated medically.[129] However, given the paucity of existing data to address this issue, this decision is one that needs to be made based on the judgment of individual clinicians on a case-by-case basis.

SUMMARY

Primary aldosteronism is a relatively common, yet often undiagnosed, cause of hypertension that is associated with substantial morbidity and mortality even independent of its effect on blood pressure. In this article, we have discussed the most updated knowledge of this condition and shared our suggested practical diagnostic and treatment approaches based on the most recent available data. Future prospective and interventional studies are necessary to enhance the recognition of earlier and more subtle forms of autonomous aldosteronism and to identify individualized therapies to improve the care of patients with primary aldosteronism.

REFERENCES

1. Barrett KV, McCurley AT, Jaffe IZ. Direct contribution of vascular mineralocorticoid receptors to blood pressure regulation. Clin Exp Pharmacol Physiol 2013;40(12):902–9.
2. Brilla CG, Weber KT. Mineralocorticoid excess, dietary sodium, and myocardial fibrosis. J Lab Clin Med 1992;120(6):893–901.
3. Diaz-Otero JM, Fisher C, Downs K, et al. Endothelial mineralocorticoid receptor mediates parenchymal arteriole and posterior cerebral artery remodeling during angiotensin II-induced hypertension. Hypertension 2017;70(6):1113–21.
4. Kim SK, McCurley AT, DuPont JJ, et al. Smooth muscle cell-mineralocorticoid receptor as a mediator of cardiovascular stiffness with aging. Hypertension 2018; 71(4):609–21.
5. Martinez DV, Rocha R, Matsumura M, et al. Cardiac damage prevention by eplerenone: comparison with low sodium diet or potassium loading. Hypertension 2002;39(2 Pt 2):614–8.
6. McCurley A, Pires PW, Bender SB, et al. Direct regulation of blood pressure by smooth muscle cell mineralocorticoid receptors. Nat Med 2012;18(9):1429–33.
7. Mueller KB, Bender SB, Hong K, et al. Endothelial mineralocorticoid receptors differentially contribute to coronary and mesenteric vascular function without modulating blood pressure. Hypertension 2015;66(5):988–97.
8. Pitt B, Zannad F, Remme WJ, et al. The effect of spironolactone on morbidity and mortality in patients with severe heart failure. Randomized Aldactone Evaluation Study Investigators. N Engl J Med 1999;341(10):709–17.
9. Rocha R, Stier CT Jr, Kifor I, et al. Aldosterone: a mediator of myocardial necrosis and renal arteriopathy. Endocrinology 2000;141(10):3871–8.
10. Tesch GH, Young MJ. Mineralocorticoid receptor signaling as a therapeutic target for renal and cardiac fibrosis. Front Pharmacol 2017;8:313.
11. Funder JW, Carey RM, Mantero F, et al. The management of primary aldosteronism: case detection, diagnosis, and treatment: an endocrine society clinical practice guideline. J Clin Endocrinol Metab 2016;101(5):1889–916.
12. Vaidya A, Mulatero P, Baudrand R, et al. The expanding spectrum of primary aldosteronism: implications for diagnosis, pathogenesis, and treatment. Endocr Rev 2018;39(6):1057–88.
13. Monticone S, Burrello J, Tizzani D, et al. Prevalence and clinical manifestations of primary aldosteronism encountered in primary care practice. J Am Coll Cardiol 2017;69(14):1811–20.
14. Mosso L, Carvajal C, Gonzalez A, et al. Primary aldosteronism and hypertensive disease. Hypertension 2003;42(2):161–5.
15. Omura M, Saito J, Yamaguchi K, et al. Prospective study on the prevalence of secondary hypertension among hypertensive patients visiting a general outpatient clinic in Japan. Hypertens Res 2004;27(3):193–202.
16. Rossi GP, Bernini G, Caliumi C, et al, PAPY Study Investigators. A prospective study of the prevalence of primary aldosteronism in 1,125 hypertensive patients. J Am Coll Cardiol 2006;48(11):2293–300.

17. Baudrand R, Guarda FJ, Torrey J, et al. Dietary sodium restriction increases the risk of misinterpreting mild cases of primary aldosteronism. J Clin Endocrinol Metab 2016;101(11):3989–96.
18. Calhoun DA, Nishizaka MK, Zaman MA, et al. Hyperaldosteronism among black and white subjects with resistant hypertension. Hypertension 2002;40(6):892–6.
19. Carey RM, Calhoun DA, Bakris GL, et al, American Heart Association Professional/Public Education and Publications Committee of the Council on Hypertension; Council on Cardiovascular and Stroke Nursing; Council on Clinical Cardiology; Council on Genomic and Precision Medicine; Council on Peripheral Vascular Disease; Council on Quality of Care and Outcomes Research; and Stroke Council. Resistant hypertension: detection, evaluation, and management: a scientific statement from the American Heart Association. Hypertension 2018;72(5):e53–90.
20. Nishizaka MK, Pratt-Ubunama M, Zaman MA, et al. Validity of plasma aldosterone-to-renin activity ratio in African American and white subjects with resistant hypertension. Am J Hypertens 2005;18(6):805–12.
21. Williams B, MacDonald TM, Morant SV, et al. British Hypertension Society programme of Prevention and Treatment of Hypertension With Algorithm based Therapy Study Group. Endocrine and haemodynamic changes in resistant hypertension, and blood pressure responses to spironolactone or amiloride: the PATHWAY-2 mechanisms substudies. Lancet Diabetes Endocrinol 2018; 6(6):464–75.
22. Catena C, Colussi G, Nadalini E, et al. Cardiovascular outcomes in patients with primary aldosteronism after treatment. Arch Intern Med 2008;168(1):80–5.
23. Milliez P, Girerd X, Plouin PF, et al. Evidence for an increased rate of cardiovascular events in patients with primary aldosteronism. J Am Coll Cardiol 2005; 45(8):1243–8.
24. Mulatero P, Monticone S, Bertello C, et al. Long-term cardio- and cerebrovascular events in patients with primary aldosteronism. J Clin Endocrinol Metab 2013; 98(12):4826–33.
25. Savard S, Amar L, Plouin PF, et al. Cardiovascular complications associated with primary aldosteronism: a controlled cross-sectional study. Hypertension 2013; 62(2):331–6.
26. Rossi GP, Cesari M, Cuspidi C, et al. Long-term control of arterial hypertension and regression of left ventricular hypertrophy with treatment of primary aldosteronism. Hypertension 2013;62(1):62–9.
27. Rossi GP, Maiolino G, Flego A, et al, PAPY Study Investigators. Adrenalectomy lowers incident atrial fibrillation in primary aldosteronism patients at long term. Hypertension 2018;71(4):585–91.
28. Chen W, Li F, He C, et al. Elevated prevalence of abnormal glucose metabolism in patients with primary aldosteronism: a meta-analysis. Ir J Med Sci 2014; 183(2):283–91.
29. Hanslik G, Wallaschofski H, Dietz A, et al, participants of the German Conn's Registry. Increased prevalence of diabetes mellitus and the metabolic syndrome in patients with primary aldosteronism of the German Conn's Registry. Eur J Endocrinol 2015;173(5):665–75.
30. Fallo F, Veglio F, Bertello C, et al. Prevalence and characteristics of the metabolic syndrome in primary aldosteronism. J Clin Endocrinol Metab 2006;91(2):454–9.
31. Monticone S, D'Ascenzo F, Moretti C, et al. Cardiovascular events and target organ damage in primary aldosteronism compared with essential hypertension:

a systematic review and meta-analysis. Lancet Diabetes Endocrinol 2018;6(1): 41–50.

32. Reincke M, Rump LC, Quinkler M, et al, Participants of German Conn's Registry. Risk factors associated with a low glomerular filtration rate in primary aldosteronism. J Clin Endocrinol Metab 2009;94(3):869–75.

33. Ribstein J, Du Cailar G, Fesler P, et al. Relative glomerular hyperfiltration in primary aldosteronism. J Am Soc Nephrol 2005;16(5):1320–5.

34. Rossi GP, Bernini G, Desideri G, et al, PAPY Study Investigators. Renal damage in primary aldosteronism: results of the PAPY Study. Hypertension 2006;48(2): 232–8.

35. Sechi LA, Novello M, Lapenna R, et al. Long-term renal outcomes in patients with primary aldosteronism. JAMA 2006;295(22):2638–45.

36. Hundemer GL, Baudrand R, Brown JM, et al. Renin phenotypes characterize vascular disease, autonomous aldosteronism, and mineralocorticoid receptor activity. J Clin Endocrinol Metab 2017;102(6):1835–43.

37. Hundemer GL, Curhan GC, Yozamp N, et al. Renal outcomes in medically and surgically treated primary aldosteronism. Hypertension 2018;72(3):658–66.

38. Reincke M, Fischer E, Gerum S, et al, German Conn's Registry-Else Kröner-Fresenius-Hyperaldosteronism Registry. Observational study mortality in treated primary aldosteronism: the German Conn's registry. Hypertension 2012;60(3): 618–24.

39. Ruhle BC, White MG, Alsafran S, et al. Keeping primary aldosteronism in mind: deficiencies in screening at-risk hypertensives. Surgery 2019;165(1):221–7.

40. Baudrand R, Guarda FJ, Fardella C, et al. Continuum of renin-independent aldosteronism in normotension. Hypertension 2017;69(5):950–6.

41. Markou A, Pappa T, Kaltsas G, et al. Evidence of primary aldosteronism in a predominantly female cohort of normotensive individuals: a very high odds ratio for progression into arterial hypertension. J Clin Endocrinol Metab 2013;98(4): 1409–16.

42. Vasan RS, Evans JC, Larson MG, et al. Serum aldosterone and the incidence of hypertension in nonhypertensive persons. N Engl J Med 2004;351(1):33–41.

43. Brown JM, Robinson-Cohen C, Luque-Fernandez MA, et al. The spectrum of subclinical primary aldosteronism and incident hypertension: a cohort study. Ann Intern Med 2017;167(9):630–41.

44. Young WF. Primary aldosteronism: renaissance of a syndrome. Clin Endocrinol (Oxf) 2007;66(5):607–18.

45. Stowasser M, Ahmed AH, Pimenta E, et al. Factors affecting the aldosterone/renin ratio. Horm Metab Res 2012;44(3):170–6.

46. Rye P, Chin A, Pasieka J, et al. Unadjusted plasma renin activity as a "First-Look" test to decide upon further investigations for primary aldosteronism. J Clin Hypertens (Greenwich) 2015;17(7):541–6.

47. Guo Z, Poglitsch M, McWhinney BC, et al. Aldosterone LC-MS/MS assay-specific threshold values in screening and confirmatory testing for primary aldosteronism. J Clin Endocrinol Metab 2018;103(11):3965–73.

48. Byrd JB, Turcu AF, Auchus RJ. Primary aldosteronism. Circulation 2018;138(8): 823–35.

49. Vaidya A, Malchoff CD, Auchus RJ, et al. An individualized approach to the evaluation and management of primary aldosteronism. Endocr Pract 2017;23(6): 680–9.

50. Young W. Diagnosis of primary aldosteronism. Waltham (MA): UpToDate. Available at: https://www.uptodate.com. Accessed January 23, 2019.

51. Maiolino G, Rossitto G, Bisogni V, et al. Quantitative value of aldosterone-renin ratio for detection of aldosterone-producing adenoma: the aldosterone-renin ratio for primary aldosteronism (AQUARR) study. J Am Heart Assoc 2017;6(5). https://doi.org/10.1161/JAHA.117.005574.

52. Morera J, Reznik Y. Management of endocrine disease: the role of confirmatory tests in the diagnosis of primary aldosteronism. Eur J Endocrinol 2018. https://doi.org/10.1530/EJE-18-0704.

53. Ahmed AH, Cowley D, Wolley M, et al. Seated saline suppression testing for the diagnosis of primary aldosteronism: a preliminary study. J Clin Endocrinol Metab 2014;99(8):2745–53.

54. Stowasser M, Ahmed AH, Cowley D, et al. Comparison of seated with recumbent saline suppression testing for the diagnosis of primary aldosteronism. J Clin Endocrinol Metab 2018;103(11):4113–24.

55. Song Y, Yang S, He W, et al, Chongqing Primary Aldosteronism Study (CONPASS). Confirmatory tests for the diagnosis of primary aldosteronism: a prospective diagnostic accuracy study. Hypertension 2018;71(1):118–24.

56. Kempers MJ, Lenders JW, van Outheusden L, et al. Systematic review: diagnostic procedures to differentiate unilateral from bilateral adrenal abnormality in primary aldosteronism. Ann Intern Med 2009;151(5):329–37.

57. Lim V, Guo Q, Grant CS, et al. Accuracy of adrenal imaging and adrenal venous sampling in predicting surgical cure of primary aldosteronism. J Clin Endocrinol Metab 2014;99(8):2712–9.

58. Nanba AT, Nanba K, Byrd JB, et al. Discordance between imaging and immunohistochemistry in unilateral primary aldosteronism. Clin Endocrinol (Oxf) 2017;87(6):665–72.

59. Young WF, Stanson AW, Thompson GB, et al. Role for adrenal venous sampling in primary aldosteronism. Surgery 2004;136(6):1227–35.

60. Williams TA, Lenders JWM, Mulatero P, et al, Primary Aldosteronism Surgery Outcome (PASO) Investigators. Outcomes after adrenalectomy for unilateral primary aldosteronism: an international consensus on outcome measures and analysis of remission rates in an international cohort. Lancet Diabetes Endocrinol 2017;5(9):689–99.

61. Kupers EM, Amar L, Raynaud A, et al. A clinical prediction score to diagnose unilateral primary aldosteronism. J Clin Endocrinol Metab 2012;97(10):3530–7.

62. Riester A, Fischer E, Degenhart C, et al. Age below 40 or a recently proposed clinical prediction score cannot bypass adrenal venous sampling in primary aldosteronism. J Clin Endocrinol Metab 2014;99(6):E1035–9.

63. Dekkers T, Prejbisz A, Kool LJS, et al, SPARTACUS Investigators. Adrenal vein sampling versus CT scan to determine treatment in primary aldosteronism: an outcome-based randomised diagnostic trial. Lancet Diabetes Endocrinol 2016;4(9):739–46.

64. Beuschlein F, Mulatero P, Asbach E, et al. The SPARTACUS trial: controversies and unresolved issues. Horm Metab Res 2017;49(12):936–42.

65. Rossi GP, Funder JW. Adrenal venous sampling versus computed tomographic scan to determine treatment in primary aldosteronism (The SPARTACUS Trial): a critique. Hypertension 2017;69(3):396–7.

66. Young WF Jr. Diagnosis and treatment of primary aldosteronism: practical clinical perspectives. J Intern Med 2019;285(2):126–48.

67. El Ghorayeb N, Mazzuco TL, Bourdeau I, et al. Basal and post-ACTH aldosterone and its ratios are useful during adrenal vein sampling in primary aldosteronism. J Clin Endocrinol Metab 2016;101(4):1826–35.

68. Kline G, Leung A, So B, et al. Application of strict criteria in adrenal venous sampling increases the proportion of missed patients with unilateral disease who benefit from surgery for primary aldosteronism. J Hypertens 2018;36(6):1407–13.
69. Lethielleux G, Amar L, Raynaud A, et al. Influence of diagnostic criteria on the interpretation of adrenal vein sampling. Hypertension 2015;65(4):849–54.
70. Rossi GP, Auchus RJ, Brown M, et al. An expert consensus statement on use of adrenal vein sampling for the subtyping of primary aldosteronism. Hypertension 2014;63(1):151–60.
71. Takeda Y, Umakoshi H, Takeda Y, et al, JPAS Study Group. Impact of adrenocorticotropic hormone stimulation during adrenal venous sampling on outcomes of primary aldosteronism. J Hypertens 2018. https://doi.org/10.1097/HJH.0000000000001964.
72. Wolley MJ, Gordon RD, Ahmed AH, et al. Does contralateral suppression at adrenal venous sampling predict outcome following unilateral adrenalectomy for primary aldosteronism? A retrospective study. J Clin Endocrinol Metab 2015;100(4):1477–84.
73. Faillot S, Assie G. Endocrine tumours: the genomics of adrenocortical tumors. Eur J Endocrinol 2016;174(6):R249–65.
74. Monticone S, Buffolo F, Tetti M, et al. Genetics in endocrinology: the expanding genetic horizon of primary aldosteronism. Eur J Endocrinol 2018;178(3):R101–11.
75. Prada ETA, Burrello J, Reincke M, et al. Old and new concepts in the molecular pathogenesis of primary aldosteronism. Hypertension 2017;70(5):875–81.
76. Seccia TM, Caroccia B, Gomez-Sanchez EP, et al. The biology of normal zona glomerulosa and aldosterone-producing adenoma: pathological implications. Endocr Rev 2018;39(6):1029–56.
77. Zennaro MC, Boulkroun S, Fernandes-Rosa F. Genetic causes of functional adrenocortical adenomas. Endocr Rev 2017;38(6):516–37.
78. Mulatero P, Tizzani D, Viola A, et al. Prevalence and characteristics of familial hyperaldosteronism: the PATOGEN study (Primary Aldosteronism in TOrino-GENetic forms). Hypertension 2011;58(5):797–803.
79. Lifton RP, Dluhy RG, Powers M, et al. A chimaeric 11 beta-hydroxylase/aldosterone synthase gene causes glucocorticoid-remediable aldosteronism and human hypertension. Nature 1992;355(6357):262–5.
80. Litchfield WR, Coolidge C, Silva P, et al. Impaired potassium-stimulated aldosterone production: a possible explanation for normokalemic glucocorticoid-remediable aldosteronism. J Clin Endocrinol Metab 1997;82(5):1507–10.
81. Mulatero P, Veglio F, Pilon C, et al. Diagnosis of glucocorticoid-remediable aldosteronism in primary aldosteronism: aldosterone response to dexamethasone and long polymerase chain reaction for chimeric gene. J Clin Endocrinol Metab 1998;83(7):2573–5.
82. Pallauf A, Schirpenbach C, Zwermann O, et al. The prevalence of familial hyperaldosteronism in apparently sporadic primary aldosteronism in Germany: a single center experience. Horm Metab Res 2012;44(3):215–20.
83. Carss KJ, Stowasser M, Gordon RD, et al. Further study of chromosome 7p22 to identify the molecular basis of familial hyperaldosteronism type II. J Hum Hypertens 2011;25(9):560–4.
84. Sukor N, Mulatero P, Gordon RD, et al. Further evidence for linkage of familial hyperaldosteronism type II at chromosome 7p22 in Italian as well as Australian and South American families. J Hypertens 2008;26(8):1577–82.

85. Fernandes-Rosa FL, Daniil G, Orozco IJ, et al. A gain-of-function mutation in the CLCN2 chloride channel gene causes primary aldosteronism. Nat Genet 2018; 50(3):355–61.

86. Scholl UI, Stolting G, Schewe J, et al. CLCN2 chloride channel mutations in familial hyperaldosteronism type II. Nat Genet 2018;50(3):349–54.

87. Choi M, Scholl UI, Yue P, et al. K+ channel mutations in adrenal aldosterone-producing adenomas and hereditary hypertension. Science 2011;331(6018): 768–72.

88. Hattangady NG, Olala LO, Bollag WB, et al. Acute and chronic regulation of aldosterone production. Mol Cell Endocrinol 2012;350(2):151–62.

89. Oki K, Plonczynski MW, Luis Lam M, et al. Potassium channel mutant KCNJ5 T158A expression in HAC-15 cells increases aldosterone synthesis. Endocrinology 2012;153(4):1774–82.

90. Daniil G, Fernandes-Rosa FL, Chemin J, et al. CACNA1H mutations are associated with different forms of primary aldosteronism. EBioMedicine 2016;13: 225–36.

91. Korah HE, Scholl UI. An update on familial hyperaldosteronism. Horm Metab Res 2015;47(13):941–6.

92. Scholl UI, Stolting G, Nelson-Williams C, et al. Recurrent gain of function mutation in calcium channel CACNA1H causes early-onset hypertension with primary aldosteronism. Elife 2015;4:e06315.

93. Scholl UI, Goh G, Stolting G, et al. Somatic and germline CACNA1D calcium channel mutations in aldosterone-producing adenomas and primary aldosteronism. Nat Genet 2013;45(9):1050–4.

94. Eckle VS, Shcheglovitov A, Vitko I, et al. Mechanisms by which a CACNA1H mutation in epilepsy patients increases seizure susceptibility. J Physiol 2014; 592(4):795–809.

95. Pinggera A, Lieb A, Benedetti B, et al. CACNA1D de novo mutations in autism spectrum disorders activate Cav1.3 L-type calcium channels. Biol Psychiatry 2015;77(9):816–22.

96. Pinggera A, Mackenroth L, Rump A, et al. New gain-of-function mutation shows CACNA1D as recurrently mutated gene in autism spectrum disorders and epilepsy. Hum Mol Genet 2017;26(15):2923–32.

97. Splawski I, Yoo DS, Stotz SC, et al. CACNA1H mutations in autism spectrum disorders. J Biol Chem 2006;281(31):22085–91.

98. Nanba K, Omata K, Else T, et al. Targeted molecular characterization of aldosterone-producing adenomas in White Americans. J Clin Endocrinol Metab 2018;103(10):3869–76.

99. Nanba K, Omata K, Gomez-Sanchez CE, et al. Genetic characteristics of aldosterone-producing adenomas in blacks. Hypertension 2019;73(4):885–92.

100. Arnesen T, Glomnes N, Stromsoy S, et al. Outcome after surgery for primary hyperaldosteronism may depend on KCNJ5 tumor mutation status: a population-based study from Western Norway. Langenbecks Arch Surg 2013;398(6): 869–74.

101. Ip JC, Pang TC, Pon CK, et al. Mutations in KCNJ5 determines presentation and likelihood of cure in primary hyperaldosteronism. ANZ J Surg 2015;85(4): 279–83.

102. Kitamoto T, Suematsu S, Matsuzawa Y, et al. Comparison of cardiovascular complications in patients with and without KCNJ5 gene mutations harboring aldosterone-producing adenomas. J Atheroscler Thromb 2015;22(2):191–200.

103. Lenzini L, Rossitto G, Maiolino G, et al. A meta-analysis of somatic KCNJ5 K(+) channel mutations in 1636 patients with an aldosterone-producing adenoma. J Clin Endocrinol Metab 2015;100(8):E1089–95.

104. Rossi GP, Cesari M, Letizia C, et al. KCNJ5 gene somatic mutations affect cardiac remodelling but do not preclude cure of high blood pressure and regression of left ventricular hypertrophy in primary aldosteronism. J Hypertens 2014;32(7):1514–21 [discussion: 22].

105. Boulkroun S, Samson-Couterie B, Dzib JF, et al. Adrenal cortex remodeling and functional zona glomerulosa hyperplasia in primary aldosteronism. Hypertension 2010;56(5):885–92.

106. Nishimoto K, Nakagawa K, Li D, et al. Adrenocortical zonation in humans under normal and pathological conditions. J Clin Endocrinol Metab 2010;95(5): 2296–305.

107. Nishimoto K, Tomlins SA, Kuick R, et al. Aldosterone-stimulating somatic gene mutations are common in normal adrenal glands. Proc Natl Acad Sci U S A 2015;112(33):E4591–9.

108. Omata K, Anand SK, Hovelson DH, et al. Aldosterone-producing cell clusters frequently harbor somatic mutations and accumulate with age in normal adrenals. J Endocr Soc 2017;1(7):787–99.

109. Nanba K, Vaidya A, Williams GH, et al. Age-related autonomous aldosteronism. Circulation 2017;136(4):347–55.

110. Omata K, Satoh F, Morimoto R, et al. Cellular and genetic causes of idiopathic hyperaldosteronism. Hypertension 2018;72(4):874–80.

111. Nanba K, Vaidya A, Rainey WE. Aging and adrenal aldosterone production. Hypertension 2018;71(2):218–23.

112. Cogswell ME, Loria CM, Terry AL, et al. Estimated 24-hour urinary sodium and potassium excretion in US adults. JAMA 2018;319(12):1209–20.

113. Kalogeropoulos AP, Georgiopoulou VV, Murphy RA, et al. Dietary sodium content, mortality, and risk for cardiovascular events in older adults: the health, aging, and body composition (Health ABC) study. JAMA Intern Med 2015;175(3): 410–9.

114. Parthasarathy HK, Menard J, White WB, et al. A double-blind, randomized study comparing the antihypertensive effect of eplerenone and spironolactone in patients with hypertension and evidence of primary aldosteronism. J Hypertens 2011;29(5):980–90.

115. Wu VC, Chueh SJ, Chen L, et al. Risk of new-onset diabetes mellitus in primary aldosteronism: a population study over 5 years. J Hypertens 2017;35(8): 1698–708.

116. Wu VC, Wang SM, Chang CH, et al. Long term outcome of aldosteronism after target treatments. Sci Rep 2016;6:32103.

117. Hundemer GL, Curhan GC, Yozamp N, et al. Cardiometabolic outcomes and mortality in medically treated primary aldosteronism: a retrospective cohort study. Lancet Diabetes Endocrinol 2018;6(1):51–9.

118. Hundemer GL, Curhan GC, Yozamp N, et al. Incidence of atrial fibrillation and mineralocorticoid receptor activity in patients with medically and surgically treated primary aldosteronism. JAMA Cardiol 2018;3(8):768–74.

119. Duncan JL 3rd, Fuhrman GM, Bolton JS, et al. Laparoscopic adrenalectomy is superior to an open approach to treat primary hyperaldosteronism. Am Surg 2000;66(10):932–5 [discussion: 5–6].

120. Meria P, Kempf BF, Hermieu JF, et al. Laparoscopic management of primary hyperaldosteronism: clinical experience with 212 cases. J Urol 2003;169(1):32–5.

121. Rossi H, Kim A, Prinz RA. Primary hyperaldosteronism in the era of laparoscopic adrenalectomy. Am Surg 2002;68(3):253–6 [discussion: 6–7].
122. Blumenfeld JD, Sealey JE, Schlussel Y, et al. Diagnosis and treatment of primary hyperaldosteronism. Ann Intern Med 1994;121(11):877–85.
123. Harris DA, Au-Yong I, Basnyat PS, et al. Review of surgical management of aldosterone secreting tumours of the adrenal cortex. Eur J Surg Oncol 2003;29(5): 467–74.
124. Lo CY, Tam PC, Kung AW, et al. Primary aldosteronism. Results of surgical treatment. Ann Surg 1996;224(2):125–30.
125. Meyer A, Brabant G, Behrend M. Long-term follow-up after adrenalectomy for primary aldosteronism. World J Surg 2005;29(2):155–9.
126. Stowasser M, Klemm SA, Tunny TJ, et al. Response to unilateral adrenalectomy for aldosterone-producing adenoma: effect of potassium levels and angiotensin responsiveness. Clin Exp Pharmacol Physiol 1994;21(4):319–22.
127. Sukor N, Kogovsek C, Gordon RD, et al. Improved quality of life, blood pressure, and biochemical status following laparoscopic adrenalectomy for unilateral primary aldosteronism. J Clin Endocrinol Metab 2010;95(3):1360–4.
128. Velema M, Dekkers T, Hermus A, et al, SPARTACUS Investigators. Quality of life in primary aldosteronism: a comparative effectiveness study of adrenalectomy and medical treatment. J Clin Endocrinol Metab 2018;103(1):16–24.
129. Omata K, Yamazaki Y, Nakamura Y, et al. Genetic and histopathologic intertumor heterogeneity in primary aldosteronism. J Clin Endocrinol Metab 2017;102(6): 1792–6.

Low-Renin Hypertension

Shobana Athimulam, MBBS[a], Natalia Lazik, MD, PhD[b],
Irina Bancos, MD[a],*

KEYWORDS

- Low-renin hypertension • Primary aldosteronism • Liddle syndrome
- Gordon syndrome • Apparent mineralocorticoid excess syndrome
- Glucocorticoid-resistance syndrome
- Mineralocorticoid receptor– activating mutation • CYP11B1 and CYP17 deficiency

KEY POINTS

- Approximately 30% of patients with arterial hypertension display low renin concentrations.
- Low-renin hypertension occurs because of inherent genetic syndromes, acquired somatic mutations, and endogenous and exogenous factors.
- Differentiation of the subtypes of low-renin hypertension is important in tailoring therapy accordingly.

INTRODUCTION

Hypertensive patients can be classified as affected by low-, normal-, or high-renin hypertension based on plasma renin activity or direct renin concentration.[1] Low-renin hypertension affects 30% of patients with hypertension.[2,3] The most common cause of low-renin hypertension is primary aldosteronism, which presents with suppressed renin but elevated aldosterone concentrations. Low-renin hypertension with low aldosterone represents a wide spectrum of disorders, which includes hereditary monogenic forms, secondary to either endogenous or exogenous factors, and essential forms.[4–7] When evaluating a patient with low-renin hypertension, measurement of plasma aldosterone and potassium concentrations are followed by workup for differential diagnosis (**Fig. 1** and **Table 1**).

Funding: James A. Ruppe Career Development Award in Endocrinology to I. Bancos, Robert and Elizabeth Strickland Career Development Award within the Division of Endocrinology, Metabolism, Diabetes and Nutrition to I. Bancos, Advancement in Medicine Catalyst award to I. Bancos.
a Division of Endocrinology, Diabetes, Metabolism and Nutrition, Mayo Clinic, 200 1st Street Southwest, Rochester, MN 55905, USA; b Department of Internal Medicine, Mayo Clinic, 200 1st Street Southwest, Rochester, MN 55905, USA
* Corresponding author.
E-mail address: bancos.irina@mayo.edu

Endocrinol Metab Clin N Am 48 (2019) 701–715
https://doi.org/10.1016/j.ecl.2019.08.003
0889-8529/19/© 2019 Elsevier Inc. All rights reserved.

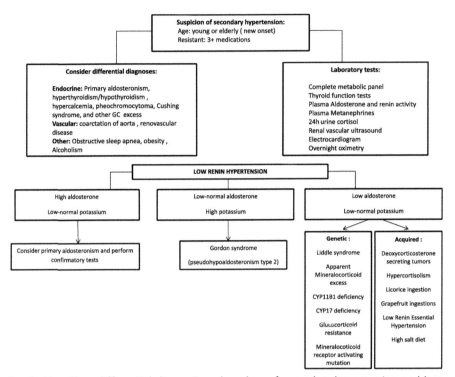

Fig. 1. Algorithm: differential diagnosis and workup of secondary hypertension and low-renin hypertension.

The renin-angiotensin-aldosterone system has a vital role in regulating fluid balance alongside sodium (Na^+) and potassium (K^+) homeostasis. Renin secretion stimulated by renal hypofiltration and/or by activation of the sympathetic nervous system leads to cleavage of angiotensinogen to generate angiotensin II which, in turn, stimulates aldosterone production from adrenal zona-glomerulosa.[8–11]

Evaluation of the renin status in patients with hypertension is based on measurement of either plasma renin activity or direct renin concentrations. Renin plasma activity can be measured by the radioimmunoassay that quantifies angiotensin I generated as a function of time[1] or directly through liquid mass spectrometry.[12] The direct renin concentration is measured by the chemiluminescent immunometric method.[13] Overall, plasma renin activity measured by radioimmunoassay and direct renin concentrations measured by the chemiluminescent method demonstrate a good correlation,[14] and either can be used, as recommended by the 2016 Endocrine Society guidelines.[11] This review addresses the different conditions that present with low-renin hypertension, discussing an appropriate diagnostic approach and highlighting the genetic subtypes within familial forms.

LOW-RENIN ESSENTIAL HYPERTENSION

Low-renin hypertension is a multifactorial disease that is more common in older adults and individuals of African descent.[15] Several mechanisms have been implicated in the development of low-renin hypertension, including molecular mechanisms as well as exogenous causes, such as medications. Reduction in nephrons (e.g., in diabetic

Table 1
Causes, characteristics, and management of low-renin hypertension

Cause	Prevalence[a]	Inheritance	Genetics	Pathogenesis	ALDO	K	Other	Comments on clinical Presentation	Management
Low-renin essential hypertension	20%–30%	Multifactorial	Multifactorial	High-sodium diet	↑	↓/↔	Metabolic alkalosis ↓Mg ↓Kidney function	Obstructive sleep apnea, obesity, metabolic syndrome, neuromuscular and cardiac symptoms	Low-sodium diet, electrolyte replacement, antihypertensive management
Primary aldosteronism	6%–10%	Varies	Sporadic *KCNJ5*, *CACNA1D*, *ATP1A1*, *ATP2B3*	Chronic activation of MR by aldosterone-stimulating somatic mutations	↑	↓/↔		Variable: mild to resistant hypertension. Occasionally associated with heart and kidney disease	• Adrenalectomy (unilateral adenoma) • MR antagonist in bilateral adrenal disease or not a surgical candidate
Cushing syndrome (usually ectopic)	Rare	—	—	Hypercortisolism-induced MR activation	↑	↓	Metabolic alkalosis ↑Glucose ↑Cholesterol	Proximal myopathy, metabolic syndrome, insomnia, psychiatric symptoms, easy bruising, striae, abdominal fat redistribution, osteoporosis	Surgical removal of ACTH-secreting neuroendocrine tumor or bilateral adrenalectomy
Licorice	Variable	—	—	Inhibition of 11β-HSD2, direct effect on MR	↓	↓	Increase in cortisol-to-cortisone ratio	Hypertension, and muscle weakness	Discontinuation of licorice ingestion
Grapefruit	Variable	—	—	Inhibition of 11β-HSD2	↓	↓	Increase in cortisol-to-cortisone ratio	Borderline hypertension	Discontinuation of grapefruit ingestion
DOC-secreting tumors	Very rare	—	—	Malignant adrenal mass secreting DOC	↓	↓	+/– Androgen hypersecretion	↑ Urinary tetrahydrodeoxycorticosterone • Virilization in females • Feminization in men	Surgical resection of tumor
Liddle syndrome	0.9%–6%	AD	SCNN1A, SCNN1B, SCNN1G	↑ENaC expression → Na reabsorption	↓	↓	Metabolic alkalosis	Early-onset hypertension	ENaC blockers (amiloride, triamterene) ↓Sodium diet

(continued on next page)

Table 1
(continued)

Cause	Prevalence[a]	Inheritance	Genetics	Pathogenesis	ALDO	K	Other	Comments on clinical Presentation	Management
Gordon syndrome/pseudohypoaldosteronism type 2	Very rare	AD/AR	WNK1, WNK4, CUL3, KLHL3	• Thiazide-sensitive Na-Cl cotransporter → increase in Na reabsorption • Reduced expression of renal outer medulla K$^+$ channel (ROMK)	↓	↑	Metabolic acidosis, hyperchloremia ± hypercalciuria	Mutations in CUL3, KLHL3: earlier onset, more severe hyperkalemia	Thiazide diuretics
CYP11B1 congenital adrenal hyperplasia	Very rare	AR	CYP11B1	Impaired conversion of 11-deoxycortisol to cortisol, leading to increase in ACTH and DOC, and adrenal androgens	↓	↓	Androgen excess, cortisol deficiency	Virilization of females, accelerated growth, premature closure of growth plates	Glucocorticoid replacement therapy, +/– MR antagonist
CYP17 congenital adrenal hyperplasia	Very rare	AR	CYP17A1	Impaired conversion of pregnenolone and progesterone to 17-OH forms. Increase in DOC-activating MR	↓	↓	Androgen and cortisol deficiency	Primary amenorrhea, lack of secondary sexual characteristics in females	Glucocorticoid replacement, +/– MR antagonist and replacement of sex steroids
Apparent mineralocorticoid excess syndrome	Very rare	AR	HSD11B2	Impaired HSD11B2 → cortisol activation of MR	↓	↓		Severe-mild phenotypes: hypertension	MR antagonist, dexamethasone
MR-activating mutation	Very rare	AD	NR3C2	MR is activated by progesterone and spironolactone	↓	↓		• Early-onset hypertension • Exacerbation in pregnancy	Amiloride Finerenone Spironolactone is contraindicated
Glucocorticoid-resistance syndrome	Very rare	AR	NR3C1	Glucocorticoid receptor resistance with hypercortisolism-induced MR activation, ACTH hypersecretion	↓/↔	↓	Metabolic alkalosis Increased androgens	Fatigue (cortisol deficiency) Hirsutism Absence of Cushingoid features	Dexamethasone, MR antagonists

Abbreviations: ↑, high; ↓, low; ↔, normal; 11β-HSD2, 11β-hydroxysteroid dehydrogenase type 2; ACTH, corticotropin (adrenocorticotropic hormone); AD, autosomal dominant; ALDO, aldosterone; AR, autosomal recessive; Cl⁻, chloride; DOC, deoxycorticosterone; ENaC, epithelial sodium channel; K⁺, potassium; MR, mineralocorticoid receptor; Na, sodium.

a Prevalence, based on hypertensive populations.

nephropathy), chronic glomerulonephritis, unilateral nephrectomy, and aging may also induce a low-renin and low-aldosterone status.[2] Stress was also reported to cause corticotropin (ACTH)-mediated aldosterone hypersecretion and contribute to the development of low-renin hypertension.[16]

The most common causes of low-renin hypertension are a high-sodium diet (aldosterone concentrations will be suppressed) and drugs known to interfere with the renin-angiotensin-aldosterone system.[2,17–19] Nonsteroidal anti-inflammatory drugs and cyclooxygenase-2 inhibitors exert their inhibitory effect by suppression of intrarenal prostaglandin and renin production and by reducing sodium excretion and inducing volume expansion,[20] whereas β-blockers and centrally acting agents, such as clonidine and methyldopa, reduce the activation of the renin-angiotensin-aldosterone system.[17] Interestingly, unfractionated heparin was reported to strongly inhibit aldosterone production.[18]

It has also been hypothesized that single-nucleotide polymorphisms or rare variants in the same genes causing monogenic forms could also contribute to the development of low-renin essential hypertension by enhancing Na^+ reabsorption, but without causing the classic monogenic syndromes, representing phenotypes with a milder spectrum of the classic forms.[21] In particular, patients of African descent with low-renin hypertension demonstrate a high frequency of the pThr594Met substitution.[22] These observations are supported by improvement in blood-pressure control in patients of African descent with low-renin hypertension treated with amiloride when compared with those treated following standard guidelines.[23]

Minor alterations in 11BHSD2 may also play a role in the development of low-renin hypertension. Patients with essential hypertension may have a prolonged half-life of plasma cortisol, reflecting HSD11B2 activity, compared with normotensive controls.[24] There is a significant correlation between serum cortisol/cortisone ratio and age,[25] suggesting an age-related 11BHSD2 dysfunction, which can partly account for the low-renin phenotype observed in the older population. Furthermore, salt-sensitive hypertension has also been correlated with a decreased HSD11B2 activity, which is explained by blood-pressure response to thiazide diuretic therapy.[26,27]

PRIMARY ALDOSTERONISM

Primary aldosteronism is characterized by autonomous hypersecretion of aldosterone from the adrenal glands. This condition can be either unilateral or bilateral, and occur sporadically or present as a familial condition. Patients with primary aldosteronism present with suppressed renin, normal or elevated aldosterone concentrations, and hypokalemia (occurring in circa 10%–40% of patients).[11] Chronic activation of the mineralocorticoid receptor (MR) by autonomous excessive production of aldosterone leads to increased Na^+ reabsorption within the distal nephron, resulting in compensatory chronic suppression of renin production by the juxtaglomerular apparatus.

At present, primary aldosteronism is considered the most common form of endocrine hypertension, accounting for up to 20% of cases of resistant hypertension[28] and around 6% of the general hypertensive population.[29] Patients with primary aldosteronism present with an increased risk of cardiovascular and metabolic diseases in comparison with patients with essential hypertension.[30]

Endocrine Society clinical practice guidelines recommend evaluation for primary aldosteronism (with measurements of aldosterone and renin concentrations) in any patient with hypertension, hypokalemia, an adrenal mass, sleep apnea, or a family history of primary aldosteronism or early cardiovascular disease.[11]

In patients with suppressed renin and aldosterone concentrations of at least 10 ng/dL or higher, an aldosterone-to-renin ratio of greater than 30 is considered a positive screening test for primary aldosteronism. However, suppressed renin in the context of nonsuppressed aldosterone (>6–9 ng/dL) could suggest a milder form of primary aldosteronism and should lead to further investigation.[11]

At present, there are several investigations available to confirm or rule out the diagnosis of primary aldosteronism: (1) intravenous saline loading test; (2) fludrocortisone suppression test; (3) oral saline loading test; and (4) captopril challenge test.[11] Once the diagnosis of primary aldosteronism is confirmed, the next step is differentiation of subtype. This step involves cross-sectional adrenal imaging (such as computed tomography) and adrenal venous sampling, a reliable method to identify unilateral adenomas that require adrenalectomy versus bilateral forms that require medical management. Subtyping is important because patients with an aldosterone-producing adenoma are biochemically freed from primary aldosteronism following adrenalectomy in 94% of cases,[31] while in patients with a familial form, further diagnostic workup can be avoided by careful history taking.[32]

Almost 90% of patients affected by primary aldosteronism present with a sporadic form, which consists of either aldosterone-producing adenomas or bilateral adrenal hyperplasia. Historically these 2 conditions were considered separate entities, but over the recent years this distinction is less clear.[33,34] Four genes (KCNJ5, CACNA1D, ATP1A1, and ATP2B3) have been identified as aldosterone-stimulating somatic mutations through next-generation sequencing. These genes are involved in different ways in the maintenance of membrane potential and intracellular ion homeostasis in nearly 60% of sporadic aldosterone-producing adenomas.[35,36] Up to 6% of patients present with familial primary aldosteronism.[33,37]

HYPERCORTISOLISM

Cushing syndrome is a rare cause of secondary hypertension affecting less than 1% of patients with resistant hypertension. Cushing syndrome presents with low-renin hypertension caused by excessive glucocorticoid production saturating glucocorticoid receptors, allowing excess glucocorticoids to activate MRs, resulting in mineralocorticoid excess effects. Hypokalemia and metabolic alkalosis occur in proportion to the degree of severity of cortisol excess, and both aldosterone and renin plasma activity are low, if measured. Low-renin hypertension is more likely to occur in patients with ectopic Cushing syndrome, which is characterized by a higher degree of cortisol excess. Frequently, patients do not present with classic Cushingoid features but develop severe myopathy, bruising, hypokalemia, and hypertension.[38]

Hypertension is reported in 50% to 75% of patients of patients with hypercortisolism.[39,40] Cortisol and aldosterone are equally potent MR agonists, but cortisol is inactivated to cortisone by HSD11B2, conferring a protective mechanism to the MR from excessive cortisol stimulation. However, in a state of severe hypercortisolism, the HSD11B2 is overwhelmed, resulting in cortisol-mediated MR activation and intravascular volume expansion with low renin and aldosterone levels.[41]

The diagnosis of overt cortisol excess is confirmed using 2 of the following investigations: (1) elevated 24-h urinary free cortisol; (2) elevated midnight salivary cortisol; or (3) failure to suppress cortisol following 1-mg dexamethasone suppression test. Treatment involves removing the culprit lesion (usually the ACTH-secreting neuroendocrine tumor).[42] In severe Cushing syndrome, treatment is urgent because uncontrolled cortisol excess frequently leads to high mortality attributable to cardiovascular complications or opportunistic infections.

LIDDLE SYNDROME

Liddle syndrome, first described by Liddle in 1963 is a monogenic form of low-renin hypertension, inherited in an autosomal dominant pattern.[2] It was initially known as pseudoaldosteronism because clinically it was similar to primary aldosteronism, but plasma aldosterone concentrations were reported to be suppressed.[43] Affected patients present with early-onset hypertension, suppressed plasma renin activity, low aldosterone, hypokalemia, and metabolic alkalosis.[44]

Liddle syndrome can be confirmed by genetic sequencing to confirm germline mutations of the SCNN1A, SCNN1B, and SCNN1G genes, which encode the α, β, and γ subunit of the epithelial sodium channel (ENaC), respectively (see **Table 1**). ENaC is expressed on the epithelium of distal nephron,[45] where it is positively regulated by aldosterone and antidiuretic hormone.[46] Thus far, 31 different mutations have been described in 72 families, resulting in Liddle syndrome.[44] Most of these mutations are missense, nonsense, or frameshift, causing increased ENaC expression at the distal nephron apical membrane, with a subsequent increase in Na^+ reabsorption.

MR antagonists are not helpful in the treatment of Liddle syndrome. It neither improves hypokalemia nor arterial hypertension, as Na^+ reabsorption is independent from MR activation and the lack of response to MR antagonists is considered as an adjunctive clinical criterion to suspect the diagnosis.[2] Patients do respond to management with ENaC blockers, amiloride, or triamterene, as well as following a low-sodium diet.[44]

Liddle syndrome should be suspected in a patient with early-onset hypertension presenting with low aldosterone, low renin, and low potassium concentrations. The diagnosis of Liddle syndrome is based on gene sequencing of SCNN1A, SCNN1B, and SCNN1G, and genetic screening should also be offered to first-degree relatives of affected patients.[44]

GORDON SYNDROME

Gordon syndrome, first described in the 1960s, is a rare genetic condition comprising altered renal salt absorption. Patients affected by Gordon syndrome display hyperkalemia, which distinguishes it from other forms of low-renin hypertension that present with hypokalemia[2] (see **Table 1**). Other presenting features include low renin, along with low-normal aldosterone concentrations, metabolic acidosis, hyperchloremia, and, occasionally, hypercalciuria.

Gordon syndrome occurs secondary to mutations in WNK1, WNK4, CUL3, or KLHL3 genes, and can be inherited in either an autosomal dominant or recessive form.[47–49] The WNK (With No Lysine) kinases, encoded by WNK1 and WNK4 genes, regulate the expression of the Na^+/Cl^- cotransporter in the distal nephron, while the scaffold protein Cullin 3 and the adaptor protein Kelch 3 (encoded by the CUL3 and KLHL3 genes, respectively) are involved in the ubiquitination and proteasomal degradation of the WNK kinases.[50] The final effects of these complex interactions are upregulation of the Na^+/Cl^- cotransporter at the plasma membrane resulting in increased Na^+ reabsorption, reduced expression of renal outer medullar K^+ channel, and subsequent hyperkalemia. Patients diagnosed with Gordon syndrome may be treated with thiazide diuretics that act by inhibiting the Na^+/Cl^- cotransporter.[51]

APPARENT MINERALOCORTICOID EXCESS SYNDROME

Apparent mineralocorticoid excess syndrome is an autosomal recessive disorder that presents with a clinical phenotype of low-renin hypertension. It is caused by germline mutations of the HSD11B2 gene resulting in deficiency of HSD11B2 enzyme, which mediates the conversion of active cortisol to inactive cortisone.[52] In an unaffected individual, the MR has affinity for both aldosterone and cortisol.[53] However, it is shielded from cortisol activation by HSD11B2 activity. Impaired HSD11B2 function in patients with the apparent mineralocorticoid excess syndrome enables cortisol-induced activation of the MR, leading to hypertension.[52] Patients with classic apparent mineralocorticoid excess syndrome display failure to thrive, polyuria, polydipsia, and severe hypertension, and present with hypokalemia and low renin and aldosterone concentrations. The diagnosis of apparent mineralocorticoid excess syndrome should be considered in a case of aldosterone-independent low-renin hypertension and an increased cortisol-to-cortisone ratio in the serum or urine and/or genetic sequencing of HSD11B2.[54,55] Around 40 germline mutations have been reported since the first mutation, leading to the apparent mineralocorticoid excess syndrome described.[56] Patients born from the consanguineous marriages and endogamy, or regions with founder effect, are at higher risk.[52]

It is noteworthy that at times this condition can present in a less severe or "nonclassic" form, and may be difficult to distinguish from essential hypertension. This depends on the degree of severity of HSD11B2 deficiency[56] or heterozygosity with existent partial activity of the HSD11B2 gene.[54]

In contrast to patients with Liddle syndrome, patients diagnosed with apparent mineralocorticoid excess syndrome respond well to MR antagonists, as well as to dexamethasone, which suppresses endogenous cortisol production while not undergoing metabolism by HSD11B2.[2]

CYP11B1 DEFICIENCY CONGENITAL ADRENAL HYPERPLASIA

CYP11B1 deficiency congenital adrenal hyperplasia (CAH) is an autosomal recessive disorder and is the second most common form, occurring in 5% to 8% of patients with CAH and further occurring in 1 in 100,000 Caucasians and 1 in 6000 Moroccan Jews.[57] CYP11B1 deficiency is caused by mutations in the CYP11B1 gene,[58] which facilitates the conversion of 11-deoxycortisol to cortisol. This leads to increased ACTH secretion and abnormally elevated production of 11-dexoxycortisol, deoxycorticosterone, and adrenal androgens.[59] Depending on the severity of CYP11B1 deficiency, affected patients present with variable degrees of virilization of female external genitalia, precocious puberty in males, and premature closure of growth plates resulting in short stature in adulthood. Deoxycorticosterone in excess leads to MR activation with a subsequent increase in sodium reabsorption, volume expansion, and low-renin hypertension.[60]

Therapy is directed at replacing cortisol to reduce ACTH secretion in excess and overproduction of deoxycorticosterone and androgens. Therefore, glucocorticoid therapy is the mainstay of treatment.[58] MR antagonists can be considered as additional therapy if hypertension is uncontrolled.[58,60]

CYP17 DEFICIENCY CONGENITAL ADRENAL HYPERPLASIA

CYP17 deficiency CAH is rare, affecting 1 in 50,000, with an increased frequency in Brazil.[61,62] The lack of 17-hydroxylase activity forces steroidogenesis to corticosterone rather than cortisol via 11-deoxycorticosterone (DOC). DOC is a mineralocorticoid that is slightly less potent than aldosterone. The increase in circulating corticosterone substitutes for lack of cortisol and supplies glucocorticoid activity.[62] In parallel, increased DOC concentrations saturate the MR, displaying a clinical picture similar to patients with CYP11B1 deficiency presenting with mineralocorticoid excess.[2] Consequently, adrenal 17-OH deficiency rarely leads to adrenal crisis and is usually diagnosed based on presentation of primary amenorrhea (due to androgen deficiency) and early-onset low-renin hypertension from DOC excess.

Patients present with a reduction in cortisol and adrenal and gonadal sex steroid production. The deficiency in sex hormones results in absence of secondary sexual characteristics in adolescent females, amenorrhea, and low-renin hypertension.[58] Treatment consists of cortisol replacement therapy if needed, MR antagonists if hypertension is uncontrolled, and replacement of sex steroids.[62]

GLUCOCORTICOID-RESISTANCE SYNDROME

Glucocorticoid-resistance syndrome is caused by point mutations or deletions in the NR3C1 gene (chromosome 5q31-q32) encoding for the glucocorticoid receptor, and is inherited in an autosomal recessive manner.[63] The mutation affects either the DNA-binding or the ligand-binding domain, resulting in end-organ resistance to glucocorticoids coupled with increased ACTH and hypercortisolism without the clinical phenotype of Cushing syndrome.[64,65] The increased ACTH leads to hypersecretion of adrenal mineralocorticoids and androgens, and MR activation by cortisol excess. The most common clinical presentation consists of chronic fatigue caused by glucocorticoid deficiency, low-renin hypertension, hypokalemia, and metabolic alkalosis.[64] Low-renin hypertension occurs because of saturation of 11BHSD2 enzymatic activity.[2] Affected patients also present with alopecia in males, hirsutism in females, acne, precocious puberty, and infertility.[66,67]

Dexamethasone administration, the mainstay of therapy, activates the glucocorticoid receptor with the aim of suppressing ACTH secretion[66] and MR antagonists to control hypertension.[68]

MINERALOCORTICOID RECEPTOR–ACTIVATING MUTATION

Syndrome caused by the MR-activating mutation is a rare autosomal dominant condition, which to date has been described in one family.[69] A point mutation in the NR3C2 gene that encodes the MR results in the missense substitution of serine at codon 810. The S810L mutation displays a significant degree of constitutive activation of the mutant MR, which also is strongly activated by progesterone (during pregnancy) and unexpectedly by the MR antagonist spironolactone. The condition consists of early-onset low-renin hypertension associated with hypokalemia that worsens during pregnancy.[69] Both cortisone and 11-dehydrocorticosterone can activate the mutant MR, resulting in hypertension and hypokalemia in nonpregnant women and male patients. Because of its ability to activate the mutant MR, the use of spironolactone is contraindicated. Amiloride (which inhibits ENaC) and finerenone (a nonsteroidal selective MR antagonist) are recommended for treatment.[70]

DEOXYCORTICOSTERONE-PRODUCING ADRENAL TUMORS

DOC-producing adrenal tumors causing hypertension are very rare, and thus far approximately 10 cases have been described in the literature. These tumors are usually large and malignant. Some secrete androgens and estrogens in addition to DOC, which may cause virilization in women and feminization in men. A high level of plasma DOC or urinary tetrahydrodeoxycorticosterone, and a large adrenal tumor identified by computed tomography, confirms the diagnosis. This entity of adrenal disorder consists of low-renin hypertension with a large adrenal mass, but no aldosterone excess or clinical signs of Cushing syndrome. Surgical resection of adrenal tumor is the optimal management.[71]

LICORICE INGESTION

Licorice, the root of *Glycyrrhiza glabra*, has been used since remote antiquity for both culinary and medicinal purposes. Several studies reported both short-term and long-term consumption of significant amounts of licorice may lead to hypokalemia, hypertension, and even cardiac arrest.[72–74] The mechanism by which licorice leads to complications involves the inhibition of HSD11B2, an enzyme that converts active cortisol to inactive cortisone. Glycyrrhizin (the primary active ingredient of licorice) is hydrolyzed into glycyrrhetinic acid, which directly inhibits HSD11B2. Inhibition of HSD11B2 leads to a substantial accumulation of cortisol with subsequent MR activation. Licorice-induced pseudohyperaldosteronism is thus characterized by increased sodium retention and potassium excretion along with renin-angiotensin system suppression, leading to hypertension.[75] In addition, licorice can also bind directly to the MR, thus potentially exacerbating the pseudohyperaldosteronism syndrome.[76]

The US Food and Drug Administration has issued a warning that ingesting 40 to 50 g/d for up to 2 weeks can increase the risk of arrhythmia, and longer-term consumption can potentially lead to hypertension and pseudohyperaldosteronism.[77,78] Clinically the diagnosis of licorice overconsumption should be suspected in patients presenting with hypokalemia, hypertension, and muscle weakness that are unexplained by other causes. Additional laboratory tests may document the increase in cortisol/cortisone plasma ratio (see **Table 1**).

GRAPEFRUIT INGESTION

Naringin, along with its metabolite aglycone naringin, belong to a series of flavonoids present in grapefruit juice and are responsible for grapefruit-induced pseudohyperaldosteronism. The inhibitory effect of aglycone naringin on HSD11B2 is similar to that of licorice.[79] Prolonged consumption of grapefruit juice has been reported to induce low-renin hypertension associated with hypokalemia and to induce hyperaldosteronism associated with hypokalemia, borderline hypertension, and renin-angiotensin system suppression.[80] Discontinuation of grapefruit juice consumption for 30 days led to normalization of potassium concentrations and reduction in edema. Ingestion of 250 mL/d of grapefruit juice for 7 days was reported to lead to a significant inhibition of HSD11B2.[81] Supplements with flavonoids are available in health food stores. Thus, patients at risk need to be educated about the risks of consuming large volumes of grapefruit juice or flavonoid products.

SUMMARY

Low-renin hypertension encompasses a wide range of disorders. Measurement of direct renin concentration or plasma renin activity, aldosterone, and potassium is key to diagnosing low-renin hypertension. A detailed family history and genetic testing may aid the differential diagnosis (see **Fig. 1**). Therapy depends on the subtype of low-renin hypertension and is targeted toward normalization of hypertension.

REFERENCES

1. Sealey JE, Gordon RD, Mantero F. Plasma renin and aldosterone measurements in low renin hypertensive states. Trends Endocrinol Metab 2005;16(3):86–91.

2. Mulatero P, Verhovez A, Morello F, et al. Diagnosis and treatment of low-renin hypertension. Clin Endocrinol (Oxf) 2007;67(3):324–34.

3. Sagnella GA. Why is plasma renin activity lower in populations of African origin? J Hum Hypertens 2001;15(1):17–25.

4. Adlin EV, Marks AD, Channick BJ. The salivary sodium/potassium ratio in hypertension: relation to race and plasma renin activity. Clin Exp Hypertens A 1982; 4(9–10):1869–80.

5. Woods JW, Liddle GW, Michelakis AM, et al. Effect of an adrenal inhibitor in hypertensive patients with suppressed renin. Arch Intern Med 1969;123(4):366–70.

6. Adlin EV, Marks AD, Channick BJ. Spironolactone and hydrochlorothiazide in essential hypertension. Blood pressure response and plasma renin activity. Arch Intern Med 1972;130(6):855–8.

7. Fisher ND, Hurwitz S, Jeunemaitre X, et al. Familial aggregation of low-renin hypertension. Hypertension 2002;39(4):914–8.

8. Bock HA, Hermle M, Brunner FP, et al. Pressure dependent modulation of renin release in isolated perfused glomeruli. Kidney Int 1992;41(2):275–80.

9. DiBona GF. Neural control of the kidney: functionally specific renal sympathetic nerve fibers. Am J Physiol Regul Integr Comp Physiol 2000;279(5):R1517–24.

10. Sparks MA, Crowley SD, Gurley SB, et al. Classical Renin-Angiotensin system in kidney physiology. Compr Physiol 2014;4(3):1201–28.

11. Funder JW, Carey RM, Mantero F, et al. The management of primary aldosteronism: case detection, diagnosis, and treatment: an endocrine society clinical practice guideline. J Clin Endocrinol Metab 2016;101(5):1889–916.

12. Carter S, Owen LJ, Kerstens MN, et al. A liquid chromatography tandem mass spectrometry assay for plasma renin activity using online solid-phase extraction. Ann Clin Biochem 2012;49(Pt 6):570–9.

13. Rossi GP, Barisa M, Belfiore A, et al. The aldosterone-renin ratio based on the plasma renin activity and the direct renin assay for diagnosing aldosterone-producing adenoma. J Hypertens 2010;28(9):1892–9.

14. Burrello J, Monticone S, Buffolo F, et al. Diagnostic accuracy of aldosterone and renin measurement by chemiluminescent immunoassay and radioimmunoassay in primary aldosteronism. J Hypertens 2016;34(5):920–7.

15. Fisher ND, Hurwitz S, Ferri C, et al. Altered adrenal sensitivity to angiotensin II in low-renin essential hypertension. Hypertension 1999;34(3):388–94.

16. Markou A, Sertedaki A, Kaltsas G, et al. Stress-induced aldosterone hyper-secretion in a substantial subset of patients with essential hypertension. J Clin Endocrinol Metab 2015;100(8):2857–64.

17. Mulatero P, Rabbia F, Milan A, et al. Drug effects on aldosterone/plasma renin activity ratio in primary aldosteronism. Hypertension 2002;40(6):897–902.

18. Oster JR, Singer I, Fishman LM. Heparin-induced aldosterone suppression and hyperkalemia. Am J Med 1995;98(6):575–86.

19. Tobin MD, Raleigh SM, Newhouse S, et al. Association of WNK1 gene polymorphisms and haplotypes with ambulatory blood pressure in the general population. Circulation 2005;112(22):3423–9.

20. Gordon RD, Laragh JH, Funder JW. Low renin hypertensive states: perspectives, unsolved problems, future research. Trends Endocrinol Metabol 2005;16(3): 108–13.

21. Baudrand R, Vaidya A. The low-renin hypertension phenotype: genetics and the role of the mineralocorticoid receptor. Int J Mol Sci 2018;19(2) [pii:E546].

22. Baker EH, Dong YB, Sagnella GA, et al. Association of hypertension with T594M mutation in beta subunit of epithelial sodium channels in black people resident in London. Lancet 1998;351(9113):1388–92.

23. Akintunde A, Nondi J, Gogo K, et al. Physiological Phenotyping for Personalized Therapy of Uncontrolled hypertension in Africa. Am J Hypertens 2017;30(9): 923–30.

24. Soro A, Ingram MC, Tonolo G, et al. Evidence of coexisting changes in 11 beta-hydroxysteroid dehydrogenase and 5 beta-reductase activity in subjects with untreated essential hypertension. Hypertension 1995;25(1):67–70.

25. Campino C, Martinez-Aguayo A, Baudrand R, et al. Age-related changes in 11beta-hydroxysteroid dehydrogenase type 2 activity in normotensive subjects. Am J Hypertens 2013;26(4):481–7.

26. Lovati E, Ferrari P, Dick B, et al. Molecular basis of human salt sensitivity: the role of the 11beta-hydroxysteroid dehydrogenase type 2. J Clin Endocrinol Metab 1999;84(10):3745–9.

27. Williams TA, Mulatero P, Filigheddu F, et al. Role of HSD11B2 polymorphisms in essential hypertension and the diuretic response to thiazides. Kidney Int 2005; 67(2):631–7.

28. Calhoun DA, Nishizaka MK, Zaman MA, et al. Hyperaldosteronism among black and white subjects with resistant hypertension. Hypertension 2002;40(6):892–6.

29. Monticone S, D'Ascenzo F, Moretti C, et al. Cardiovascular events and target organ damage in primary aldosteronism compared with essential hypertension: a systematic review and meta-analysis. Lancet Diabetes Endocrinol 2018;6(1): 41–50.

30. Mulatero P, Monticone S, Bertello C, et al. Long-term cardio- and cerebrovascular events in patients with primary aldosteronism. J Clin Endocrinol Metab 2013; 98(12):4826–33.

31. Williams TA, Lenders JWM, Mulatero P, et al. Outcomes after adrenalectomy for unilateral primary aldosteronism: an international consensus on outcome measures and analysis of remission rates in an international cohort. Lancet Diabetes Endocrinol 2017;5(9):689–99.

32. Monticone S, Viola A, Rossato D, et al. Adrenal vein sampling in primary aldosteronism: towards a standardised protocol. Lancet Diabetes Endocrinol 2015;3(4): 296–303.

33. Monticone S, Else T, Mulatero P, et al. Understanding primary aldosteronism: impact of next generation sequencing and expression profiling. Mol Cell Endocrinol 2015;399:311–20.

34. Gomez-Sanchez CE, Qi X, Velarde-Miranda C, et al. Development of monoclonal antibodies against human CYP11B1 and CYP11B2. Mol Cell Endocrinol 2014; 383(1–2):111–7.

35. Choi M, Scholl UI, Yue P, et al. K+ channel mutations in adrenal aldosterone-producing adenomas and hereditary hypertension. Science 2011;331(6018): 768–72.

36. Fernandes-Rosa FL, Williams TA, Riester A, et al. Genetic spectrum and clinical correlates of somatic mutations in aldosterone-producing adenoma. Hypertension 2014;64(2):354–61.

37. Mulatero P, Tizzani D, Viola A, et al. Prevalence and characteristics of familial hyperaldosteronism: the PATOGEN study (Primary Aldosteronism in TOrino-GENetic forms). Hypertension 2011;58(5):797–803.

38. Ilias I, Torpy DJ, Pacak K, et al. Cushing's syndrome due to ectopic corticotropin secretion: twenty years' experience at the National Institutes of Health. J Clin Endocrinol Metab 2005;90(8):4955–62.
39. Cieszynski L, Berendt-Obolonczyk M, Szulc M, et al. Cushing's syndrome due to ectopic ACTH secretion. Endokrynol Pol 2016;67(4):458–71.
40. Isidori AM, Kaltsas GA, Pozza C, et al. The ectopic adrenocorticotropin syndrome: clinical features, diagnosis, management, and long-term follow-up. J Clin Endocrinol Metab 2006;91(2):371–7.
41. Isidori AM, Graziadio C, Paragliola RM, et al. The hypertension of Cushing's syndrome: controversies in the pathophysiology and focus on cardiovascular complications. J Hypertens 2015;33(1):44–60.
42. Nieman LK, Biller BM, Findling JW, et al. Treatment of Cushing's syndrome: an endocrine society clinical practice guideline. J Clin Endocrinol Metab 2015; 100(8):2807–31.
43. Liddle GWBT, Coppage WSJ. A familial renal disorder simulating primary aldosteronism but with negligible aldosterone secretion. Trans Assoc Am Phys 1963;76: 199–213.
44. Tetti M, Monticone S, Burrello J, et al. Liddle syndrome: review of the literature and description of a new case. Int J Mol Sci 2018;19(3) [pii:E812].
45. Canessa CM, Schild L, Buell G, et al. Amiloride-sensitive epithelial Na+ channel is made of three homologous subunits. Nature 1994;367(6462):463–7.
46. Hanukoglu I, Hanukoglu A. Epithelial sodium channel (ENaC) family: phylogeny, structure-function, tissue distribution, and associated inherited diseases. Gene 2016;579(2):95–132.
47. Wilson FH, Disse-Nicodeme S, Choate KA, et al. Human hypertension caused by mutations in WNK kinases. Science 2001;293(5532):1107–12.
48. Louis-Dit-Picard H, Barc J, Trujillano D, et al. KLHL3 mutations cause familial hyperkalemic hypertension by impairing ion transport in the distal nephron. Nat Genet 2012;44(4):456–60. S1-3.
49. Boyden LM, Choi M, Choate KA, et al. Mutations in kelch-like 3 and cullin 3 cause hypertension and electrolyte abnormalities. Nature 2012;482(7383):98–102.
50. O'Shaughnessy KM. Gordon syndrome: a continuing story. Pediatr Nephrol 2015; 30(11):1903–8.
51. Mayan H, Munter G, Shaharabany M, et al. Hypercalciuria in familial hyperkalemia and hypertension accompanies hyperkalemia and precedes hypertension: description of a large family with the Q565E WNK4 mutation. J Clin Endocrinol Metab 2004;89(8):4025–30.
52. New MI, Geller DS, Fallo F, et al. Monogenic low renin hypertension. Trends Endocrinol Metabol 2005;16(3):92–7.
53. Krozowski ZS, Funder JW. Renal mineralocorticoid receptors and hippocampal corticosterone-binding species have identical intrinsic steroid specificity. Proc Natl Acad Sci U S A 1983;80(19):6056–60.
54. Funder JW. Apparent mineralocorticoid excess. J Steroid Biochem Mol Biol 2017; 165(Pt A):151–3.
55. Carvajal CA, Romero DG, Mosso LM, et al. Biochemical and genetic characterization of 11 beta-hydroxysteroid dehydrogenase type 2 in low-renin essential hypertensives. J Hypertens 2005;23(1):71–7.
56. Wilson RC, Dave-Sharma S, Wei JQ, et al. A genetic defect resulting in mild low-renin hypertension. Proc Natl Acad Sci U S A 1998;95(17):10200–5.

57. Zachmann M, Tassinari D, Prader A. Clinical and biochemical variability of congenital adrenal hyperplasia due to 11 beta-hydroxylase deficiency. A study of 25 patients. J Clin Endocrinol Metab 1983;56(2):222–9.

58. El-Maouche D, Arlt W, Merke DP. Congenital adrenal hyperplasia. Lancet 2017; 390(10108):2194–210.

59. Monticone S, Losano I, Tetti M, et al. Diagnostic approach to low-renin hypertension. Clin Endocrinol (Oxf) 2018;89(4):385–96.

60. Bulsari K, Falhammar H. Clinical perspectives in congenital adrenal hyperplasia due to 11beta-hydroxylase deficiency. Endocrine 2017;55(1):19–36.

61. Costa-Santos M, Kater CE, Auchus RJ, Brazilian Congenital Adrenal Hyperplasia Multicenter Study Group. Two prevalent CYP17 mutations and genotype-phenotype correlations in 24 Brazilian patients with 17-hydroxylase deficiency. J Clin Endocrinol Metab 2004;89(1):49–60.

62. Auchus RJ. Steroid 17-hydroxylase and 17,20-lyase deficiencies, genetic and pharmacologic. J Steroid Biochem Mol Biol 2017;165(Pt A):71–8.

63. Chrousos GP, Vingerhoeds A, Brandon D, et al. Primary cortisol resistance in man. A glucocorticoid receptor-mediated disease. J Clin Invest 1982;69(6): 1261–9.

64. Nicolaides NC, Charmandari E. Chrousos syndrome: from molecular pathogenesis to therapeutic management. Eur J Clin Invest 2015;45(5):504–14.

65. Yang N, Ray DW, Matthews LC. Current concepts in glucocorticoid resistance. Steroids 2012;77(11):1041–9.

66. Roberts ML, Kino T, Nicolaides NC, et al. A novel point mutation in the DNA-binding domain (DBD) of the human glucocorticoid receptor causes primary generalized glucocorticoid resistance by disrupting the hydrophobic structure of its DBD. J Clin Endocrinol Metab 2013;98(4):E790–5.

67. Mendonca BB, Leite MV, de Castro M, et al. Female pseudohermaphroditism caused by a novel homozygous missense mutation of the GR gene. J Clin Endocrinol Metab 2002;87(4):1805–9.

68. Bouligand J, Delemer B, Hecart AC, et al. Familial glucocorticoid receptor haploinsufficiency by non-sense mediated mRNA decay, adrenal hyperplasia and apparent mineralocorticoid excess. PLoS One 2010;5(10):e13563.

69. Geller DS, Farhi A, Pinkerton N, et al. Activating mineralocorticoid receptor mutation in hypertension exacerbated by pregnancy. Science 2000;289(5476): 119–23.

70. Amazit L, Le Billan F, Kolkhof P, et al. Finerenone impedes aldosterone-dependent nuclear import of the mineralocorticoid receptor and prevents genomic recruitment of steroid receptor coactivator-1. J Biol Chem 2015;290(36): 21876–89.

71. Young WF. Endocrine hypertension. In: Gardner DG, Shoback D, editors. Greenspan's basic & clinical endocrinology. 10th edition. New York: McGraw-Hill Education; 2017.

72. Flores-Robles BJ, Sandoval AR, Dardon JD, et al. Lethal liquorice lollies (liquorice abuse causing pseudohyperaldosteronism). BMJ Case Rep 2013;2013.

73. Crean AM, Abdel-Rahman SE, Greenwood JP. A sweet tooth as the root cause of cardiac arrest. Can J Cardiol 2009;25(10):e357–8.

74. Sontia B, Mooney J, Gaudet L, et al. Pseudohyperaldosteronism, liquorice, and hypertension. J Clin Hypertens (Greenwich) 2008;10(2):153–7.

75. Stewart PM, Wallace AM, Valentino R, et al. Mineralocorticoid activity of liquorice: 11-beta-hydroxysteroid dehydrogenase deficiency comes of age. Lancet 1987; 2(8563):821–4.

76. Calo LA, Zaghetto F, Pagnin E, et al. Effect of aldosterone and glycyrrhetinic acid on the protein expression of PAI-1 and p22(phox) in human mononuclear leukocytes. J Clin Endocrinol Metab 2004;89(4):1973–6.
77. Evaluation of certain food additives. World Health Organization technical report series. 2005;928:1–156.
78. Omar HR, Komarova I, El-Ghonemi M, et al. Licorice abuse: time to send a warning message. Ther Adv Endocrinol Metab 2012;3(4):125–38.
79. Walker BR, Best R. Clinical investigation of 11 beta-hydroxysteroid dehydrogenase. Endocr Res 1995;21(1–2):379–87.
80. Palermo M, Armanini D, Delitala G. Grapefruit juice inhibits 11beta-hydroxysteroid dehydrogenase in vivo, in man. Clin Endocrinol (Oxf) 2003;59(1):143–4.
81. Lee YS, Lorenzo BJ, Koufis T, et al. Grapefruit juice and its flavonoids inhibit 11 beta-hydroxysteroid dehydrogenase. Clin Pharmacol Ther 1996;59(1):62–71.

Hypertension and Cardiovascular Mortality in Patients with Cushing Syndrome

Lynnette K. Nieman, MD

KEYWORDS

- Hypertension • Cushing syndrome • Cardiovascular disease
- Standard mortality rate

KEY POINTS

- Hypercortisolemic patients with active Cushing syndrome have an increased standardized mortality rate that is driven largely by cardiovascular disease.
- Hypertension, dyslipidemia, obesity, and diabetes are frequent comorbidities that contribute to cardiovascular risk; each should be specifically treated during Cushing syndrome evaluation and treatment.
- Hypertension in Cushing syndrome is caused in part by subnormal renal conversion of cortisol to cortisone, leading to salt retention and volume expansion.
- Hypertension is also caused by cortisol action to enhance sensitivity to vasoconstrictors and by reduced concentration of vasodilators.
- Treatment of hypertension based on pathophysiology includes mineralocorticoid antagonists, angiotensin II receptor blockers, or angiotensin-converting enzyme inhibitors; calcium channel or beta blockers are also useful.

EPIDEMIOLOGY

The sustained hypercortisolism of active Cushing syndrome is associated with an increased standardized mortality rate (SMR) of 2.8- to 16-fold that of the comparison population, depending on the report.[1] Surgical cure, with normalization of cortisol, led to the reduction of SMR compared with rates seen in the general population in most, but not all, studies.[1]

The rate of cardiovascular disease in Cushing syndrome is increased up to 5 times that of the population average.[2,3] As shown in **Table 1**, this is a major contributor to the increased mortality in patients with hypercortisolism.[1,4] In the general population, the

Disclosure Statement: The author has nothing to disclose.
Diabetes, Endocrinology and Obesity Branch, The National Institute of Diabetes and Digestive and Kidney Diseases (NIDDK), National Institutes of Health, Building 10, CRC, 1 East, Room 1-3140, 10 Center Drive, MSC 1109, Bethesda, MD 20892-1109, USA
E-mail address: NiemanL@nih.gov

Table 1
Causes of death in 253 patients with Cushing syndrome (excluding adrenal cancer and malignant ectopic ACTH secretion) compared with the expected rate in the population matched for age and sex

Cause of Death	Observed %	Expected %
Cancer	22	28
Ischemic heart disease	19	22
Stroke	17	10
Sepsis	17	
Pulmonary embolism	11	

Data from BollandMJ, Holdaway IM, Berkeley JE, et al. Mortality and morbidity in Cushing's syndrome in New Zealand. ClinEndocrinol (Oxf) 2011;75:436-442.

risk of death from heart disease, stroke, or other vascular disease doubles for every 20 mm Hg increase in systolic blood pressure and every 10 mm Hg increase in diastolic values.[5] Hypertension is present in up to 85% of adult patients with Cushing syndrome[6] and its prevalence is higher, up to 95%, in patients with ectopic adrenocorticotropic hormone (ACTH) production as a cause.[7] Thus it is likely that the presence of hypertension increases the risk of cardiovascular events in Cushing syndrome as well as the general population.[8]

RISK FACTORS

Hypertension in Cushing syndrome is associated with older age, increased body mass index (BMI), and the severity and duration of hypercortisolism. In addition to the deleterious effects of hypertension on cardiovascular function, many other risks for cardiovascular disease are common in Cushing syndrome, including a hypercoagulablestate,[9] impaired glucose tolerance, hyperlipidemia, and obesity.[10] Other risks such as smoking should be considered.

PATHOPHYSIOLOGY
Hypertension

A variety of factors are postulated to contribute to development of hypertension in endogenous Cushing syndrome (**Fig. 1**). The renal 11β-hydroxysteroid-dehydrogenase type 2 (11β-HSD2) enzyme normally converts cortisol to cortisone, thereby inactivating its ability to bind to the mineralocorticoid receptor. Because cortisol circulates at much higher levels than aldosterone, this tissue-specific inactivation allows aldosterone (rather than cortisol) to act as the major mineralocorticoid in healthy people. By contrast, in Cushing syndrome, extremely high cortisol levels saturate the renal 11β-HSD2 enzyme so that it cannot convert all cortisol to cortisone. As a result, cortisol can bind to the mineralocorticoid receptor, leading to sodium retention, volume expansion, and hypertension.[11]

There is a direct correlation between the severity of hypercortisolism and the inability to inactivate cortisol via 11β-HSD2, so that this is seen primarily in patients with hypokalemia who have cortisol levels more than 5 times the normal level.[7] However, the persistence of hypertension after administration of a mineralocorticoid antagonist suggests that other pathophysiologic mechanisms exist.[12] Furthermore, hypertension improves with administration of mifepristone, a glucocorticoid antagonist that does not bind the mineralocorticoid receptor.[13] Taken together, these data

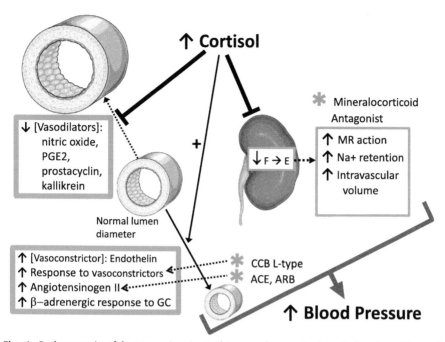

Fig. 1. Pathogenesis of hypertension in Cushing syndrome. Text indicates the effects of excess glucocorticoids (GC) on the renin-angiotensin system and other pathways involved. [ ], concentration; ↑, increased; ↓, decreased; *, indicates potential therapeutic strategies based on reversal of the pathophysiologic effect; ACE, angiotensin-converting enzyme inhibitor; ARB, angiotensin II receptor blocker; CCB, calcium channel blocker; E, cortisone; F, cortisol; MR, mineralocorticoid receptor; Na+, sodium; PGE2, prostaglandin E2.

provide strong evidence that the glucocorticoid receptor is involved directly in the pathogenesis of hypertension.

In contrast to the kidney, vascular endothelial and smooth muscle cells contain 11β-hydroxysteroid-dehydrogenase type 1 (11β-HSD1) as well as 11β-HSD2.[14] 11β-HSD1 converts inactive cortisone to cortisol, which may possibly modulate vascular sensitivity to vasoconstricting agents. Indeed, although circulating concentrations of angiotensin II are not changed in Cushing syndrome, the pressor response to this agent is increased.[15] The circulating concentration of some other vasoconstricting agents (eg, catecholamines and renin) is also not increased in Cushing syndrome.[16] However, in healthy adults, glucocorticoids increase the sensitivity to infusions of norepinephrine and phenylephrine.[17] Similarly, β-adrenoreceptor sensitivity to catecholamines is increased in patients with Cushing syndrome.[18,19]

The data presented earlier suggest that in Cushing syndrome hypertension results in part from enhanced sensitivity to vasoconstrictors. In addition, levels of endothelin-1, a potent vasoconstrictor, are elevated in hypercortisolemic patients with untreated, active Cushing syndrome.[20,21] Additional data suggest that the resulting imbalance between vasoconstriction and dilation is enhanced further by reduced levels of vasodilators, including nitric oxide,[22] prostacyclin, PGE2, and kallikrein.[23,24]

Finally, at the structural level of the airways, increased fat in the neck and abdomen and weakened muscles responsible for patency of the airways may lead to sleep apnea[25] with its increased risk of hypertension.[26]

Cardiovascular Disease

Several studies have evaluated intima-media thickness (IMT) in the carotid artery as a surrogate marker of whole body and coronary atherosclerosis. In one such study, significant carotid artery atherosclerosis was found in 8 out of 25 patients with active Cushing disease compared with 2 out of 32 subjects matched for BMI, age, and sex. These abnormalities were accompanied by a smaller lumen diameter with less distensibility of the artery and increased IMT. At 1 year after surgical cure, the rate of these abnormalities was similar in both groups but remained greater than that of age- and sex-matched control subjects.[8]

Albiger and colleagues[27] also studied carotid artery parameters in patients with Cushing syndrome who were matched with control subjects for sex, age, smoking habit, BMI, blood pressure, fasting glucose/insulin, and lipid values. The proportion of subjects with hypertension was similar in both groups. Compared with control subjects, patients with Cushing syndrome had significantly greater IMT at the common carotid, carotid bulb, and abdominal aorta but not the femoral artery. The presence of atherosclerotic plaques also was increased significantly in the patient group (14.2% vs 7.1%). Within the Cushing syndrome group, IMT showed a weak to moderate correlation with fasting glucose, homeostatic model assessment index, and waist-to-hip ratio ($r^2 = 0.37$–0.64).

A recent literature review and meta-analysis of 14 studies of 332 patients with Cushing syndrome and 462 controls largely confirmed these findings.[28] The odds ratio for an increased number of carotid plaques was increased both in patients with active hypercortisolism (odds ratio [OR]: 8.85, 95% confidence interval [CI]: 4.09–19.14; $P<.001$) and in those who are in remission (OR: 9.88, 95%CI: 2.69–36.3; $P<.001$). In this large population, age, abnormal glucose tolerance, obesity, and cortisol levels influenced the finding of increased IMT in Cushing syndrome.

Direct investigations of cardiac structure and function provide insight into the pathogenesis of cardiovascular disease. Forty-two hypercortisolemic patients with hypertension had more diastolic dysfunction than control subjects with similar age, sex, and blood pressure as judged by echocardiography[29]; this functional change was likely influenced by structural changes, which included worse midwall systolic movement and left ventricular hypertrophy (10/42) and concentric remodeling (26/42).

Abnormal echocardiographic findings were confirmed in a larger study of 70 patients and matched control subjects, both in the active phase of Cushing syndrome and during remission.[30] Left ventricular hypertrophy was more prevalent (70%) in this study, in which 42% of patients had concentric hypertrophy and 23% had concentric remodeling. Despite these abnormalities, ejection fraction was normal. After remission, the ventricular abnormalities improved but remained more prevalent than in the control group.

Because ultrasound measurements of the right heart may be inaccurate, investigators used cardiac MRI to assess function of the ventricles and left atrium in 18 patients with active Cushing syndrome and 18 healthy controls who matched for age, sex, and BMI.[31] In contrast to the Toja study, ejection fractions at all 3 locations were significantly reduced and end-diastolic left ventricular mass index was increased. All ejection fractions improved after treatment, although not all changes were statistically significant: increases occurred at the left ventricle (15%, $P = .029$), left atrium (45%, $P<.001$), and the right ventricle (11%, $P = NS$). The left ventricle mass index also decreased by 17% ($P<.001$).

Few studies have directly assessed coronary artery plaque burden. In one, calcified and noncalcified plaque were assessed using a multidetector CT coronary angiogram scan in 15 patients with ACTH-dependent Cushing syndrome, 4 of whom were eucortisolemic as a result of medical treatment or hormone cyclicity.[32] The Agatston score, representing calcified plaque and the noncalcified plaque volume, was compared with that of control subjects matched for sex, age, and BMI who had at least one risk factor for cardiovascular disease. Both noncalcified plaque volume and the Agatston score were significantly increased in the patients with Cushing syndrome, including those who were eucortisolemic.

Taken together, these studies show an increased rate of carotid, coronary, and aortic atherosclerosis in patients with active Cushing syndrome. Many of these abnormalities persist when eucortisolism is restored, but their frequency may be reduced to levels similar to that of patients without Cushing syndrome who have the same cardiovascular risk factors (eg, obesity, diabetes, hypertension).

CLINICAL FEATURES

Hypertension in Cushing syndrome is characterized by significant attenuation of the normal nocturnal decline in blood pressure during sleep.[33] This "nondipping" pattern has been attributed to hypercortisolemia with loss of the bedtime nadir in serum cortisol levels. Within the general population, nondipping is associated with an increased risk of cardiovascular events, both in hypertensive and normotensive individuals.[34] A recent literature review suggests that administration of antihypertensives at bedtime may reduce cardiovascular risk, but notes that further targeted studies with adequate statistical power are needed.[35] This approach has not been tested in a Cushing syndrome population.

ANTIHYPERTENSIVE THERAPY IN CUSHING SYNDROME

Effective medical therapy with steroidogenesis inhibitors[36] improves blood pressure in most, but not all, patients. It is well established that hypertension resolves or improves in most patients when evaluated 1 year after surgical cure of CS, when a threshold criterion of 140/90 mm Hg is used (see later discussion).[37,38] Thus treatment to normalize cortisol is the mainstay of antihypertensive treatment in Cushing syndrome. However, there is often a long delay before definitive surgery is performed, and some patients are unable to undergo surgical resection of the causative tumor, because of invasion, metastases, or inability to identify a lesion. In these cases, antihypertensive therapy should be initiated until the effects of surgery can be assessed.

Because of the multifactorial cause of hypertension in cortisol excess states, there is no one optimal approach to treatment. Thus the choice of antihypertensive may best be chosen based on the multiple causes of hypertension (see **Fig. 1**). Use of angiotensin II receptor blockers or angiotensin-converting enzyme inhibitors is recommended, based on evidence that the renin-angiotensin system is upregulated and also on a potential improvement in nitric oxide levels.[33,39–41] However, many patients require more than one medication. Spironolactone may be quite helpful, particularly in those with moderate to severe hypokalemia. Combination therapy generally does not lead to hyperkalemia. There are few data to support or refute the use of calcium channel blockers or beta blockers; clinical experience suggests that they may be useful. Hydralazine may be helpful in reducing vasoconstriction. In theory, the dual endothelin receptor antagonist aprocitentan might be useful in Cushing syndrome, but to our knowledge has not been tested in this population.[42]

As noted earlier, normalization of hypercortisolism may normalize blood pressure. However, in one study, 28% of such patients remained hypertensive 1 year after surgical cure.[38] Although the severity of hypertension did not predict hypertensive remission, a longer duration of hypertension was associated with lack of remission, possibly because of vascular remodeling. This provides an ancillary reason for aggressive treatment of hypertension before surgical cure.

However, it should not be assumed that hypertension will remit after surgery, and the time-course of remission, when it occurs, is not known. As a result, the need for antihypertensive therapy should be reevaluated in the immediate postoperative period and afterward. It is possible that the number and/or dose of medications could be reduced, as patients lose weight after cure.

PROGNOSIS

As noted earlier, the mortality rate in patients with Cushing syndrome is increased and is driven largely by cardiovascular events. The risk of cardiovascular events persists for at least 5 years after successful cure.[2] However, no study has examined the rate of events in patients in whom comorbidities of hypertension, insulin resistance, and overweight/obesity were normalized. These comorbidities usually remit within a year after surgical cure but may continue in up to 25% of patients.[3,8,38]

Data are inconsistent regarding whether the SMR normalizes after cure of Cushing syndrome. Apparent continued increases may reflect a long time frame of study during which limited treatment choices in the distant past influenced a worse overall outcome,[43] although in one large comparative study, the mortality rates differed at different sites during similar time frames. Whether this reflects an inherent difference in the patient population, local physicians' management strategies, or access to care is not clear. However, it is evident that all comorbidities should be addressed and aggressively treated, both before and after cure, to reduce cardiovascular events.[44]

Waiting for cure of Cushing syndrome by surgery is not sufficient to address cardiovascular morbidity and mortality. Each patient with active Cushing syndrome should be assessed for the presence of glucose intolerance, hypertension, dyslipidemia, and overweight/obesity (the latter almost universal). If present, each should be specifically treated with a goal to normalize the abnormality.

Ideally, surgical resection leads to cure and reduction in cardiovascular risk, but apart from cortisol-secreting adrenal adenomas, the rate of remission from surgery is less than 90% in most centers. Thus the postoperative period is an important time to reassess for improvement in metabolic comorbidities, to allow for adjustment or continuation of their medical treatments.

Most patients receiving radiation therapy for Cushing disease lose pituitary hormone function, including growth hormone. The contribution of growth hormone deficiency to cardiovascular risk and the effect of its replacement to increase or mitigate risk remain areas of active interest.[45]

Finally, the causal tumor may be occult, or Cushing syndrome may persist after surgery. These patients are often treated with steroidogenesis inhibitors, glucocorticoid antagonists, or agents to reduce ACTH secretion. Here, normalization of cortisol is essential. Reduced but persistently supraphysiologic exposure to cortisol is equivalent to a mild to moderate cortisol excess state. In other words, Cushing syndrome continues, with all its associated risks. This was illustrated by a study of mifepristone treatment in which 87% of patients had some improvement in comorbid parameters, but 20% gained weight, mean fasting glucose decreased only to 104.7 ± 37.5 mg/dL, and there was no overall significant decrease in systolic or diastolic blood pressure.[46] Thus when medical therapy is used, it is critical to adjust it to achieve clinical eucortisolism (in those on glucocorticoid antagonists) along with biochemical eucortisolism (when using other medical therapies) and additionally to address and treat all of the comorbidities associated with death.[47]

ACKNOWLEDGMENTS

This work was supported by the NIH Intramural Research Program of NIDDK.

REFERENCES

1. Clayton RN, Raskauskiene D, Reulen RC, et al. Mortality and morbidity in Cushing's disease over 50 years in Stoke-on-Trent, UK: audit and meta-analysis of literature. J Clin Endocrinol Metab 2011;96:632–42.
2. Colao A, Pivonello R, Spiezia S, et al. Persistence of increased cardiovascular risk in patients with Cushing's disease after five years of successful cure. J Clin Endocrinol Metab 1999;84:2664–72.
3. Bolland MJ, Holdaway IM, Berkeley JE, et al. Mortality and morbidity in Cushing's syndrome in New Zealand. Clin Endocrinol (Oxf) 2011;75:436–42.
4. Extabe J, Vazquez JA. Morbidity and mortality in Cushing's disease: an epidemiological approach. Clin Endocrinol (Oxf) 1994;40:479–84.
5. Whelton PK, Carey RM, Aronow WS, et al. ACC/AHA/AAPA/ABC/ACPM/AGS/APhA/ASH/ASPC/NMA/PCNAguideline for the prevention, detection, evaluation, and management of high blood pressure in adults: executive summary: a report of the American College of Cardiology/American Heart Association task force on clinical practice guidelines. Hypertension 2018;71:1269–324.
6. Mancini T, Kola B, Mantero F, et al. High cardiovascular risk in patients with Cushing's syndrome according to 1999 WHO/ISH guidelines. Clin Endocrinol (Oxf) 2004;61:768–77.
7. Stewart PM, Walker BR, Holder F. 11 beta-hydroxysteroiddehydrogense activity in Cushing's syndrome: explaining the mineralocorticoid excess state of the ectopic adrenocorticotropin syndrome. J Clin Endocrinol Metab 1995;80:3617–20.
8. Faggiano A, Pivonello R, Spiezia S, et al. Cardiovascular risk factors and common carotid artery caliber and stiffness in patients with Cushing's disease during active disease and 1 year after disease remission. J Clin Endocrinol Metab 2003;88:2527–33.
9. van der Paas R, Leebeek FW, Hofland LJ, et al. Hypercoagulability in Cushing's syndrome: prevalence, pathogenesis and treatment. Clin Endocrinol (Oxf) 2013; 78:481–8.
10. Sharma ST, Nieman LK. Cushing's syndrome: all variants, detection, and treatment. Endocrinol Metab Clin North Am 2011;40:379–91.
11. Ulick S, Wang JZ, Blumenfeld JD, et al. Cortisol inactivation overload: a mechanism of mineralocorticoid hypertension in the ectopic adrenocorticotropin syndrome. J Clin Endocrinol Metab 1992;74:963–7.
12. Bailey MA, Mullins JJ, Kenyon CJ. Mineralocorticoid and glucocorticoid receptors stimulate epithelial sodium channel activity in a mouse model of Cushing syndrome. Hypertension 2009;54:890–6.
13. Nieman LK, Chrousos GP, Kellner C, et al. Successful treatment of Cushing's syndrome with the glucocorticoid antagonist RU 486. J Clin Endocrinol Metab 1985; 61:536–40.
14. Hatakeyama H, Inaba S, Miyamori I. 11beta-hydroxysteroid dehydrogenase in cultured human vascular cells: possible role in the development of hypertension. Hypertension 1999;33:1179–84.

15. Sato A, Suzuki H, Murakami M, et al. Glucocorticoid increases angiotensin II type 1 receptor and its gene expression. Hypertension 1994;23:25–30.
16. Mangos GJ, Whitworth JA, Williamson PM. Glucocorticoids and the kidney. Nephrology 2003;8:267–73.
17. Pirpiris M, Sudhir K, Yeung S, et al. Pressor responsiveness in corticosteroid-induced hypertension in humans. Hypertension 1992;19:567–74.
18. Ritchie CM, Sheridan B, Fraser R, et al. Studies on the pathogenesis of hypertension in Cushing's disease and acromegaly. Q J Med 1990;280:855–67.
19. McKnight JA, Rooney DP, Whitehead H, et al. Blood pressure responses to phenylephrine infusions in subjects with Cushing's syndrome. J Hum Hypertens 1995; 9:855–8.
20. Kirilov G, Tomova A, Dakovska L, et al. Elevated plasma endothelin as an additional cardiovascular risk factor in patients with Cushing's syndrome. Eur J Endocrinol 2003;149:549–53.
21. Setola E, Losa M, Lanzi R, et al. Increased insulin-stimulated endothelin-1 release is a distinct vascular phenotype distinguishing Cushing's disease from metabolic syndrome. Clin Endocrinol (Oxf) 2007;66:586–92.
22. Wallerath T, Witte K, Schäfer SC, et al. Down-regulation of the expression of endothelial NO synthase is likely to contribute to glucocorticoid-mediated hypertension. Proc Natl Acad Sci U S A 1999;96:13357–62.
23. Saruta T, Suzuki H, Handa M, et al. Multiple factors contribute to the pathogenesis of hypertension in Cushing's syndrome. J Clin Endocrinol Metab 1986;62:275–9.
24. Axelrod L. Inhibition of prostacyclin production mediates permissive effect of glucocorticoids on vascular tone. Perturbations of this mechanism contribute to pathogenesis of Cushing's syndrome and Addison's disease. Lancet 1983;23: 904–6.
25. Shipley JE, Schteingart DE, Tandon R, et al. Sleep architecture and sleep apnea in patients with Cushing's disease. Sleep 1992;15:514–8.
26. Nieto FJ, Young TB, Lind BK, et al. Association of sleep-disordered breathing, sleep apnea, and hypertension in a large community-based study. Sleep Heart Health Study. JAMA 2000;283:1829–36.
27. Albiger N, Testa RM, Almoto B, et al. Patients with Cushing's syndrome have increased intimal media thickness at different vascular levels: comparison with a population matched for similar cardiovascular risk factors. Horm Metab Res 2006;38:405–10.
28. Lupoli R, Ambrosino P, Tortora A, et al. Markers of atherosclerosis in patients with Cushing's syndrome: a meta-analysis of literature studies. Ann Med 2017;49: 206–16.
29. Muiesan ML, Lupia M, Salvetti M, et al. Left ventricular structural and functional characteristics in Cushing's syndrome. J Am Coll Cardiol 2003;41:2275–9.
30. Toja PM, Branzi G, Ciambellotti F, et al. Clinical relevance of cardiac structure and function abnormalities in patients with Cushing's syndrome before and after cure. Clin Endocrinol (Oxf) 2012;76:332–8.
31. Kamenický P, Redheuil A, Roux C, et al. Cardiac structure and function in Cushing's syndrome: a cardiac magnetic resonance imaging study. J Clin Endocrinol Metab 2014;99:E2144–53.
32. Neary NM, Booker OJ, Abel BS, et al. Hypercortisolism is associated with increased coronary arterial atherosclerosis: analysis of noninvasive coronary angiography using multidetector computerized tomography. J Clin Endocrinol Metab 2013;98:2045–52.

33. Zacharieva S, Orbetzova M, Stoynev A, et al. Circadian blood pressure profile in patients with Cushing's syndrome before and after treatment. J Endocrinol Invest 2004;27:924–30.

34. Hermida RC, Ayala DE, Mojón A, et al. Blunted sleep-time relative blood pressure decline increases cardiovascular risk independent of blood pressure level–the "normotensive non-dipper" paradox. Chronobiol Int 2013;30:87–98.

35. Bowles NP, Thosar SS, Herzig MX, et al. Chronotherapy for hypertension. Curr Hypertens Rep 2018;20:97 [Erratum appears in CurrHypertens Rep 2018;21:1].

36. Fallo F, Paoletta A, Tona F, et al. Response of hypertension to conventional anti-hypertensive treatment and/or steroidogenesis inhibitors in Cushing's syndrome. J Intern Med 1993;234:595–8.

37. Raker JW. Surgical experience with the treatment of hypertension of Cushing's Syndrome. Am J Surg 1964;107:153–8.

38. Fallo F, Sonino N, Barzon L, et al. Effect of surgical treatment on hypertension in Cushing's syndrome. Am J Hypertens 1996;9:77–80.

39. Dalakos TG, Elias AN, Anderson GH Jr, et al. Evidence for an angiotensinogenic mechanism of the hypertension of Cushing's syndrome. J Clin Endocrinol Metab 1978;46:114–8.

40. Girolamo G, Gonzalez E, Livio D, et al. The effect of enalapril on PGI(2) and NO levels in hypertensive patients. Prostaglandins Leukot Essent Fatty Acids 2002;66:493–8.

41. Yagi S, Morita T, Katayama S. Combined treatment with an AT1 receptor blocker and angiotensin converting enzyme inhibitor has an additive effect on inhibiting neointima formation via improvement of nitric oxide production and suppression of oxidative stress. Hypertens Res 2004;27:129–35.

42. Sidharta PN, Melchior M, Kankam MK, et al. Single- and multiple-dose tolerability, safety, pharmacokinetics, and pharmacodynamics of the dual endothelin receptor antagonist aprocitentan in healthy adult and elderly subjects. Drug Des Devel Ther 2019;13:949–64.

43. Ntali G, Asimakopoulou A, Siamatras T, et al. Mortality in Cushing's syndrome: systematic analysis of a large series with prolonged follow-up. Eur J Endocrinol 2013;169:715–23.

44. De Leo M, Pivonello R, Auriemma RS, et al. Cardiovascular disease in Cushing's syndrome: heart versus vasculature. Neuroendocrinology 2010;92(Suppl 1):50–4.

45. Formenti AM, Maffezzoni F, Doga M, et al. Growth hormone deficiency in treated acromegaly and active Cushing's syndrome. Best Pract Res Clin Endocrinol Metab 2017;31:79–90.

46. Fleseriu M, Biller BM, Findling JW, et al. Mifepristone, a glucocorticoid receptor antagonist, produces clinical and metabolic benefits in patients with Cushing's syndrome. J Clin Endocrinol Metab 2012;97:2039–49.

47. Nieman LK, Biller BM, Findling JW, et al. Treatment of Cushing's Syndrome: an endocrine society clinical practice guideline. J Clin Endocrinol Metab 2015;100:2807–31.

Pheochromocytomas and Paragangliomas

Sergei G. Tevosian, PhD[a], Hans K. Ghayee, DO[b],*

KEYWORDS

- Pheochromocytomas • Paragangliomas • Neuroendocrine tumors
- Extra-adrenal pheochromocytoma • Hypertension

KEY POINTS

- Suspected patients with pheochomocytoma/paraganglioma (PCC/PGL) will need to have plasma metanephrines or 24 hour urine catecholamines and metanephrines checked.
- Commonly used drugs that cause false positive results in diagnosis are tricyclic antidepressants, sympathomimetics (ephedrine, albuterol, amphetamines), -blockers, and caffeine.
- Imaging modalities for PCC/PGL includes CT scans, MRI, and PET scans. Newer DOTA-TATE scans have recently been found to be helpful.
- Treatment involves surgical removal of the tumor. There are limited options for those patients with metastatic disease.
- PCC/PGL is one of the most hereditary tumors. Patients diagnosed with PCC/PGL need to be evaluated for genetic testing.

INTRODUCTION

Pheochromocytomas (PCCs) are rare neuroendocrine tumors. About 80% to 85% of these cancers arise from chromaffin cells residing in the adrenal medulla. The remaining 15% to 20% of such tumors are extra-adrenal. These extra-adrenal lesions that arise from the autonomic neural ganglia are termed paraganglioma (PGL) or sometimes called extra-adrenal PCC.[1–4] Collectively, these tumors are often abbreviated as PCC/PGL (or PPGL) in the literature. The clinical symptoms of the disease are common between the adrenal and extra-adrenal forms and are determined by excess secretion of catecholamines (norepinephrine, epinephrine, and dopamine). Hypertension is a critical and often dramatic feature of PCC/PGL, and its most prevalent reported symptom

[a] Department of Physiological Sciences, College of Veterinary Medicine, University of Florida, 1600 Southwest Archer Road, Suite H-2, Gainesville, FL 32608, USA; [b] Department of Medicine, Division of Endocrinology, University of Florida, Malcom Randall VA Medical Center, Gainesville, FL 32610, USA
* Corresponding author. Department of Medicine, Division of Endocrinology, University of Florida College of Medicine, Malcom Randall VA Medical Center, 1600 Southwest Archer Road, Suite H-2, Gainesville, FL 32608.
E-mail address: hans.ghayee@medicine.ufl.edu

Endocrinol Metab Clin N Am 48 (2019) 727–750
https://doi.org/10.1016/j.ecl.2019.08.006
0889-8529/19/Published by Elsevier Inc.
endo.theclinics.com

(with a sensitivity of 80.7%).[5,6] However, given the rare occurrence of this cancer, in patients undergoing screening for hypertension, the prevalence of PCC/PGL ranges from 0.1% to 0.6%.[1,7–9] Still, patients frequently come to the attention of the endocrinologist when PCC/PGL is suspected as a secondary cause of hypertension.[10,11] This article summarizes current clinical approaches to patients with PCC/PGL.

GENETICS OF PHEOCHROMOCYTOMAS AND PARAGANGLIOMAS

PCC/PGL is one of the most hereditary tumors (reviewed in[12–14]), with germline mutations associated with PCC/PGL being present in neurofibromatosis (NF-1), multiple endocrine neoplasia (MEN2a and MEN2b), von Hippel–Lindau (VHL), and familial PGL syndromes.[3] Moreover, about 30% of the sporadic cases of PCC/PGL are found to harbor a known gene mutation. Early analysis of PCC/PGL tumors focused on the MEN2A and MEN2B syndromes. In fact, historical and genetic analysis confirmed that the first reported PCC was described in a patient with MEN2A.[15,16] Patients with MEN2A also present with medullary thyroid carcinoma and hyperparathyroidism. Similar to patients with MEN2A, patients with MEN2B syndrome develop PCC and medullary thyroid carcinoma; however, instead of hyperparathyroidism, they are burdened with neuromas (reviewed in[17]). Patients with NF-1 have also been recognized to have PCC in addition to neurofibromas.[18] Patients with VHL syndrome are known to have pancreatic cysts, PCC, angiomas, and renal cell carcinomas.[19]

Although renal cell carcinoma is caused by germline mutations in the VHL tumor suppressor gene, it is also found in carriers of mutations in the enzymes of the tricarboxylic acid cycle, such as succinate dehydrogenase (SDHx) subunit genes and fumarate hydratase (FH). Succinate dehydrogenase is involved in oxidative phosphorylation and the tricarboxylic acid cycle of mitochondrial complex II. SDHx gene mutations are inherited as autosomal dominant and act in a tumor suppressor-like fashion.[20,21] SDHB-associated PCC/PGL arise owing to inactivating mutations in the SDHB gene, located on chromosome 1p35 to 36. This syndrome is commonly caused by tumors localized to the skull base, neck, mediastinum, abdomen, pelvis, and adrenal medulla.[22,23] Patients with this mutation are at increased risk for malignant PGL as well as renal cell carcinoma and papillary thyroid cancer.[12,23,24] The other key SDHx mutation that can be seen in patients with hypertension is the SDHD mutation. This gene is located on chromosome 11q23. These tumors are mostly nonsecreting and are associated with parasympathetic PGLs at skull base and neck (head and neck PCC/PGL).[25] However, adrenal location for SDHD-associated tumors was also reported[26,27] Interestingly, penetrance of SDHD-associated disease is parent-of-origin dependent and the disease is only manifested when paternally inherited.[23,25]

There is now a better appreciation of how genetic testing improves outcomes in the management of PCC/PGL.[28] The study by Buffet and colleagues[28] demonstrated the critical importance of identifying the genetic cause of PCC/PGL (eg, SDHx or a VHL mutation) for the practical management, clinical outcome, and increasing survival of the patients. Knowing a patient's genetic predisposition ultimately resulted in the more systematic follow-up and an informed change in the management taking into account their increased genetic risk. A comprehensive work from The Cancer Genome Atlas Program has recognized that there are several clusters of gene mutations that cause PCC/PGL.[29] Cluster 1 is associated with a pseudohypoxia pathway. These tumors activate a gene expression program associated with hypoxic conditions even under normal oxygen pressure. Tumors from cluster 1 secrete norepinephrine or dopamine only, as they do not express the phenylethanolamine-N-methyl transferase (PNMT) enzyme. Within the adrenal gland, PNMT is present and converts norepinephrine to epinephrine. PNMT expression is limited to the adrenal gland, brain, and organ of Zuckerkandl. Cortisol produced from the adrenal cortex stimulates PNMT activity in the adrenal medulla, which is critical for converting norepinephrine into epinephrine.[30] In contrast, PGL tumors do not express PNMT and secrete norepinephrine or dopamine. Examples of genetic mutations associated with these PGLs include *EGLN1*, *HIF2*, *SDHx*, *FH*, *MDH2*, and *VHL* (**Fig. 1**).

Cluster 2 tumors are associated with kinase signaling. Examples of such tumors include tumors harboring *RET* gene mutations (MEN2A and MEN2B syndromes), *NF-1*, and *TMEM127*. Tumors from cluster 2 secrete both epinephrine and norepinephrine as they express PNMT. Cluster 3 is associated with alteration in Wnt signaling pathway. The somatic genetic alterations that belong to this cluster are *MAML3* fusion genes, which are clinically associated with an aggressive and metastatic form of disease. The fourth cluster described by the consortium was a cortical admixture group of tumors that include tumors harboring the MYC-associated factor

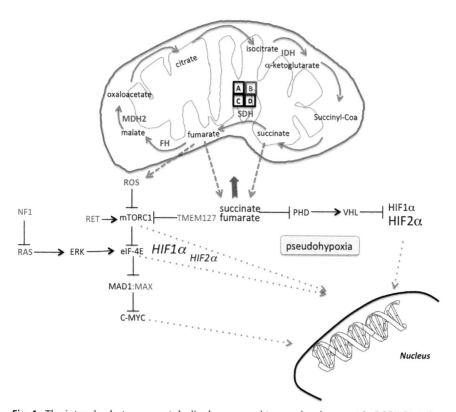

Fig. 1. The interplay between metabolic changes and tumor development in PCC/PGL. Mitochondrial genes involved in PCC/PGL development are shown in bold red; proteins involved in PCC/PGL are shown in red and pathways in orange. *c-MYC*, MYC proto-oncogene; *eIF-4E*, eukaryotic initiation factor 4E; *ERK*, extracellular signal-regulated kinase; *FH*, fumarate hydroxylase; *IDH*, isocitrate dehydrogenase; *MAD1*, mitotic arrest-deficient 1; *MAX*, Myc-associated factor X; *MDH2*, malate dehydrogenase; *mTORC1*, mammalian target of rapamycin complex 1; *NF1*, neurofibromin 1; *PHD*, prolyl hydroxylase domain protein; *RAS*, rat sarcoma oncogene; *RET*, rearranged during transfection proto-oncogene; *ROS*, reactive oxygen species; *SDH*, succinate dehydrogenase; *sα*, hypoxia-inducible factor alpha; *TMEM127*, trans-membrane protein 127; *VHL*, von Hippel-Lindau protein.

X gene (*MAX*) mutations. MAX-mutated tumors tend to secrete predominantly norepinephrine compared with epinephrine, likely because their PNMT level is low. Investigators have also noted that the expression level of PNMT seems to be intermediate between cluster 1 and cluster 2 in both the MAML3 fusion protein and *MAX*-associated tumors.[31] Given an ever-increasing number of gene mutations associated with PCC/PGL, genetic screening in all patients with PCC/PGL merits consideration, including patient counseling, where applicable.[2,32]

HOW PHEOCHROMOCYTOMAS AND PARAGANGLIOMAS CAUSE HYPERTENSION

Different types of PCC/PGL do not normally demonstrate distinctive patterns of hypertension, because the surge of catecholamines may be both continuous and intermittent (reviewed in[33]). These patterns lead to variations in the clinical picture where both sustained or paroxysmal hypertension could be observed.[5] Still, different catecholamines produce different vasoactive effects and in some cases these could be informative. Norepinephrine stimulation of α-receptors results in vasoconstriction, volume contraction and elevation of blood pressure (**Fig. 2**, top panel), whereas β2-receptor activation (predominantly from epinephrine) results in skeletal muscle vasodilatation and consequently postural hypotension.[34,35] Depending on the type of catecholamines produced, PCC/PGL may be grouped into noradrenergic phenotype—predominantly norepinephrine secreting (as seen in cluster 1 gene mutations) with sustained hypertension, and the adrenergic phenotype—mainly epinephrine secreting (as seen in cluster 2 gene mutations) with paroxysmal symptoms.[5] Hypertension has traditionally been thought to be uncommon in patients with purely dopamine-producing tumors. However, newer data from evaluating patients with head and neck PGLs with high 3-methoxytyramine levels (a breakdown product of dopamine) indicated that these patients have hypertension.[36,37]

CLINICAL PRESENTATION

It is widely believed that PCC/PGLs largely retain their differentiated state, endocrine function, and regulatory hormonal control. Episodic catecholamine surge by the PCC/PGL results in the classic triad of headache, sweating, and palpitations, a so-called PCC/PGL triad, also known as an attack, that may be diagnostically relevant. Although idiopathic attacks may occur in some cases, there can be multiple triggers for this characteristic disease presentation that include anesthesia, tumor manipulation, postural change, and exercise. Attacks can also be caused by different medications such as antidepressants, β-blockers, opioid analgesics, metoclopramide, and sympathomimetics.[2,5,34] Episodes of hormonal surge may also lead to a form of catecholaminergic cardiomyopathy (Takotsubo cardiomyopathy). The mechanism of this disease is not clear and both direct damage to the myocytes owing to excess catecholamines or indirect ischemic injury owing to microvascular dysfunction have been proposed.[38] A patient's first presentation could be with heart failure.[35,39] In pregnant women, the first presentation often comes with preeclampsia or eclampsia secondary to excess hormone release triggered by the pressure of enlarging gravid uterus on the tumor.[40,41]

Paroxysmal (approximately 48%) or persistent (approximately 29%) hypertension is detected in most patients with PCC/PGL and the episode can often result from mere manipulation of the tumor during surgery.[6,42] Normotension is present in about approximately 13% of patients who come to clinical attention owing to hereditary syndromes or incidental findings on imaging studies and are often asymptomatic.[10] It is important to emphasize that most patients presenting with severe hypertension or

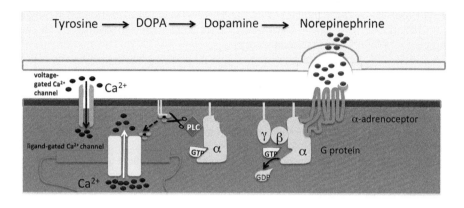

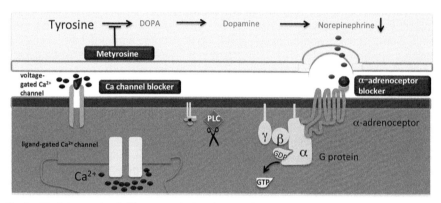

Fig. 2. (*Top*) Sympathetic-like control of BP by catecholamines in PCC/PGL. Elevated levels of catecholamines released from PCC/PGL (mostly norepinephrine) bind to α1- and α2-adreno-ceptors in the smooth muscle vasculature. These adrenoceptors are coupled with G-proteins that activate phospholipase C enzyme (PLC). PLC splits a membrane-bound phospholipid phosphatidylinositol bisphosphate (PIP2) into 2 important second messenger molecules, inositol 1,4,5-trisphosphate (IP_3) and diacylglycerol (DAG). IP_3 diffuses in the cytosol where it binds to its receptor, a ligand-gated Ca^{2+} channel located in the endoplasmic reticulum (or sarcoplasmic reticulum of the muscle). Stimulation of a receptor promotes the release of the Ca^{2+} into cytosol and causes the smooth muscle to contract. Another signaling molecule that results from the PIP2 hydrolyses, DAG, is lipid-soluble and remains in the membrane where it activates protein kinase C (PKC, not shown). Stimulation of α1-adrenoceptors causes vasoconstriction upon stimulation, leading to higher BP and increase in heart and breathing rate. (*Bottom*) Preoperative treatment options normally include α-adrenoceptor and calcium-channel blockers, which decrease Ca^{2+}-channels permeability and prevents cal-cium from entering the cytosol, thereby constricting blood vessels. Blockage of calcium en-try relaxes and widens blood vessels. In addition, metyrosine (Demser), an inhibitor of the tyrosine hydroxylase, a rate-limiting enzyme in catecholamine biosynthesis, decreases cate-cholamine synthesis and therefore decreases catecholamine-induced vasoconstriction of the vessels. (*Adapted from* Malaza G, Brofferio A, Lin F, et al. Ivabradine in catecholamine-induced tachycardia in a patient with paraganglioma. N Engl J Med 2019;380(13):1284-6.)

episodic attacks do not necessarily have PCC/PGL. Similarly, a classic signature of catecholamine excess may be completely missing in patients with rare dopamine-secreting tumors. Other diseases that resemble PCC/PGL symptomatically include hypoglycemia, carcinoid syndrome, mast cell diseases, essential hypertension, panic attacks, and cardiac arrhythmias. All of these entities should be considered in the differential diagnosis of PCC/PGL (reviewed in[43]). As a result, the expedient and accurate diagnosis of PCC/PGL is quite challenging.

PCC/PGL is diagnosed at all ages and exhibits no gender preference. The age of presentation is important, because it is likely to be informative with respect to the tumor secretion phenotype and an underlying genetic cause.[10,44] An established mutation or hereditary syndrome usually manifests at a younger age than sporadic disease. With increased referrals for genetic testing, older patients who would have otherwise been considered to have a sporadic mutation are being diagnosed with familial syndromes. Many times, older patients do not exhibit typical signs or symptoms, and tumors are often discovered serendipitously in patients with critical vascular illness, for example, stroke or heart failure with no obvious cause.[45] Hypertension can lead to a vasospasm and neurologic manifestations, such as stroke and seizures.[46] Large tumors are more commonly present in association with cardiovascular disease.[47,48]

Another challenge that could further complicate the diagnoses could arise owing to other hormones secreted in parallel with catecholamines, or induced by their excess. Some of these hormones are adrenocorticotrophic hormone that can cause Cushing's syndrome, parathyroid hormone-related peptide that can provoke hypercalcemia, vasopressin, vasoactive intestinal peptide promoting diarrhea, and growth hormone–releasing hormone that can cause acromegaly.[49–52] Catecholamines can induce abnormally high calcitonin and inhibition of insulin release, causing hyperglycemia or overt diabetes mellitus.[46] Fortunately, surgical removal of the tumor, if possible, normally alleviates these conditions. However, immediately after surgery, these patients may be at high risk for hypoglycemia because the decrease in catecholamine levels results in insulin release from the islet cells of the pancreas.

Historically, PCC/PGL came to attention in patients with symptomatic disease. However, increased use and availability of diagnostic imaging resulted in PCC/PGL being found during a hormonal evaluation for adrenal incidentalomas.[53,54] Because more patients are being evaluated by genetic counselors, diagnostic follow-up leads to tumor discovery in relatives of a patient with a known genetic mutation. Incidentally discovered tumors tend to be asymptomatic and smaller on average compared with tumors causing symptomatic disease. PCC/PGL is often associated with genetic syndromes such as MEN type 2 (MEN 2A and MEN 2B), NF-1, SDHx, and VHL syndrome. It is important for a clinician to recognize these conditions and evaluate these patients for the presence of PCC/PGL[10] (**Table 1**).

DIAGNOSIS
Who Should Be Evaluated for Pheochromocytomas and Paragangliomas?

Although clinicians are increasingly faced with the PCC/PGL in the setting of an incidentally discovered adrenal mass (eg,[55]), PCC/PGL are often diagnosed via a biochemical analysis of hormonal concentrations, followed by anatomic localization of the tumor(s). As described elsewhere in this article, PCC/PGL comes to the attention of an endocrinologist encountering patients exhibiting classic adrenergic spells (PCC/PGL triad). Subjects with a known family history (eg, *NF1*, *MEN2*, *SDHx*, and *VHL*) or those exhibiting symptoms or diagnosed for familial syndromes associated with catecholamine-secreting tumors should also be evaluated for PCC/PGL.[10,56]

Biochemical Diagnosis

The biochemical diagnosis remains the mainstay of PCC/PGL diagnosis (**Fig. 3**). Catecholamine excess indicative of an excess secreting tissue (a tumor) can be

Table 1
Genetic syndromes and clinical manifestations associated with PCC/PGL

VHL syndrome (*VHL*) VHL mutations	(PCC ~20%; ~5% malignant), angiomas, renal cell carcinoma, pancreatic cysts
MEN (type 2) syndrome (*RET*) mutations Type 2a (type 2); MEN 2A	MTC, PCC, hyperparathyroidism
MEN (type 2) syndrome (*RET*) mutations Type 2b (Type 3); MEN2B	MTC, PCC, marfanoid habitus, mucosal neuromas
NF (type 1) (*NF1*) mutations	PCC (<5%; 20% bilateral) neurofibromas, café-au-lait spots, Lisch nodules (iris hamartomas)
Succinate Dehydrogenase complex subunits B, D, C, A, AF2 (*SDHB, SDHD, SDHC, SDHA, SDHAF2*) mutations	PCC/PGL, renal cancers, GIST; pituitary adenomas
(*TMEM27*) mutations	PCC and rare renal cancers
(*MAX*) mutations	PCC/PGL
(*KIF1B*) mutations	PCC and neuroblastoma
(*EGLN1*) mutations	PCC and congenital erythrocytosis
Malate dehydrogenase (*MDH2*) mutations	PCC/PGL
Fumarate hydratase (*FH*) mutations	Rare PCC/PGL, cutaneous and uterine leiomyomas, type 2 papillary renal carcinoma
Pacak-Zhuang Syndrome (*HIF2* also known as *EPAS1*) alpha activating mutations	Somatostatinomas, PGLs, polycythemia
Carney triad (unknown genetics)	Pulmonary chondromas, GIST, extra-adrenal PGLs; in addition patients may have: adrenal cortical adenoma and esophageal leiomyoma
Carney-Stratakis syndrome (dyad) (*SDHC, SDHD, SDHB*) mutations	GIST, PGLs

Abbreviations: GIST, gastrointestinal stromal tumors; MTC, medullary thyroid carcinoma.

established by measuring levels of catecholamine (dopamine, norepinephrine, and epinephrine) metabolite products (normetanephrine for norepinephrine and metanephrine for epinephrine) in the plasma or urine.[57,58] Measuring 24-hour urine catecholamine level is important in PGL patients who do not produce norepinephrine and additional catecholamine measurements can be useful for diagnosis of dopamine-producing tumors.[59] The 2016 European Endocrine Society guidelines recommend the addition of 3-methoxytyramine test for diagnosis and follow-up of patients with PGLs; however, this test is not easily available in the United States.[37,60]

The biochemical pathway leading to the production of various catecholamines is summarized in **Fig. 4**. It begins with the conversion of tyrosine (either dietary or synthesized through hepatic phenylalanine route) into 3,4-dihydroxyphenylalanine (DOPA). This reaction is catalyzed by tyrosine hydroxylase, a rate-limiting enzyme specific for the adrenal medulla and catecholaminergic nerve terminals of the brain and sympathetic nervous system. DOPA is converted to dopamine, which becomes hydroxylated to form norepinephrine. Norepinephrine is an active hormone in some neurons of the brain and in peripheral sympathetic neurons, and it is released into circulation or the neuronal synaptic cleft upon activation. Importantly, in the chromaffin

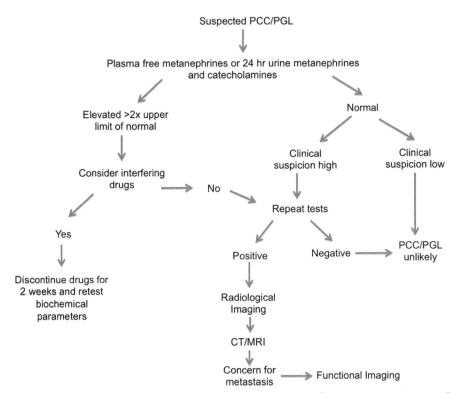

Fig. 3. A schematic diagnostic algorithm upon suspicion of PCC/PGL. CT, computed tomography.

cells of the adrenal medulla and in some neurons of central and peripheral system, PNMT (discussed elsewhere in this article) converts norepinephrine to epinephrine (adrenaline). Norepinephrine is removed from the synaptic cleft by reuptake through the norepinephrine transporter.

Most of the hormone is metabolized within the hormone-producing neuronal cells. The hormone that escapes into the bloodstream has a very short half-life and is taken up by non-neuronal cells. The turnover of norepinephrine and epinephrine by non-neuronal tissue and the adrenal medulla occurs mostly by the action of catechol-O-methyltransferase, which converts norepinephrine to normetanephrine and epinephrine to metanephrine that are known collectively as O-methylated metabolites. These metabolites are in turn oxidized by monoamine oxidase to vanillylmandelic acid. Alternatively, norepinephrine and epinephrine may be metabolized by monoamine oxidase first and later converted into vanillylmandelic acid by catechol-O-methyltransferase.[46]

Although catecholamines are secreted intermittently and have a fairly short half-life, their O-methylated derivatives are produced continuously inside tumor cells and remain relatively more stable in plasma; furthermore, the plasma metanephrine concentration is mostly independent of sympathoadrenal excitation.[61–63] Measurement of plasma high-performance liquid chromatography–fractionated metanephrines has excellent sensitivity (96%–100%) and specificity (85%–89%) as well as measuring of urinary metanephrines (sensitivity, 92%–97%; specificity, 86%–95%).[61–65] Plasma fractionated metanephrines compared with urinary metabolites seem to be less

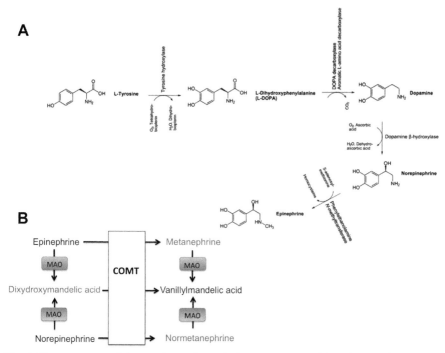

Fig. 4. The enzymes and the products of catecholamine synthesis (*A*) and degradation (*B*) in human cells. COMT, catechol-O-methyltransferase; DOPGAL, 3,4-dihydroxyphenylglycolaldehyde; MAO, monoamine oxidase.

affected by the concurrent use of medications (such as α- and β-blockers). An analysis of urinary vanillylmandelic acid is no longer recommended owing to reports of false-negative results.[2]

Medications (tricyclic antidepressants, levodopa, amphetamines, phenoxybenzamine, and reserpine), illness, and stress can influence concentrations of metanephrines and normetanephrines in the plasma[1,46,66] (**Table 2**); in the past, acetaminophen presence was considered to be a concern, but this is not supported by the new data for example.[67] Hence, stress-causing conditions should ideally be alleviated in advance of testing. Drugs and caffeinated beverages are known to affect

Table 2	
Medications often responsible for false positive results in PCC/PGL diagnosis	
Medication	High Metabolite Level (False Positive Result for PCC/PGL diagnoses)
α-Blockers	Norepinephrine, normetanephrine
Caffeine	Norepinephrine, epinephrine
Cocaine	Norepinephrine, epinephrine
Levodopa	Norepinephrine
MAO inhibitors	Normetanephrine, metanephrine
Sympathomimetics (ephedrine, albuterol, amphetamines)	Norepinephrine, epinephrine, Normetanephrine, metanephrine
Tricyclic antidepressants	Norepinephrine, normetanephrine

Abbreviation: MAO, monoamine oxidase.

catecholamine levels and these should be avoided or discontinued before biochemical testing.[46,63]

Interpretation of the results and diagnosis should take into consideration the initial level of suspicion and the degree (fold) of increase in the hormone levels. PCC/PGL in patients with cluster 2 mutations such as MEN2A, MEN2B, NF-1, and TMEM127 predominantly secrete epinephrine and metanephrine, whereas tumors within cluster 2 mutations such as SDHx, VHL, EPAS, and EGLN1 are norepinephrine and normetanephrine producing owing to lack of PNMT expression.[61,62] Additionally, PCC/PGL in patients with MEN2 normally have higher tyrosine hydroxylase activity compared with patients with VHL syndrome, accounting for higher levels of catecholamines and metabolites in MEN2 patients. Most clinicians agree that a 3- to 4-fold increase in the normetanephrine levels is affirmative of the diagnoses in a high-risk patient (eg, the one with a genetic predisposition); however, any elevation of metanephrine fraction should be carefully followed, and measurements repeated and not discarded as a false positive.[67] Similarly, normal level of metabolites in a low-risk patient could be used to exclude PCC/PGL.[64,66] The opposite outcome—positive results in a low-risk patient and negative test in a high index of suspicion patient (eg, the one with established hereditary disorder)—requires further studies before a definitive conclusion can be reached.[65] If the urine and plasma metanephrines results are ambiguous, a dynamic testing using the clonidine suppression test may be helpful for patients with norepinephrine-secreting tumors.

Localization

Diagnostic localization of a PCC/PGL is traditionally attempted only once the fact of catecholamine excess has been biochemically established. However, the quality and frequency of abdominal diagnostic imaging increase the chances for the incidental discovery of adrenal neoplasia. As a practical matter, most (approximately 85%) hormone-secreting tumors are found in the adrenal glands. The patient's age, presence of a family history, and plasma/urine hormonal levels are important in predicting the type and location of the tumor; a younger age and familial syndromes may signal extra-adrenal and/or multifocal locations.

Both computed tomography (CT) scanning and MRI are the mainstays for adrenal imaging used as the primary test for localization of catecholamine-secreting tumors. With tumors surgically confirmed, it was estimated that the sensitivity for MRI and CT to detect catecholamine-secreting tumors are 98% and 89%, respectively.[65] On CT, lipid-rich benign cortical adrenal adenomas are characterized by low unenhanced attenuation values (<10 Hounsfield units) with a rapid washout (>50% at 10 minutes) after administration of contrast medium. These tumors are usually round, homogeneous, are small (<3 cm in size), and unilateral.[68,69] In contrast, PCC almost always appear on CT scans as having high attenuation on contrast CT (>10 Hounsfield units) with less than 50% washout at 10 minutes after administration of contrast medium,[46] although some PCC may exhibit high washout (for example[70]). On MRI, lipid-rich cortical adenomas show no or only mild enhancement; in contrast, PCC/PGL show high signal intensity, especially on T2-weighted images.

If the CT scan and/or MRI fail to detect the tumor, or if there is concern that the patient has metastatic disease owing to large primary tumor size, functional localization can be attempted using a number of detecting modalities described here. This imaging takes advantage of the specific properties of the PCC/PGL related to its distinctive biochemical characteristics (reviewed in[71]).

A. PET scanning. This technology uses several radiolabeled ligands that target synthesis and metabolism of catecholamines and can be used to locate PCC/PGL tumors. The ^{18}F isotope-labeled compounds, such as ^{18}F-3, 4-dihydroxyphenylalanine (DOPA), ^{18}F-fluorodopamine (18F-FDA), or ^{18}F-fluoro-2-deoxy-D-glucose (18F-FDG) have been described in the literature; however, 18F-FDG PET is most commonly used.

B. ^{123}I-metaiodobenzylguanidine (MIBG) scintigraphy. This method uses MIBG, a norepinephrine analog with a high affinity for the norepinephrine transporter to localize the tumor.[72] It has been demonstrated that MIBG preferentially accumulates in catecholamine-producing tumors and scintigraphic localization using either ^{123}I-MIBG or ^{131}I-MIBG isotopes has been suggested for tumor localization where the results of CT/MRI studies were ambiguous. The reported sensitivity of the test is 81%, with a specificity of 99%.[73,74] Between the 2 radioisotopes, ^{123}I-MIBG is normally preferred over ^{131}I-MIBG because it allows obtaining higher quality images with a lower risk of radiation exposure.[75] Medications such as labetalol, antidepressants, and prochlorperazine are known to interfere with ^{123}I-MIBG uptake. It is recommended to discontinue these drugs 48 to 72 hours before imaging and to use an iodide preparation to protect the thyroid gland.[76] Some studies argue that there is insufficient evidence of MIBG scintigraphy value in improving diagnostic outcomes and it should be restricted to cases where radiopharmaceutical MIBG-based therapy (discussed elsewhere in this article) is to follow.[77]

C. Somatostatin receptor imaging. This approach relies on the presence of somatostatin receptors in PCC/PGL tumors.[78] ^{68}Ga-DOTATATE PET/CT scans are now being considered, especially if the tumor expresses somatostatin receptors, to detect PCC/PGL lesions as commonly seen in other types of neuroendocrine tumors such as carcinoid. This test is also instrumental for establishing the presence of functional somatostatin receptors in the tumor, which is particularly important in metastatic disease.

As with the biochemical tests, the choice of the best diagnostic imaging approach is dictated by the type of tumor. Nonfunctional imaging (CT scans and MRI) provides reasonable sensitivity and are applicable to both metastatic and nonmetastatic disease. ^{18}F-FDG is more sensitive than CT scans/MRI in detecting metastases to bone (93.7% vs 76.7%).[79–81] A new diagnostic modality for tumors expressing somatostatin receptors is ^{68}Ga-DOTATATE PET/CT imaging. In patients with malignant PCC/PGL, this approach seems to be very promising when compared with other available modalities, for example, PET or MIBG scans.[82–86] Studies are now actively being conducted to identify which subset of patients will benefit from DOTATATE imaging over other types of imaging modalities.

DISEASE MANAGEMENT
Surgery

Surgical excision remains the mainstay of management for PCC/PGL. Tumor removal not only drastically reduces the immediate negative consequences of catecholamine excess, but also leads to regression of chronic vascular and myocardial abnormalities. Evaluation of carotid intima-media thickness and left ventricular mass index in patients with PCC/PGL 5 years subsequent to tumor removal demonstrated significant improvement.[87] A comprehensive preoperative management of blood pressure is required to prevent perioperative cardiovascular complications. Several weeks of α-blockade are necessary before surgical resection of PCC/PGL. Because these patients are often volume depleted, it is important they are well-hydrated.[2,34,88,89]

Initial management normally includes an α-blocker. Phenoxybenzamine is commonly prescribed owing to its long duration of action (**Fig. 5, Table 3**). To counteract the tachycardia and postural hypotension sometimes resulting from the α-blocker use, β-blockers can be added on only after several days after α-blockers have been started to avoid a hypertensive crisis as a result of unopposed α-receptor stimulation. A medication such as labetalol that has action on both α- and β-receptors, also should not be started initially in a patient with PCC/PGL. Patients with PCC/PGL need at least 4:1 α- to β-blockade, and drugs such as labetalol have a 1:7 ratio α- to β-blockade. That is why it is extremely important to apply α-blocking agents first.[90] Calcium channel blockers should also be considered to block catecholamine-mediated calcium influx into vascular smooth muscle for controlling hypertension and tachyarrhythmias.[91]

The therapeutic targets of preoperative management are blood pressure less than 130/80 mm Hg and systolic pressure of greater than 90 mm Hg.[2] The advantages of perioperative management of hypertension using selective or nonselective α-blockers remain inconclusive and further studies are needed.[92–94] In any case, selective α-blocker such as doxazosin is often administered in cases where phenoxybenzamine is not well tolerated[2,34,95] (see **Fig. 2**, bottom). To better control blood pressure, calcium channel blockers or other antihypertensive agents (eg, tyrosine hydroxylase inhibitor, metyrosine[96]) could be added (see **Table 3**). Although it is necessary to take all appropriate precautions to stabilize blood pressure, peri-operative hemodynamic instability remains a major challenge.[97] Higher risk for blood pressure volatility should be anticipated in cases with larger tumor size and greater urinary/plasma metanephrine levels.[98,99]

Laparoscopic surgery is the preferred approach for PCC/PGL tumor resection.[100] As is the case with all minimally invasive approaches, this method is predictably associated with benefits for the patient (eg, shorter mean operative time and subsequent length of stay, diminished requirement for intensive care, reduced blood loss and required pain management) compared with open surgery.[95,101] Postoperative complications are more common in patients who have a history of coronary disease, experience longer duration of surgery, and blood pressure instability during surgery.[102,103]

Preoperative α-blocker therapy

Phenoxybenzamine or other alpha-blockers; adjust dose depending on patient's blood pressure and heart rate

↓

If a patient is tachycardic, consider ß-blockers only AFTER α-blocker is already in place for several days. Calcium channel blockers can be added to help with hypertension. Consider tyrosine hydroxylase inhibitor, if blood pressure remains uncontrolled

↓

Perioperatively, the patient will need plenty of intravenous fluids along with alpha blockers

Fig. 5. A schematic preoperative algorithm for PCC/PGL.

Table 3

Common outpatient medications for management of hypertension in patients with PCC/PGL

Drug	Mechanism	Dosing	Side Effects
α-blockers			
Phenoxybenzamine	Nonselective α-blocker	Oral: Initially 10 mg twice daily, gradually increasing every other day to doses ranging between 20 and 60 mg. Some cases may require higher dosing than 60 mg/d.	Nasal congestion, tachycardia, orthostasis, nausea, and retrograde ejaculation
Doxazosin	α$_1$-adrenergic blocker	1–16 mg/d in divided doses 1–3 times/d	Priapism, orthostasis, edema
Terazosin	α$_1$-adrenergic blocker	1–5 mg/d (maximum dose 20 mg/d)	Edema, orthostasis, and tachycardia
Prazosin	α$_1$-adrenergic blocker	2–15 mg/d in 2–3 divided doses	Edema, orthostasis, and tachycardia
Calcium channel blockers			
Verapamil	Calcium channel blocker	120–240 mg once daily (sustained release orally)	Bradycardia, constipation, edema
Nicardipine	Calcium channel blocker	Oral: 30–60 mg twice daily	Edema, tachycardia, nausea, and sweats
Amlodipine	Calcium channel blocker	5–10 mg daily	Edema, tachycardia, headache
β-blockers			
Propranolol	Nonselective β-blocker	40–240 mg/d in 2–3 divided doses	Bradycardia, fatigue, asthma exacerbation
Metoprolol	Cardio-selective β-blocker	50–400 mg/d in 2 divided doses	Bradycardia, fatigue, asthma exacerbation
Catecholamine synthesis inhibitor			
Metyrosine (tyrosine hydroxylase inhibitor)	Tyrosine hydroxylase inhibitor	Oral: 250 mg 4 times a day; may be increased by 250–500 mg daily up to 4 g/d in divided doses	Extrapyramidal side effects and crystalluria

Open surgery is mostly recommended for large tumors (>6 cm) and multifocal PCC/ PGL. Adrenalectomy and adrenocortical-sparing surgery may be performed in bilateral disease and where tumors are small.[2] Intraoperative monitoring should be performed by an anesthesiologist with experience in assisting in PCC/PGL surgeries.[104] Phentolamine therapy is a preferred route for managing hypertensive crisis, with β-blockade and other agents sometimes used to control cardiac arrhythmias (**Table 4**). Hypotension is often observed postoperatively and is normally sufficiently relieved by intravenous fluid therapy. Hypoglycemia could be managed through glucose administration.[2,34,95]

Palliative Management of Malignant Pheochromocytomas and Paragangliomas

Palliative surgery

Decreasing the tumor burden reduces disease severity and alleviates the symptoms owing to a decrease in hormonal synthesis from the tumor. Major risk factors are determined by the tumor type and genetic makeup. Additional factors contributing to aggressive course and excess mortality include old age, dopamine secretion, large tumor size and extensive metastases. For patients with malignant disease, open surgery is preferred because it allows for more extensive exploration, lymph node clearance, and resection of metastasis.

Palliative chemotherapy

Chemotherapy remains only partially effective in patients with malignant PCC/PGL (**Fig. 6**). It has been reported that treatment with a combination of cyclophosphamide, vincristine and dacarbazine chemotherapy led to partial response in 37% of 50 patients from 4 studies.[105] Partial response based on the reduction in catecholamine output had been observed in 40% of the 35 patients who were assessed. Only 4%

Table 4
Management of urgent hypertension in patients with PCC/PGL

Drug	Mechanism	Dosing	Side Effects
Phentolamine	Nonselective α-blocker	Bolus doses of 2.5–5 mg intravenously as required	Orthostasis, tachycardia and priapism
Nicardipine	Calcium channel blocker	Intravenous: start initially, 5 mg/h infusion; titrate 2.5 mg/h every 5 min (rapid titration) to 15 min (gradual titration); maximum dose is 15 mg/h; may decrease after reaching BP goal	Edema, headache, tachycardia
Nitroglycerine infusion	Nitric oxide precursor	5–100 μg/min (for hypertensive crisis)	Orthostasis, headache, tachycardia
Sodium nitroprusside infusion	Nitric oxide precursor	Intravenous: initially, 0.3–0.5 μg/kg/min; titration, increase in increments of 0.5 μg/kg/min to blood pressure target; maximum dose 10 μg/kg/min	Hypotension and cyanide toxicity
Ivabradine	Pacemaker I_f current inhibitor	5 mg orally twice a day; maximum dose 7.5 mg orally twice a day	Luminous phenomena, bradycardia, headache, dizziness

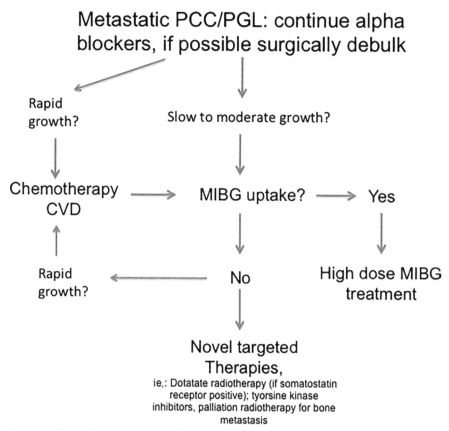

Fig. 6. A schematic management algorithm for malignant PCC/PGL. CVD, cyclophospha-mide, vincristine, and dacarbazine.

of patients achieved a complete response based on tumor volume; also, toxicity led to termination of therapy in several cases. In an attempt to take advantage of the angio-genic and proliferative pathways that are activated by the genetic alterations driving PCC/PGL, angiogenic inhibitors (eg, sunitinib) have been explored in the clinic, with several of them in current clinical trials.[106–108] Considering that the mammalian target of rapamycin (mTOR) signaling pathway has been implicated through TMEM127 gene mutations,[109] other chemotherapeutic agents such as mTOR inhibitor everolimus have been tried, but so far not proven to be effective.[110] Dual mTORC1 mTORC2 inhibitors are currently being explored.[111] Other chemotherapeutic agents under current inves-tigation for patients with malignant PCC/PGL disease include hypoxia-inducible fac-tor-2 antagonists[112] and temozolomide.[113]

Other approaches taking advantage of diagnostic nuclear medicine have evolved into viable treatment options for patients with metastatic disease. For example, it stands to reason that MIBG can be used not only for detecting tumors (discussed else-where in this article), but, owing to its carrying a radioactive [135]I moiety, this compound can emit radiation, induce irreparable DNA damage, and promote apoptosis in cancer cells that import MIBG through their norepinephrine transporters.[114] However, unlike its established diagnostic use, a clinical role for MIBG itself was uncertain, with only 30% of patients with PCC/PGL experiencing improvement.[115]

One reason for MIBG-limited therapeutic application is an isotope exchange manufacturing method that is used for its synthesis.[116] That process inevitably leads to a mixture of isotope-labeled (hot) and unlabeled (cold) MIBG, where the unlabeled molecule is present in large excess. Cold MIBG likely competes with labeled MIBG for binding to the transporters, interfering with the uptake of active MIBG and decreasing treatment efficacy. Low specific activity of MIBG (approximately 1.59 MBq/μg) necessitates large therapeutic quantities of the compound necessary to achieve an effect.[117] At these concentrations, nonspecific effects of excess MIBG start interfering with the norepinephrine signaling and can lead to adverse cardiovascular incidents upon administration.[118]

To convert MIBG into a therapeutically promising compound, iobenguane was developed. Unlike the original compound, iobenguane ^{131}I is manufactured in a way that contains only ^{131}I-labeled molecules. It can produce a much higher radioactive (approximately 92.5 MBq/μg) dose at much lower concentration. It has been reported that iobenguane ^{131}I carries lower cardiovascular risk that classic MIBG.[119] In a trial that included 68 patients, iobenguane (Azedra) was tested for a primary outcome of at least a 50% decrease in antihypertension medications for 6 months. The secondary end point was overall tumor response measured by imaging. The study met the primary end point, with 17 of 68 patients (25%) experiencing 50% or greater reduction in all antihypertensive medication for at least 6 months. Overall tumor response was achieved in 15 of the patients (22%) studied.[120] As a result, the US Food and Drug Administration approved high-dose iobenguane for patients with metastatic PCC/PGL in 2018 (see **Fig. 6**).

Future Directions in Pheochromocytoma and Paraganglioma Treatment

Currently, clinical approaches and medicine specifically tailored toward treatment of malignant PCC/PGL starting to emerge as logical extensions of the successful diagnostic methods, improvement of existing therapies, or a combination of these strategies (reviewed in[121]). Similar to the MIBG-iobenguane paradigm, successful tumor detection using somatostatin receptor ligands (ie, ^{68}Ga-DOTATATE) offers the foundation for the related treatment strategy. So far the response rates using this type of compounds, ^{177}Lu-DOTATATE and ^{90}Y-DOTATE, in patients with PCC/PGL have been promising and further studies that involve larger patient cohorts are needed.[122–125] As newer nuclear medicine strategies are being used for treatment of metastatic PCC/PGL, it is important to be even more vigilant in controlling hemodynamic parameters. The possibility of severe hypertension and tachycardia should be considered as the tumor-produced catecholamines continue to increase, even in the patient who is well-medicated with α-blocker. An example of such a case was recently described in a patient who received ^{177}Lu-DOTATATE treatment for metastatic PCC/PGL. The patient experienced severe hypertension and tachycardia that were difficult to control with a conventional comprehensive approach, including α-blockers, calcium channel blockers, metyrosine, and β-blockers. The patient's tachycardia was finally controlled with ivabradine (Corlanor), an inhibitor of the cyclic nucleotide–gated channel residing in the sinoatrial node. Ivabradine acted to slow the sinoatrial node in the heart and lowered the heart rate.[91]

Despite recent progress in understanding the genetic and metabolic basis of PCC/PGL, no practical guidelines based on these advances have been developed for treatment of patients with malignant PCC/PGL,[126–129] and currently therapeutic approaches available for malignant disease remain noncurative. However, constantly improving fundamental knowledge of the disease provides the much-needed hope for the impending breakthrough in mechanism-guided approach for this rare cancer.

The disease associated with a germline mutation of the succinate dehydrogenase subunit B (SDHB) attracts particular attention since it is found in approximately 30% of patients with malignant PCC/PGL.[130] Tumors harboring SDHB mutations develop abnormal robust vasculature, DNA hypermethylation and upregulate genes associated with epithelial-to-mesenchymal transition, which likely promotes their dissemination.[131–134] Importantly, these tumors upregulate glucose transporters and activate glucose phosphorylation to support their metabolic needs.[135] Glucose dependence of *SDHB*-associated PCC/PGLs promotes their identification by FDG-PET.[136] FDG-PET is also an excellent read-out for the treatment success or otherwise, as reduction in glucose uptake correlates well with overall response rate in these tumors.

It is tempting to speculate that combined therapies (including those targeting universal cancer aspects of the malignant PCC/PGL) may deliver a higher rate of response and sustainable progress. The multiple drug regimen will have to be meticulously calibrated to obtain the best response while minimizing the toxicity. It is also likely that our constantly improving knowledge of PCC/PGLs will inform generation of novel, more refined and personalized approaches founded in better understanding of tumor genetics and uncover new biochemical targets to control both tumor growth and catecholamine production.

ACKNOWLEDGMENTS

This work was supported by the Gatorade Trust through funds by the University of Florida, Department of Medicine to HKG.

REFERENCES

1. Jain A, Baracco R, Kapur G. Pheochromocytoma and paraganglioma-an update on diagnosis, evaluation, and management. Pediatr Nephrol 2019. https://doi.org/10.1007/s00467-018-4181-2.
2. Lenders JW, Duh QY, Eisenhofer G, et al. Pheochromocytoma and paraganglioma: an endocrine society clinical practice guideline. J Clin Endocrinol Metab 2014;99(6):1915–42.
3. Lenders JW, Eisenhofer G, Mannelli M, et al. Phaeochromocytoma. Lancet 2005; 366(9486):665–75.
4. Tsirlin A, Oo Y, Sharma R, et al. Pheochromocytoma: a review. Maturitas 2014; 77(3):229–38.
5. Soltani A, Pourian M, Davani BM. Does this patient have Pheochromocytoma? a systematic review of clinical signs and symptoms. J Diabetes Metab Disord 2015;15:6.
6. Zuber SM, Kantorovich V, Pacak K. Hypertension in pheochromocytoma: characteristics and treatment. Endocrinol Metab Clin North Am 2011;40(2): 295–311, vii.
7. Anderson GH Jr, Blakeman N, Streeten DH. The effect of age on prevalence of secondary forms of hypertension in 4429 consecutively referred patients. J Hypertens 1994;12(5):609–15.
8. Omura M, Saito J, Yamaguchi K, et al. Prospective study on the prevalence of secondary hypertension among hypertensive patients visiting a general outpatient clinic in Japan. Hypertens Res 2004;27(3):193–202.
9. Sinclair AM, Isles CG, Brown I, et al. Secondary hypertension in a blood pressure clinic. Arch Intern Med 1987;147(7):1289–93.
10. Bravo EL, Tagle R. Pheochromocytoma: state-of-the-art and future prospects. Endocr Rev 2003;24(4):539–53.

11. Viera AJ, Neutze DM. Diagnosis of secondary hypertension: an age-based approach. Am Fam Physician 2010;82(12):1471–8.
12. Crona J, Lamarca A, Ghosal S, et al. Genotype-phenotype correlations in pheochromocytoma and paraganglioma. Endocr Relat Cancer 2019. https://doi.org/10.1530/ERC-19-0024.
13. Erlic Z, Rybicki L, Peczkowska M, et al. Clinical predictors and algorithm for the genetic diagnosis of pheochromocytoma patients. Clin Cancer Res 2009; 15(20):6378–85.
14. Neumann HP, Bausch B, McWhinney SR, et al. Germ-line mutations in nonsyndromic pheochromocytoma. N Engl J Med 2002;346(19):1459–66.
15. Neumann HP, Vortmeyer A, Schmidt D, et al. Evidence of MEN-2 in the original description of classic pheochromocytoma. N Engl J Med 2007;357(13):1311–5.
16. Sisson JC, Giordano TJ, Raymond VM, et al. First description of parathyroid disease in multiple endocrine neoplasia 2A syndrome. Endocr Pathol 2008;19(4): 289–93.
17. Elisei R, Matrone A, Valerio L, et al. Fifty years after the first description, the MEN 2B syndrome diagnosis is still late: description of two recent cases. J Clin Endocrinol Metab 2018;104(7):2520–6.
18. Antonio JR, Goloni-Bertollo EM, Tridico LA. Neurofibromatosis: chronological history and current issues. An Bras Dermatol 2013;88(3):329–43.
19. Richard S, Gardie B, Couve S, et al. Von Hippel-Lindau: how a rare disease illuminates cancer biology. Semin Cancer Biol 2013;23(1):26–37.
20. Bayley JP, Devilee P, Taschner PE. The SDH mutation database: an online resource for succinate dehydrogenase sequence variants involved in pheochromocytoma, paraganglioma and mitochondrial complex II deficiency. BMC Med Genet 2005;6:39.
21. Baysal BE, Ferrell RE, Willett-Brozick JE, et al. Mutations in SDHD, a mitochondrial complex II gene, in hereditary paraganglioma. Science 2000;287(5454): 848–51.
22. Ghayee HK, Havekes B, Corssmit EP, et al. Mediastinal paragangliomas: association with mutations in the succinate dehydrogenase genes and aggressive behavior. Endocr Relat Cancer 2009;16(1):291–9.
23. Neumann HP, Pawlu C, Peczkowska M, et al. Distinct clinical features of paraganglioma syndromes associated with SDHB and SDHD gene mutations. JAMA 2004;292(8):943–51.
24. Young AL, Baysal BE, Deb A, et al. Familial malignant catecholamine-secreting paraganglioma with prolonged survival associated with mutation in the succinate dehydrogenase B gene. J Clin Endocrinol Metab 2002;87(9):4101–5.
25. Astuti D, Douglas F, Lennard TW, et al. Germline SDHD mutation in familial phaeochromocytoma. Lancet 2001;357(9263):1181–2.
26. Eng C, Kiuru M, Fernandez MJ, et al. A role for mitochondrial enzymes in inherited neoplasia and beyond. Nat Rev Cancer 2003;3(3):193–202.
27. Kadiyala S, Khan Y, de Miguel V, et al. SDHD mutation and pheochromocytoma. AACE Clin Case Rep 2018;4(3):e187.
28. Buffet A, Ben Aim L, Leboulleux S, et al. Positive impact of genetic test on the management and outcome of patients with paraganglioma and/or pheochromocytoma. J Clin Endocrinol Metab 2019;104(4):1109–18.
29. Fishbein L, Leshchiner I, Walter V, et al. Comprehensive molecular characterization of pheochromocytoma and paraganglioma. Cancer cell 2017;31(2):181–93.
30. Wurtman RJ, Axelrod J. Adrenaline synthesis: control by the pituitary gland and adrenal glucocorticoids. Science 1965;150(3702):1464–5.

31. Fishbein L, Wilkerson MD. Chromaffin cell biology: inferences from The Cancer Genome Atlas. Cell Tissue Res 2018;372(2):339–46.
32. Raygada M, King KS, Adams KT, et al. Counseling patients with succinate dehydrogenase subunit defects: genetics, preventive guidelines, and dealing with uncertainty. J Pediatr Endocrinol Metab 2014;27(9–10):837–44.
33. Pappachan JM, Tun NN, Arunagirinathan G, et al. Pheochromocytomas and hypertension. Curr Hypertens Rep 2018;20(1):3.
34. Pappachan JM, Raskauskiene D, Sriraman R, et al. Diagnosis and management of pheochromocytoma: a practical guide to clinicians. Curr Hypertens Rep 2014;16(7):442.
35. Ross JJ, Desai AS, Chutkow WA, et al. Interactive medical case. A crisis in late pregnancy. N Engl J Med 2009;361(20):e45.
36. Eisenhofer G, Peitzsch M. Laboratory evaluation of pheochromocytoma and paraganglioma. Clin Chem 2014;60(12):1486–99.
37. Rao D, Peitzsch M, Prejbisz A, et al. Plasma methoxytyramine: clinical utility with metanephrines for diagnosis of pheochromocytoma and paraganglioma. Eur J Endocrinol 2017;177(2):103–13.
38. Zhang R, Gupta D, Albert SG. Pheochromocytoma as a reversible cause of cardiomyopathy: analysis and review of the literature. Int J Cardiol 2017;249:319–23.
39. Dawson DK. Acute stress-induced (takotsubo) cardiomyopathy. Heart 2018;104(2):96–102.
40. Ghayee HK, Wyne KL, Yau FS, et al. The many faces of pheochromocytoma. J Endocrinol Invest 2008;31(5):450–8.
41. Santos DR, Barbisan CC, Marcellini C, et al. Pheochromocytoma and pregnancy: a case report and review. J Bras Nefrol 2015;37(4):496–500.
42. Zelinka T, Eisenhofer G, Pacak K. Pheochromocytoma as a catecholamine producing tumor: implications for clinical practice. Stress 2007;10(2):195–203.
43. Young WF Jr, Maddox DE. Spells: in search of a cause. Mayo Clin Proc 1995;70(8):757–65.
44. Smythe GA, Edwards G, Graham P, et al. Biochemical diagnosis of pheochromocytoma by simultaneous measurement of urinary excretion of epinephrine and norepinephrine. Clin Chem 1992;38(4):486–92.
45. Cooper ME, Goodman D, Frauman A, et al. Phaeochromocytoma in the elderly: a poorly recognised entity? Br Med J 1986;293(6560):1474–5.
46. Melmed S, Polonsky K, Larsen P, et al. Williams textbook of endocrinology. Philadelphia: Saunders/Elsevier; 2011.
47. Liao WB, Liu CF, Chiang CW, et al. Cardiovascular manifestations of pheochromocytoma. Am J Emerg Med 2000;18(5):622–5.
48. Yu R, Nissen NN, Bannykh SI. Cardiac complications as initial manifestation of pheochromocytoma: frequency, outcome, and predictors. Endocr Pract 2012;18(4):483–92.
49. Mune T, Katakami H, Kato Y, et al. Production and secretion of parathyroid hormone-related protein in pheochromocytoma: participation of an alpha-adrenergic mechanism. J Clin Endocrinol Metab 1993;76(3):757–62.
50. O'Brien T, Young WF Jr, Davila DG, et al. Cushing's syndrome associated with ectopic production of corticotrophin-releasing hormone, corticotrophin and vasopressin by a phaeochromocytoma. Clin Endocrinol 1992;37(5):460–7.
51. Onozawa M, Fukuhara T, Minoguchi M, et al. Hypokalemic rhabdomyolysis due to WDHA syndrome caused by VIP-producing composite pheochromocytoma: a case in neurofibromatosis type 1. Jpn J Clin Oncol 2005;35(9):559–63.

52. Sakuma I, Higuchi S, Fujimoto M, et al. Cushing syndrome due to ACTH-secreting pheochromocytoma, aggravated by glucocorticoid-driven positive-feedback loop. J Clin Endocrinol Metab 2016;101(3):841–6.

53. Rogowski-Lehmann N, Geroula A, Prejbisz A, et al. Missed clinical clues in patients with pheochromocytoma/paraganglioma discovered by imaging. Endocrine Connect 2018. https://doi.org/10.1530/EC-18-0318.

54. Zeiger MA, Thompson GB, Duh QY, et al. The American Association of Clinical Endocrinologists and American Association of Endocrine Surgeons medical guidelines for the management of adrenal incidentalomas. Endocr Pract 2009; 15(Suppl 1):1–20.

55. Gruber LM, Hartman RP, Thompson GB, et al. Pheochromocytoma characteristics and behavior differ depending on method of discovery. J Clin Endocrinol Metab 2019;104(5):1386–93.

56. Firth J. Endocrinology: phaeochromocytoma. Clin Med 2019;19(1):68–71.

57. Kvetnansky R, Sabban EL, Palkovits M. Catecholaminergic systems in stress: structural and molecular genetic approaches. Physiol Rev 2009;89(2):535–606.

58. van Berkel A, Lenders JW, Timmers HJ. Diagnosis of endocrine disease: biochemical diagnosis of phaeochromocytoma and paraganglioma. Eur J Endocrinol 2014;170(3):R109–19.

59. Young WF Jr. Clinical practice. The incidentally discovered adrenal mass. N Engl J Med 2007;356(6):601–10.

60. Plouin PF, Amar L, Dekkers OM, et al. European Society of Endocrinology Clinical Practice Guideline for long-term follow-up of patients operated on for a phaeochromocytoma or a paraganglioma. Eur J Endocrinol 2016;174(5):G1–10.

61. Eisenhofer G, Huynh TT, Hiroi M, et al. Understanding catecholamine metabolism as a guide to the biochemical diagnosis of pheochromocytoma. Rev Endocr Metab Disord 2001;2(3):297–311.

62. Eisenhofer G, Walther MM, Huynh TT, et al. Pheochromocytomas in von Hippel-Lindau syndrome and multiple endocrine neoplasia type 2 display distinct biochemical and clinical phenotypes. J Clin Endocrinol Metab 2001;86(5): 1999–2008.

63. Lenders JW, Pacak K, Walther MM, et al. Biochemical diagnosis of pheochromocytoma: which test is best? JAMA 2002;287(11):1427–34.

64. Sawka AM, Jaeschke R, Singh RJ, et al. A comparison of biochemical tests for pheochromocytoma: measurement of fractionated plasma metanephrines compared with the combination of 24-hour urinary metanephrines and catecholamines. J Clin Endocrinol Metab 2003;88(2):553–8.

65. Sawka AM, Prebtani AP, Thabane L, et al. A systematic review of the literature examining the diagnostic efficacy of measurement of fractionated plasma free metanephrines in the biochemical diagnosis of pheochromocytoma. BMC Endocr Disord 2004;4(1):2.

66. Eisenhofer G, Goldstein DS, Walther MM, et al. Biochemical diagnosis of pheochromocytoma: how to distinguish true- from false-positive test results. J Clin Endocrinol Metab 2003;88(6):2656–66.

67. Dobri GA, Bravo E, Hamrahian AH. Pheochromocytoma: pitfalls in the biochemical evaluation. Expert Rev Endocrinol Metab 2014;9(2):123–35.

68. Korobkin M, Brodeur FJ, Francis IR, et al. CT time-attenuation washout curves of adrenal adenomas and nonadenomas. AJR Am J Roentgenol 1998;170(3): 747–52.

69. Szolar DH, Korobkin M, Reittner P, et al. Adrenocortical carcinomas and adrenal pheochromocytomas: mass and enhancement loss evaluation at delayed contrast-enhanced CT. Radiology 2005;234(2):479–85.
70. Canu L, Van Hemert JAW, Kerstens MN, et al. CT characteristics of pheochromocytoma: relevance for the evaluation of adrenal incidentaloma. J Clin Endocrinol Metab 2019;104(2):312–8.
71. Taieb D, Pacak K. Molecular imaging and theranostic approaches in pheochromocytoma and paraganglioma. Cell Tissue Res 2018;372(2):393–401.
72. Ilias I, Shulkin B, Pacak K. New functional imaging modalities for chromaffin tumors, neuroblastomas and ganglioneuromas. Trends Endocrinol Metab 2005; 16(2):66–72.
73. Brink I, Hoegerle S, Klisch J, et al. Imaging of pheochromocytoma and paraganglioma. Fam Cancer 2005;4(1):61–8.
74. Jalil ND, Pattou FN, Combemale F, et al. Effectiveness and limits of preoperative imaging studies for the localisation of pheochromocytomas and paragangliomas: a review of 282 cases. French Association of Surgery (AFC), and The French Association of Endocrine Surgeons (AFCE). Eur J Surg 1998; 164(1):23–8.
75. Lynn MD, Shapiro B, Sisson JC, et al. Pheochromocytoma and the normal adrenal medulla: improved visualization with I-123 MIBG scintigraphy. Radiology 1985;155(3):789–92.
76. Solanki KK, Bomanji J, Moyes J, et al. A pharmacological guide to medicines which interfere with the biodistribution of radiolabelled meta-iodobenzylguanidine (MIBG). Nucl Med Commun 1992;13(7):513–21.
77. Rao D, van Berkel A, Piscaer I, et al. Impact of 123 I-MIBG scintigraphy on clinical decision making in pheochromocytoma and paraganglioma. J Clin Endocrinol Metab 2019. https://doi.org/10.1210/jc.2018-02355.
78. Ilias I, Chen CC, Carrasquillo JA, et al. Comparison of 6-18F-fluorodopamine PET with 123I-metaiodobenzylguanidine and 111in-pentetreotide scintigraphy in localization of nonmetastatic and metastatic pheochromocytoma. J Nucl Med 2008;49(10):1613–9.
79. Chew SL. Diagnosis: imaging of pheochromocytomas and paragangliomas. Nat Rev Endocrinol 2010;6(4):193–4.
80. Timmers HJ, Chen CC, Carrasquillo JA, et al. Staging and functional characterization of pheochromocytoma and paraganglioma by 18F-fluorodeoxyglucose (18F-FDG) positron emission tomography. J Natl Cancer Inst 2012;104(9): 700–8.
81. Timmers HJ, Chen CC, Carrasquillo JA, et al. Comparison of 18F-fluoro-L-DOPA, 18F-fluoro-deoxyglucose, and 18F-fluorodopamine PET and 123I-MIBG scintigraphy in the localization of pheochromocytoma and paraganglioma. J Clin Endocrinol Metab 2009;94(12):4757–67.
82. Cuccurullo V, Mansi L. Toward tailored medicine (and beyond): the phaeochromocytoma and paraganglioma model. Eur J Nucl Med Mol Imaging 2012;39(8): 1262–5.
83. Janssen I, Chen CC, Millo CM, et al. PET/CT comparing (68)Ga-DOTATATE and other radiopharmaceuticals and in comparison with CT/MRI for the localization of sporadic metastatic pheochromocytoma and paraganglioma. Eur J Nucl Med Mol Imaging 2016;43(10):1784–91.
84. Janssen I, Chen CC, Taieb D, et al. 68Ga-DOTATATE PET/CT in the localization of head and neck paragangliomas compared with other functional imaging modalities and CT/MRI. J Nucl Med 2016;57(2):186–91.

85. Maurice JB, Troke R, Win Z, et al. A comparison of the performance of (6)(8)Ga-DOTATATE PET/CT and (1)(2)(3)I-MIBG SPECT in the diagnosis and follow-up of phaeochromocytoma and paraganglioma. Eur J Nucl Med Mol Imaging 2012; 39(8):1266–70.

86. Tan TH, Hussein Z, Saad FF, et al. Diagnostic performance of (68)Ga-DOTATATE PET/CT, (18)F-FDG PET/CT and (131)I-MIBG scintigraphy in mapping metastatic pheochromocytoma and paraganglioma. Nucl Med Mol Imaging 2015;49(2): 143–51.

87. Majtan B, Zelinka T, Rosa J, et al. Long-term effect of adrenalectomy on cardiovascular remodeling in patients with pheochromocytoma. J Clin Endocrinol Metab 2017;102(4):1208–17.

88. Challis BG, Casey RT, Simpson HL, et al. Is there an optimal preoperative management strategy for phaeochromocytoma/paraganglioma? Clin Endocrinol 2017;86(2):163–7.

89. Romero M, Kapur G, Baracco R, et al. Treatment of hypertension in children with catecholamine-secreting tumors: a systematic approach. J Clin Hypertens 2015;17(9):720–5.

90. Pacak K. Preoperative management of the pheochromocytoma patient. J Clin Endocrinol Metab 2007;92(11):4069–79.

91. Malaza G, Brofferio A, Lin F, et al. Ivabradine in catecholamine-induced tachycardia in a patient with paraganglioma. N Engl J Med 2019;380(13):1284–6.

92. Li J, Yang CH. Improvement of preoperative management in patients with adrenal pheochromocytoma. Int J Clin Exp Med 2014;7(12):5541–6.

93. Randle RW, Balentine CJ, Pitt SC, et al. Selective versus non-selective alpha-blockade prior to laparoscopic adrenalectomy for pheochromocytoma. Ann Surg Oncol 2017;24(1):244–50.

94. van der Zee PA, de Boer A. Pheochromocytoma: a review on preoperative treatment with phenoxybenzamine or doxazosin. Neth J Med 2014;72(4):190–201.

95. Galati SJ, Said M, Gospin R, et al. The Mount Sinai clinical pathway for the management of pheochromocytoma. Endocr Pract 2015;21(4):368–82.

96. Perry RR, Keiser HR, Norton JA, et al. Surgical management of pheochromocytoma with the use of metyrosine. Ann Surg 1990;212(5):621–8.

97. Plouin PF, Duclos JM, Soppelsa F, et al. Factors associated with perioperative morbidity and mortality in patients with pheochromocytoma: analysis of 165 operations at a single center. J Clin Endocrinol Metab 2001;86(4):1480–6.

98. Aksakal N, Agcaoglu O, Sahbaz NA, et al. Predictive factors of operative hemodynamic instability for pheochromocytoma. Am Surg 2018;84(6):920–3.

99. Namekawa T, Utsumi T, Kawamura K, et al. Clinical predictors of prolonged postresection hypotension after laparoscopic adrenalectomy for pheochromocytoma. Surgery 2016;159(3):763–70.

100. Worrest TC, Gilbert EW, Sheppard BC. Pheochromocytoma: 20years of improving surgical care. Am J Surg 2019;217(5):967–9.

101. Heger P, Probst P, Huttner FJ, et al. Evaluation of open and minimally invasive adrenalectomy: a systematic review and network meta-analysis. World J Surg 2017;41(11):2746–57.

102. Bai S, Yao Z, Zhu X, et al. Risk factors for postoperative severe morbidity after pheochromocytoma surgery: a single center retrospective analysis of 262 patients. Int J Surg 2018;60:188–93.

103. Brunaud L, Nguyen-Thi PL, Mirallie E, et al. Predictive factors for postoperative morbidity after laparoscopic adrenalectomy for pheochromocytoma: a multicenter retrospective analysis in 225 patients. Surg Endosc 2016;30(3):1051–9.

104. Schuttler J, Westhofen P, Kania U, et al. Quantitative assessment of catecholamine secretion as a rational principle of anesthesia management in pheochromocytoma surgery. Anasthesiol Intensivmed Notfallmed Schmerzther 1995; 30(6):341–9 [in German].
105. Niemeijer ND, Alblas G, van Hulsteijn LT, et al. Chemotherapy with cyclophosphamide, vincristine and dacarbazine for malignant paraganglioma and pheochromocytoma: systematic review and meta-analysis. Clin Endocrinol 2014; 81(5):642–51.
106. Ayala-Ramirez M, Chougnet CN, Habra MA, et al. Treatment with sunitinib for patients with progressive metastatic pheochromocytomas and sympathetic paragangliomas. J Clin Endocrinol Metab 2012;97(11):4040–50.
107. Jimenez C, Cabanillas ME, Santarpia L, et al. Use of the tyrosine kinase inhibitor sunitinib in a patient with von Hippel-Lindau disease: targeting angiogenic factors in pheochromocytoma and other von Hippel-Lindau disease-related tumors. J Clin Endocrinol Metab 2009;94(2):386–91.
108. Joshua AM, Ezzat S, Asa SL, et al. Rationale and evidence for sunitinib in the treatment of malignant paraganglioma/pheochromocytoma. J Clin Endocrinol Metab 2009;94(1):5–9.
109. Qin Y, Yao L, King EE, et al. Germline mutations in TMEM127 confer susceptibility to pheochromocytoma. Nat Genet 2010;42(3):229–33.
110. Oh DY, Kim TW, Park YS, et al. Phase 2 study of everolimus monotherapy in patients with nonfunctioning neuroendocrine tumors or pheochromocytomas/paragangliomas. Cancer 2012;118(24):6162–70.
111. Giubellino A, Bullova P, Nolting S, et al. Combined inhibition of mTORC1 and mTORC2 signaling pathways is a promising therapeutic option in inhibiting pheochromocytoma tumor growth: in vitro and in vivo studies in female athymic nude mice. Endocrinology 2013;154(2):646–55.
112. Chen W, Hill H, Christie A, et al. Targeting renal cell carcinoma with a HIF-2 antagonist. Nature 2016;539(7627):112–7.
113. Hadoux J, Favier J, Scoazec JY, et al. SDHB mutations are associated with response to temozolomide in patients with metastatic pheochromocytoma or paraganglioma. Int J Cancer 2014;135(11):2711–20.
114. Bhatia KS, Ismail MM, Sahdev A, et al. 123I-metaiodobenzylguanidine (MIBG) scintigraphy for the detection of adrenal and extra-adrenal phaeochromocytomas: CT and MRI correlation. Clin Endocrinol 2008;69(2):181–8.
115. van Hulsteijn LT, Niemeijer ND, Dekkers OM, et al. (131)I-MIBG therapy for malignant paraganglioma and phaeochromocytoma: systematic review and meta-analysis. Clin Endocrinol 2014;80(4):487–501.
116. Vallabhajosula S, Nikolopoulou A. Radioiodinated metaiodobenzylguanidine (MIBG): radiochemistry, biology, and pharmacology. Semin Nucl Med 2011; 41(5):324–33.
117. Vaidyanathan G, Zalutsky MR. No-carrier-added synthesis of meta-[131I]iodobenzylguanidine. Appl Radiat Isot 1993;44(3):621–8.
118. Gonias S, Goldsby R, Matthay KK, et al. Phase II study of high-dose [131I]metaiodobenzylguanidine therapy for patients with metastatic pheochromocytoma and paraganglioma. J Clin Oncol 2009;27(25):4162–8.
119. Barrett JA, Joyal JL, Hillier SM, et al. Comparison of high-specific-activity ultratrace 123/131I-MIBG and carrier-added 123/131I-MIBG on efficacy, pharmacokinetics, and tissue distribution. Cancer Biother Radiopharm 2010;25(3): 299–308.

120. Pryma DA, Chin BB, Noto RB, et al. Efficacy and safety of high-specific-activity ^{131}I-MIBG therapy in patients with advanced pheochromocytoma or paraganglioma. J Nucl Med 2019;60(5):623–30.

121. Nolting S, Grossman A, Pacak K. Metastatic phaeochromocytoma: spinning towards more promising treatment options. Exp Clin Endocrinol Diabetes 2019; 127(2–03):117–28.

122. Forrer F, Riedweg I, Maecke HR, et al. Radiolabeled DOTATOC in patients with advanced paraganglioma and pheochromocytoma. Q J Nucl Med Mol Imaging 2008;52(4):334–40.

123. Kong G, Grozinsky-Glasberg S, Hofman MS, et al. Efficacy of peptide receptor radionuclide therapy for functional metastatic paraganglioma and pheochromocytoma. J Clin Endocrinol Metab 2017;102(9):3278–87.

124. Nastos K, Cheung VTF, Toumpanakis C, et al. Peptide receptor radionuclide treatment and (131)I-MIBG in the management of patients with metastatic/progressive phaeochromocytomas and paragangliomas. J Surg Oncol 2017; 115(4):425–34.

125. van Essen M, Krenning EP, Kooij PP, et al. Effects of therapy with [177Lu-DOTA0, Tyr3]octreotate in patients with paraganglioma, meningioma, small cell lung carcinoma, and melanoma. J Nucl Med 2006;47(10):1599–606.

126. Dahia PL. Pheochromocytoma and paraganglioma pathogenesis: learning from genetic heterogeneity. Nat Rev Cancer 2014;14(2):108–19.

127. Favier J, Amar L, Gimenez-Roqueplo AP. Paraganglioma and phaeochromocytoma: from genetics to personalized medicine. Nat Rev Endocrinol 2015;11(2): 101–11.

128. Jimenez P, Tatsui C, Jessop A, et al. Treatment for malignant pheochromocytomas and paragangliomas: 5 years of progress. Curr Oncol Rep 2017; 19(12):83.

129. Plouin PF, Fitzgerald P, Rich T, et al. Metastatic pheochromocytoma and paraganglioma: focus on therapeutics. Horm Metab Res 2012;44(5):390–9.

130. Gimenez-Roqueplo AP, Favier J, Rustin P, et al. Mutations in the SDHB gene are associated with extra-adrenal and/or malignant phaeochromocytomas. Cancer Res 2003;63(17):5615–21.

131. Dahia PL, Ross KN, Wright ME, et al. A HIF1alpha regulatory loop links hypoxia and mitochondrial signals in pheochromocytomas. PLoS Genet 2005;1(1): 72–80.

132. Letouze E, Martinelli C, Loriot C, et al. SDH mutations establish a hypermethylator phenotype in paraganglioma. Cancer cell 2013;23(6):739–52.

133. Loriot C, Burnichon N, Gadessaud N, et al. Epithelial to mesenchymal transition is activated in metastatic pheochromocytomas and paragangliomas caused by SDHB gene mutations. J Clin Endocrinol Metab 2012;97(6):E954–62.

134. Loriot C, Domingues M, Berger A, et al. Deciphering the molecular basis of invasiveness in Sdhb-deficient cells. Oncotarget 2015;6(32):32955–65.

135. van Berkel A, Rao JU, Kusters B, et al. Correlation between in vivo 18F-FDG PET and immunohistochemical markers of glucose uptake and metabolism in pheochromocytoma and paraganglioma. J Nucl Med 2014;55(8):1253–9.

136. Timmers HJ, Kozupa A, Chen CC, et al. Superiority of fluorodeoxyglucose positron emission tomography to other functional imaging techniques in the evaluation of metastatic SDHB-associated pheochromocytoma and paraganglioma. J Clin Oncol 2007;25(16):2262–9.

Pseudopheochromocytoma

Divya Mamilla, MBBS[a], Melissa K. Gonzales, BS[a],
Murray D. Esler, MB, PhD[b,c], Karel Pacak, MD, PhD, DSc[d],*

KEYWORDS

- Pseudopheochromocytoma • Pheochromocytoma • Hypertension • Spell
- Paroxysm

KEY POINTS

- Pseudopheochromocytoma is difficult for both the patients and the doctors treating them, as there is limited information to suggest an explanation for the symptoms they suffer from. The clinical manifestations are similar but not identical to those with excess circulating catecholamines.
- The potential mechanism involved in creating the patient's symptoms includes augmented cardiovascular responsiveness to catecholamines along with heightened sympathetic nervous stimulation.
- A successful management plan can be achieved by strong collaboration between a hypertension specialist and a psychiatrist or a psychologist with expertise in cognitive-behavioral panic management.

INTRODUCTION

Pseudopheochromocytoma (pseudoPHEO) is an uncommon disorder usually manifested by severe symptomatic paroxysmal episodes of hypertension (with or without tachyarrhythmia) documented by a physician or by home blood monitoring in no particular setting or trigger, similar to a clinical picture of pheochromocytoma (PHEO), and also having symptoms/signs of nervousness/anxiety, flushing, profuse sweating, palpitations, and headache. Other significant but much less common

Disclosure Statement: The authors have nothing to disclose.
Funding: This article was supported by the *Eunice Kennedy Shriver* National Institute of Child Health and Human Development, National Institutes of Health.
[a] Section on Medical Neuroendocrinology, *Eunice Kennedy Shriver* National Institute of Child Health and Human Development, National Institutes of Health, 10 Center Drive, Bethesda, MD 20892, USA; [b] Baker IDI Heart and Diabetes Institute, 75 Commercial Road, Melbourne, VIC 3004, Australia; [c] Dobney Hypertension Centre, Royal Perth Hospital Campus, University of Western Australia, Rear 50 Murray St, Perth, WA 6000, Australia; [d] Section on Medical Neuroendocrinology, *Eunice Kennedy Shriver* NICHD, NIH, Building 10, CRC, 1E-3140, 10 Center Drive, MSC-1109, Bethesda, MD 20892-1109, USA
* Corresponding author.
E-mail address: karel@mail.nih.gov

Endocrinol Metab Clin N Am 48 (2019) 751–764
https://doi.org/10.1016/j.ecl.2019.08.004
endo.theclinics.com

manifestations may include chest pain, nausea, vomiting, dizziness, paleness, and pseudoseizures.[1] Thus, clinical presentations of pseudoPHEO are similar to that of PHEO, particularly symptoms accompanied by recurrent peaks in blood pressure, but showing no anatomic and biochemical abnormality (exceptions may apply), owing possibly to altered function of the autonomic nervous system or abnormal disposition of catecholamines released from neurons within the brain. Normal plasma catecholamine concentration (some evidence of mild to moderate catecholamine excess may be present) and the absence of an adrenal tumor on imaging studies are useful to delineate pseudoPHEO from a typical PHEO. However, some reports have documented the presence of either elevated plasma dopamine (DA) sulfate levels or increased plasma epinephrine (EPI) levels.[2,3] Thus, pseudoPHEO is infrequently associated with an unknown etiology, unidentified pathophysiologic mechanisms, and in some patients with ineffective treatment using antihypertensive medications. Nevertheless, the presence of some amplified cardiovascular responses has shown a possible link between the autonomic nervous system and the pathogenesis of pseudoPHEO.[3] For a differential diagnosis associated with sustained/episodic secondary hypertension, a physician should always consider renovascular disease, primary aldosteronism, renal parenchymal disease, obstructive sleep apnea, hyperthyroidism, Cushing syndrome, carcinoid syndrome, systemic mastocytosis, panic attacks, and anxiety.[4] Management of these patients is often complex and frustrating to both physicians and patients given the repeated blood-pressure surges on a background of either normal baseline blood pressure or sustained hypertension. Because of a possible link to sympathetic nervous system (SNS) overactivity, patients respond well to medications that reduce this overactivity. Anxiolytics, antidepressants, and psychotherapy also play an important role in managing these patients. Severe and long-lasting episodes of paroxysms may require the administration of intravenous agents such as labetalol or nitroprusside, but only in a hospital setting.

This review focuses on patients in whom a diagnosis of PHEO has been excluded but who still present with symptoms that resemble catecholamine excess, called pseudoPHEO.

PATHOGENESIS

In general, the pathogenesis of pseudoPHEO is poorly understood. Initially, patients with this disorder were described as presenting with altered function of the autonomic nervous system or abnormalities in the disposition of catecholamines and their subsequent action on target organs. This proposal was initially made by Page in 1935,[5] when he described a group of women with paroxysmal hypertension and symptoms of flushing, sweating, and palpitations. These symptoms were suggested to be secondary to panic attacks, resulting in "irritation" of sympathetic and parasympathetic centers in diencephalon. Much later, in the 1980s, Kuchel[1] determined elevated DA levels to be a marker of heightened SNS activation among pseudoPHEO patients. In one of his retrospective studies, he demonstrated that among patients mimicking symptoms of PHEO, there was a substantial increase in plasma DA sulfate levels without a corresponding increase in free EPI, norepinephrine (NE), and DA concentration.[2] Therefore, increased DA sulfate levels were hypothesized to be a reservoir of free DA, which when produced in surges caused episodic hypertension and symptoms resembling the presence of PHEO. However, there was a problem with this hypothesis because an increase in circulating DA levels does not cause an increase in blood pressure or heart rate. Moreover, in 2008 Sharabi and colleagues[3] reported that patients with pseudoPHEO appeared to have amplified cardiovascular responsiveness to catecholamines with enhanced adrenal gland release of EPI in response to sympathetic nervous stimulation. Thus, one could hypothesize that an increased affinity and subsequent stimulation of adrenoceptors by catecholamines or a short catecholamine burst from the SNS could be one of the potential causes behind pseudoPHEO pathogenesis (**Fig. 1**). As stated previously, although elevated catecholamine and/or metanephrine levels are not typical for pseudoPHEO, some studies showed that patients with pseudoPHEO had higher baseline plasma EPI/metanephrine concentrations.[3] Moreover, these patients had a 6-fold increase in plasma EPI levels after sympathetic stimulation with glucagon, although some of these responses can sometimes be seen in normal individuals. These patients also showed a greater decrease in blood pressure after administration of trimethaphan (a nicotinic ganglion blocker inhibiting sympathoneural release of NE) and a greater increase in blood pressure relative to the changes in plasma NE after receiving yohimbine, an α-adrenoceptor agonist stimulating release of this neurotransmitter. Another potentially interesting and well-thought-out mechanism of pseudoPHEO etiology reported by Mann[6] proposes that the SNS is composed of 2 limbs, the adrenal and the neural. Different stressors can stimulate one limb of the SNS more than the other. Stimulation of the adrenal limb results in increased secretion of EPI from the adrenal glands, causing increased heart rate and cardiac output, whereas stimulation of the neural limb causes increased NE release from sympathetic nerve endings in vascular smooth muscle and, thus, increased peripheral resistance without a corresponding increase in heart rate. Moreover, for unknown reasons, one limb dominates over the other in different patients with pseudoPHEO.[6] Because most patients with pseudoPHEO do not have elevated catecholamine and metanephrine levels, one may view this mechanism as possibly existing, but as a very transient and quick one, therefore not leaving a solid, proven trace of

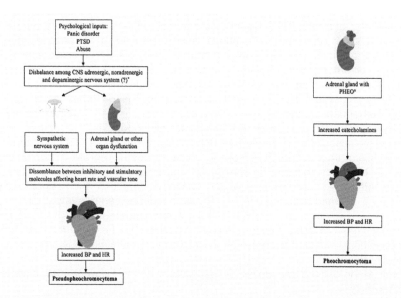

Fig. 1. Pathogenesis of pseudopheochromocytoma. *Probable sudden and brisk increase in their activity. #Extra-adrenal pheochromocytoma is known as paraganglioma. BP, blood pressure; CNS, central nervous system; HR, heart rate; PHEO, pheochromocytoma; PTSD, post-traumatic stress disorder.

elevated plasma or urinary catecholamines/metanephrine levels. Nevertheless, if measured during a paroxysm of hypertension and/or palpitations, elevated levels of these biomarkers could be detected (but almost impossible to detect outside a hospital setting). However, in patients with episodes of hypertension/tachyarrhythmia lasting for longer periods of time and negative catecholamine and metanephrine levels (usually when they present to a hospital or urgent care), such episodes cannot be explained by catecholamine release. Other mechanisms, perhaps including imbalance of central autonomic centers and catecholamines, must be considered and elucidated in the future, with one possibility being the use of specific functional brain imaging.

CLINICAL PRESENTATION

PseudoPHEO is frequently a diagnosis of exclusion requiring careful screening for PHEO before the final diagnosis is made. Currently, the extent of influence and pathogenesis of psychological factors on the severe acute elevation in blood pressure is unexplained.[7] In a group of 21 patients with pseudoPHEO, Mann[6,7] described that they typically presented with paroxysmal or episodic hypertension, which was accompanied by physical symptoms such as headache, lightheadedness, dizziness, nausea, diaphoresis, chest pain, and palpitations. The proportion of these paroxysmal events usually extended from every day to less than once per month, and the duration of each episode could last from a few minutes to a few hours, followed by intense fatigue lasting for several days.[6,7] Between the episodes, blood pressure was reported to be normal or mildly elevated. Episodic hypertension was considered to be either newly developed or already established by episodic paroxysms of high blood pressure (between episodes, the blood pressure is often normal but can be elevated in patients who also have underlying sustained hypertension, or low if antihypertensive agents are prescribed to pseudoPHEO patients who are otherwise normotensive between episodes). The studies from Cornell University and the National Institutes of Health (NIH) described the fear of recurrent attacks without warning, with debilitating clinical manifestations causing restriction of activities resulting in significant disruptions to productivity and normal quality of life.[3,7] It also seems to be more common among younger women, aged 40 to 50 years, as per our experience at the NIH (Karel Pacak, unpublished observations).[7] Mostly these patients are unable to identify a trigger to these paroxysms, such as emotional disturbances or another psychic component. A thorough psychosocial analysis often reveals a history of abuse or trauma in the past, often as long ago as childhood.[7,8] In 2015, Mann[8] nicely described the association of emotions among those with pseudoPHEO: (1) history of severe abuse or trauma and (2) personality characterized by repressive coping style ie, lifelong tendency to cope unemotionally with stress.[8,9] It is also important to assess whether the syndrome is secondary to another condition, such as obstructive sleep apnea, or medications such as tricyclic antidepressants, sympathomimetic agents, and reboxetine, all of which can increase sympathetic activity. However, these conditions are usually accompanied by positive biochemistry for PHEO.[10,11] Other conditions with similar presentation include systematic mastocytosis, cocaine use, and reninoma.[12]

Overall, Mann defined pseudoPHEO associated with the following distinctive features (**Table 1**):

- Abrupt onset of paroxysmal hypertension
- Elevated blood pressure associated with physical symptoms such as headache, lightheadedness, flushing, diaphoresis, chest pain, and palpitations (commonly seen in patients with PHEO)

Table 1
Characteristics of pseudopheochromocytoma

Clinical features	1. Sudden-onset hypertensive paroxysms 2. Associated physical symptoms: chest pain, headache, lightheadedness, diaphoresis, nausea, palpitations, flushing, dyspnea, and weakness 3. Episodes not triggered by emotional distress or panic 4. History of severe trauma or abuse
Biochemistry[a]	Plasma catecholamines: EPI, NE, and DA: WNL Plasma metanephrines: NMN and MN: WNL 24 hour urine catecholamines: EPI, NE, and DA: WNL 24 hour urine metanephrines: NMN and MN: WNL
Diagnosis	1. Clonidine-suppression test not needed if there is less suspicion for pheochromocytoma, based on biochemical evaluation 2. Anatomic/functional imaging, if needed, to rule out pheochromocytoma/paraganglioma

Abbreviations: DA, dopamine; EPI, epinephrine; MN, metanephrine; NE, norepinephrine; NMN, normetanephrine; WNL, within normal limits.
[a] Occasionally, patients with diagnosis of pseudopheochromocytoma may have elevated epinephrine levels.

- Episodes not provoked by emotional distress and panic; however, during an episode, the distressing physical symptoms do incite a dread of dying
- Negative biochemical testing performed to rule out PHEO
- Evidence of characteristic psychological background revealing a history of abuse, trauma, or a defensive personality

DIFFERENTIAL DIAGNOSIS
Pheochromocytoma

The diagnosis of PHEO must be exempted among all patients with unprovoked paroxysmal hypertension (**Table 2**).[7] PHEOs are rare catecholamine-secreting neuroendocrine tumors stemming from chromaffin cells of the adrenal medulla.[13] PseudoPHEO

Table 2
Differential diagnosis of pseudopheochromocytoma

Endocrine	Pheochromocytoma, hyperthyroidism, carcinoid, systemic mastocytosis, hypoglycemia, insulinoma, menopausal syndrome, adrenal medullary hyperplasia, Cushing syndrome, primary aldosteronism, reninoma
Pharmacologic	Tricyclic antidepressants, monoamine oxidase inhibitors + ingestion of tyramine, illicit drugs (e.g., cocaine), alcohol withdrawal, abrupt clonidine withdrawal, ingestion of sympathomimetics
Cardiovascular	Ischemic heart disease, arrhythmias, baroreflex failure, renovascular disease, postural orthostatic tachycardia syndrome, hyperdynamic β-adrenergic circulatory state
Neurologic	Migraine headache, cluster headache, stroke, diencephalic autonomic epilepsy, meningioma, hypertensive encephalopathy
Other	Preeclampsia or eclampsia, labile hypertension, obstructive sleep apnea, anxiety or panic disorder, anxiety, post-traumatic stress disorder, acute intermittent porphyria, recurrent idiopathic anaphylaxis, vasculitis

Adapted from Eisenhofer G, Sharabi Y, Pacak K. Unexplained symptomatic paroxysmal hypertension in pseudopheochromocytoma: a stress response disorder? Ann N Y Acad Sci 2008;1148:469–78.

mimics the presentation of PHEO from the presence of paroxysmal hypertension along with other signs such as headache, palpitations, sweating, dizziness, and anxiety.[7] In most patients with PHEO, catecholamines are episodically and markedly elevated.[14,15] Rarely is PHEO accompanied by a truly negative biochemical testing profile. Therefore, to confirm the diagnosis of PHEO, initial biochemical testing with measurement of plasma or urinary metanephrines is performed.[16] Findings of normal levels of plasma or urinary normetanephrine (NMN) and metanephrine (and at some centers, also plasma methoxytyramine) virtually excludes the presence of PHEO, with no further testing for tumor deemed necessary.[17] False-positive tests and equivocal catecholamine levels in both plasma and urine are ruled out using a clonidine-suppression test[16] (in many instances, repeating metanephrines fasting in the morning after 30 min of rest will show normal results, avoiding the hassle of going through a dynamic test, which may be preserved for those who continue to have elevated normetanephrine levels). Modest elevations in catecholamines are seen occasionally among patients with pseudoPHEO resulting from the activation of the SNS.[6] Concurrent use of medication (NE reuptake inhibitors, tricyclic antidepressants, β-adrenoceptor blockers, monoamine oxidase inhibitors, and recreational drugs including cold and antihistamine medications) and certain foods and drinks (caffeine-containing products, cereals, and amine-rich foods such as cheese and bananas) can also increase catecholamines and metanephrines and therefore result in modest elevations in their levels.[18,19] In 2014, Endocrine Society Clinical Practice Guidelines recommended the use of imaging studies to locate PHEOs and paragangliomas once there is clear biochemical evidence. When biochemical evidence to determine the presence of PHEO is excluded, further workup is redundant. Such patients are advised to undergo a meticulous examination to find out other possible causes of their symptoms and signs that closely resemble PHEO. Some of these are discussed later.

The clonidine-suppression test, introduced by Bravo and colleagues,[20] works on the principle that clonidine, a central α2-adrenoceptor agonist, suppresses the normal neurogenically mediated release of catecholamine.[21] However, it does not affect the autonomous secretion of catecholamines from the tumor cells. Thus, the result can be highly predictive of PHEO when interpreting its effects on plasma NE and NMN. Blood pressure and heart rate need to be monitored (to avoid a precipitous drop in blood pressure and heart rate) every 5 minutes for 20 minutes before administration of clonidine, then every 15 minutes for 3 hours subsequently. In addition, blood should be drawn before then 3 hours after clonidine administration to measure the concentration of plasma catecholamines and metanephrines. Therefore, after administration of clonidine, if plasma NE is suppressed (ie, concentration below the upper limit or a 50% reduction from baseline) or if plasma NMN is suppressed (ie, concentration below the upper limit or <40% from baseline), either of these results would suggest the absence of PHEO.[22] Antihypertensive and antidepressant medication must be avoided because these may result in false-positive test results or a severe hypotensive response to clonidine. If the patient develops hypotension during the clonidine-suppression test, this can be treated by using normal saline.

Panic Disorder

The presentation of pseudoPHEO is identical to that of panic disorder, with common physical symptoms including chest pain, palpitations, dizziness, weakness, and dyspnea. Most of these symptoms are common to those described in the *Diagnostic and Statistical Manual of Mental Disorders*, 5th edition (DSM-5) criteria to indicate panic disorder.[23] However, the major difference between these 2 conditions is that blood-pressure elevation in panic disorder is not as high as it is in pseudoPHEO.[24] Also, paroxysmal hypertension is characterized by extreme blood-pressure elevation in the absence of fear or panic. Few patients experience only fear in reaction to physical symptoms.[6] Moreover, headache, the most commonly reported symptom in patients with pseudoPHEO, is not among the symptoms used to define panic disorder from the DSM-5. Wilkinson and colleagues[25] found a marked increase in sympathetic nerve burst amplitude during a panic attack. They reported a large increase in plasma EPI secretion during spontaneous panic attacks with smaller increase in NE spillover. However, Villacres and colleagues[26] reported an increase in baseline plasma EPI levels with normal NE levels among those with panic disorder. By contrast, in 2007 Esler's group[27] suggested the role of increased brain serotonin turnover (approximately 4 times higher) in patients with panic disorder. Therefore, both disorders are related: pseudoPHEO is dominated by autonomic manifestations and panic disorder by emotional ones.

Labile Hypertension

PseudoPHEO differs strongly from labile hypertension. In the latter, blood-pressure fluctuation is attributed to either stress or emotional distress by both the physician and the patient.[28] Patients are aware that their blood pressure is elevated, for example, when they are stressed. The clinical definition of labile hypertension is derived by observing patients experiencing transient but substantial increases in blood pressure, which may be accompanied by symptoms such as headache, palpitations, or flushing, which resolve spontaneously without requiring any intervention. However, at times they may present as clinical dilemmas specifically in patients experiencing marked elevation before a medical or surgical procedure.[29] Usually, blood-pressure fluctuation is a normal phenomenon. Moreover, a normal lability is potentially harmful in certain medical conditions such as chronic aortic dissection or Marfan syndrome, and possibly in patients with recurrent nonhypertensive cerebral hemorrhage from amyloid angiopathy.[30] Therefore, in these patients prophylactic management becomes a necessity.

Post-traumatic Stress Disorder

Post-traumatic stress disorder (PTSD), included under trauma-related stress disorders in DSM-5, requires that the person be subjected to a potentially traumatic event causing significant impact on his or her social and occupational functioning for at least 1 month, without any other medical conditions or effects of toxic drugs.[31] The traumatic event and its impact are usually well appreciated by the patients. However, severe elevation of blood pressure is not frequently observed among patients with PTSD.[6] Moreover, in 1987 Kosten and colleagues[32] documented the elevation of both EPI and NE among PTSD patients, citing psychological factors as the underlying mechanism responsible for elevation of both hormones.

Baroreceptor Reflex Failure

The baroreceptor reflex is characterized by the buffering of abrupt changes in blood pressure while preventing the rise or fall of blood pressure through adjustments in heart rate, cardiac contractility, and vascular tone. Baroreceptor reflex failure is caused by an underlying condition such as accidental injury, neck surgery, or irradiation, and is associated with both hypertension and hypotension.[33] Common symptoms observed in these patients include paroxysmal hypertension, tachycardia, diaphoresis, headaches, and emotional instability.[34] By comparison, pseudoPHEO is described with the presence of paroxysmal hypertension and other associated symptoms as mentioned earlier. These patients have normal hemodynamic responses to the

Valsalva maneuver.[23] Baroreflex failure can be ruled out using appropriate diagnostic tests to determine baroreflex function. Also, the pressor episodes in baroreceptor reflex failure are occasionally associated with increased plasma NE from unrestrained activation of the SNS.[34] At times, the bouts of hypertension and associated symptoms of pseudoPHEO are eliminated with psychotherapeutic and psychopharmacologic intervention, thus arguing strongly against baroreceptor failure as a cause.[7]

MANAGEMENT

Treatment of a patient diagnosed with pseudoPHEO is demanding and should be focused on 2 important aspects: (1) control of blood pressure and (2) therapy for one of the most common causes of panic disorder (pseudoPHEO is an ill-defined clinical syndrome having variable clinical characteristics and multiple causes, one of which is panic disorder) or anxiety state.[35] However, there are no adequate clinical treatment trials nor recommendations or guidelines to treat these patients. Therefore, a combination of antihypertensive drugs, psychotropic drugs, and psychological intervention is used for treatment (**Table 3**).

Antihypertensive Drugs

Acute management
Approaches to acute management of pseudoPHEO depend on the severity of the increase in blood pressure, associated symptoms, and the presence or absence of significant comorbidities that put an individual at risk of an acute cerebrovascular or cardiovascular event. Blood pressure higher than 220/120 mm Hg can be considered severe (cutoff could be lower or higher depending on factors such as age, symptoms,

Table 3
Management of pseudopheochromocytoma

	Acute Management	Preventive Management
Antihypertensive medication	Severe increase in blood pressure: IV labetalol bolus 10–20 mg, increase the dose by 20–40 mg every 10 min up to a maximum dose of 200–300 mg IV nicardipine drip at 5 mg/h (only in hospital setting) Mild to moderate increase in blood pressure: Clonidine 0.1 mg or amlodipine 2.5 mg PO	α-Adrenoceptor antagonist: Doxazosin Terazosin Combined α- and β-adrenoceptor antagonist: carvedilol 25 mg once or twice daily Avoid anxiety, nervousness, related situations Enough sleep, good diet, environment Avoid stress, etc
Psychopharmacologic agent	Rapid-acting anxiolytic: Alprazolam 0.25–0.5 mg PO together with either PO or IV antihypertensive medication	SSRI: Citalopram 10 mg PO Paroxetine 10 mg PO Benzodiazepine: Clonazepam 0.5–1 mg PO (long-acting) or alprazolam 0.25–0.5 mg PO
Psychological/ psychiatric intervention	Reassurance and psychological awareness	

Abbreviations: IV, intravenous; PO, by mouth; SSRI, selective serotonin reuptake inhibitor.

routine blood-pressure measurement values, and underlying comorbidities). It is advised to evaluate and manage a patient with marked blood-pressure elevation associated with a comorbid condition in an emergency unit. To control an intense increase in blood pressure (especially longer lasting) requires use of rapidly acting intravenous medications such as labetalol, sodium nitroprusside, or nicardipine in a hospital setting.[6] When using labetalol, it is given at a bolus dose of 10 to 20 mg, followed by 20 to 40 mg every 10 minutes up to a maximum dose of 200 to 300 mg. If nicardipine is chosen as a first-line agent, it is given at a dose of 5 mg/h with a maximum dose of 30 mg/h.[36] A short-acting anxiolytic agent such as alprazolam is also given intravenously to modulate the associated symptoms of anxiety.[6,7] However, for patients with a less severe increase in blood pressure, no associated comorbidities, and treatment requiring special care in office or at home, a regimen consisting of alprazolam (0.25–0.50 mg) and clonidine (0.10 mg, single dose) per oral dose is preferred. Combination of these 2 medications usually lowers the blood pressure in 60 to 90 minutes.[37] Oral labetalol is not preferred because of its uncertain bioavailability.[38] Often, pseudoPHEO patients have a hypertensive emergency, which is stabilized or normalized without intervention or a visit to the emergency room. Such individuals are usually advised to sit in a quiet environment and use mechanisms to "destress," including meditation or deep breathing. A repeat blood-pressure measurement is conducted 30 minutes later. If the blood pressure remains elevated, it is recommended to take either a dose of 0.1 mg of clonidine or 2.5 mg of amlodipine, or a low-dose anxiolytic agent orally, depending on the requirements of the individual patient.[28]

Preventive management

Chronic and preventive management depends on the frequency and severity of paroxysms and its effect on day-to-day activities. Angiotensin-converting enzyme inhibitors (ACEI), angiotensin-receptor blockers (ARBs), and diuretics are not very efficient in preventing the episodes of SNS-driven paroxysmal hypertension. Also, monotherapy with either α- or β-adrenoceptor blocker would not be beneficial to reduce the SNS-mediated blood-pressure reactivity. A well-tolerated approach would be a combination of α-adrenoceptor blocker and β-adrenoceptor blockers.[39] However, both carvedilol and labetalol with combined α- and β-adrenoceptor blocker properties have unpredictable bioavailability. Therefore, an α-adrenoceptor blocker such as doxazosin or terazosin combined with a β-adrenoceptor blocker such as atenolol or metoprolol seems to be preferable.[6] Also, Garcha and Cohen[28] reported that transdermal clonidine is useful in preventing paroxysmal episodes of hypertension, although long-term use of a centrally acting α-adrenoceptor agonist is not feasible in view of the commonly associated side effect of fatigue. Other centrally active sympathetic suppressants available outside the United States are rilmenidine and moxonidine, with no systemic trials to demonstrate their efficacy among patients with pseudoPHEO. Moreover, individuals who are normotensive in between paroxysms do not require an antihypertensive regimen because of the risk of inducing iatrogenic hypotension and the absence of proven benefit.[37] Therefore, management of these patients is difficult because paroxysmal episodes of hypertension often occur several times a week, causing restrictions in lifestyle. These patients can be managed by prescribing antidepressant medication if the patient is agreeable. However, patients with chronic and sustained hypertension are treated similarly to patients with essential hypertension with no paroxysmal episodes (according to the guidelines dictated by American College of Cardiology/American Heart Association). Also, for patients with mild or infrequent paroxysms, treatment is limited to acute management at the time of paroxysms and reassurance. The use of antihypertensive medication is never prescribed on an as-needed basis. However, in this specific situation, it could be effective to manage hypertensive paroxysm in a patient who is otherwise normotensive at baseline. Moreover, if the initial episode of paroxysmal hypertension is associated with neurologic symptoms such as slurring of speech, weakness, or blurred vision, the patient should seek care from an emergency room.[28]

Psychopharmacologic Agents

There is no compelling evidence to advocate the use of an antihypertensive regimen for prevention of paroxysmal hypertension. Moreover, the use of antihypertensive agents is limited by the presence of normal blood pressure between paroxysms. The efficacy of alternatives such as antidepressants and anxiolytics was proposed given the similarity of symptoms from pseudoPHEO to those of panic disorder and anxiety state.[6,28] There is only anecdotal evidence regarding the type or duration of this aspect of therapy, but resolution of symptoms with treatment often occurs in a short period of time in this selected population.[7,29,40]

Acute management

Rapid-acting anxiolytics such as alprazolam may be used to swiftly terminate attacks of paroxysmal hypertension in some patients. As mentioned earlier, it is given at a dose of 0.25 to 0.50 mg to those patients with a less severe increase in blood pressure. Occasionally it is used in combination with antihypertensive medications, such as clonidine, to manage the significant component of anxiety associated with these paroxysms.[6]

Preventive management

The use of antidepressant medications, such as selective serotonin reuptake inhibitors (SSRIs) (paroxetine or citalopram) or tricyclic antidepressants (desipramine), is potent in reducing the frequency or eliminating paroxysms, particularly in patients who do not acknowledge an emotional trigger associated with them.[7] Garcha and Cohen[28] reported the success of using low doses of SSRIs, such as 10 mg of citalopram or paroxetine daily. A notable response is appreciated by the patients in about 3 weeks. Mild improvement in symptoms requires titration of the dose up to 20 mg daily. Alternatively, with tricyclic antidepressants such as desipramine, 10 to 25 mg is also useful in curbing these episodes of paroxysms. Recently a study published by Vaclavik and colleagues[41] reported the efficacy of using sertraline in the management of patients with paroxysmal hypertension, which led to significant clinical improvement in 75% and complete regression of symptoms in almost half of the patients. At times, use of anxiolytics in conjunction with antidepressants is helpful not only in preventing the hypertensive paroxysms but also in improving the quality of life among these patients. For longer-acting anxiolytics such as clonazepam, 0.5 to 1.0 mg twice daily can also be helpful in reducing these events.[6,28] The treatment of panic attacks and anxiety associated with pseudo-PHEO is similar; specifically, clonazepam and an SSRI can be given for long-term treatment along with cognitive-behavioral treatment described later.[35] It should also be noted that SSRIs are also cytochrome P450 enzyme inhibitors, thus interacting with other psychopharmacologic drugs and medications for medical illness. These reactions are more commonly seen with paroxetine than with sertraline or fluoxetine.[42] Thus, these medications can be used for chronic management. Moreover, many patients are reluctant to commit to long-term treatment with a psychotropic agent because of the associated social stigma of using these medications for psychological cause. An acceptable approach would be to begin an antidepressant agent among those patients with extremely severe hypertensive paroxysms, greater than 220/120 mm Hg, or with compromised ability to function. At times, delaying the initiation of an antidepressant agent allows for a trial of psychological intervention.[6]

Psychological Intervention

Antihypertensive agents and psychopharmacologic agents may control but might not cure pseudoPHEO. Psychological intervention provides an attractive alternative treatment among those patients who are considering a potential association between pseudoPHEO and emotional factors. However, many patients with repressed emotions related to severe trauma are unable to consider such a possibility. In 1999, Mann[7] reported the effectiveness of different treatment modalities among 21 patients with pseudoPHEO who had a mean follow-up of 9 months. A successful outcome was achieved in 13 of 15 evaluable patients. Three of the successfully treated patients responded to psychological intervention alone, whereas the remaining 10 responded to pharmacologic therapy, 7 of whom received antidepressant therapy and all of whom received therapy with α- and β-adrenoceptor blockers.[7] Treatment modality with this intervention includes reassurance and psychological awareness. A physician's confident reassurance that the disorder can be treated and that a catastrophic event or death during a paroxysm is unlikely could reduce associated terror and, possibly, the number and severity of the attacks. Awareness of repressed emotions behind this disorder is also helpful in reducing or eliminating the paroxysms without any psychotherapy. Later, psychotherapy may be helpful in processing the emotions that arise. Unfortunately, most patients who can repress overwhelming emotions related to unspeakable trauma will defend against awareness and continue to repress such emotions. Furthermore, patients with no history of trauma but a lifelong tendency to repress emotions are resistant to psychotherapy.[6,28] The treatment of panic attacks and anxiety among those who address these issues along with other symptoms of pseudoPHEO includes a combination of psychoeducation contributing to symptom induction, stress-reducing techniques such as paced breathing, addressing catastrophic cognitions and health anxiety caused by the alarming symptoms during the episodes, and deliberate induction of symptoms, thereby desensitizing the patient and reducing avoidance behavior.[35] Mann[6] reported in 2008 that the wisest course of action for treatment among such patients would be to offer a detailed description of the disease while providing reassurance that the disorder can be favorably managed along with restoration of normal life. At first, a patient's desire for treatment with psychotherapy and psychological discussion needs to be addressed. If he or she cannot see the connection between the disorder and trauma/repressed emotions, these therapies should be withheld.[28]

OBSTACLES TO SUCCESSFUL TREATMENT

Multiple difficulties can arise while treating a patient diagnosed with pseudoPHEO. Barriers to treatment with antihypertensive agents include: (1) ineffectiveness of ACEIs, ARBs, and diuretics; (2) normal blood pressure between paroxysms; and (3) antihypertensive agents unable to prevent paroxysms. One major obstacle to the use of antidepressants is the patient's refusal to try them because it implies a psychological cause. Finally, many patients, especially those not experiencing distress, hesitate being treated with psychological intervention because these could trigger emotions related to events from the past that might still be affecting them. At times, the mere implication of symptoms relating to an emotional component can cause enough distress to discourage the patient from seeking follow-up care. Therefore, patients with pseudoPHEO must be approached sensitively.

SUMMARY

This review helps to illustrate how perplexing and difficult it can be for clinicians to reach a diagnosis and establish an appropriate course of therapy for a patient with unexplained symptomatic paroxysmal hypertension. The implications associated with mental health along with the cost of health care in terms of diagnostic workups, ineffectual treatments, long-term medical care, and lost productivity are clearly much higher in patients with pseudoPHEO than for patients with PHEO.

REFERENCES

1. Kuchel O. Pseudopheochromocytoma. Hypertension 1985;7(1):151–8.
2. Kuchel O. Increased plasma dopamine in patients presenting with the pseudo-pheochromocytoma quandary: retrospective analysis of 10 years' experience. J Hypertens 1998;16(10):1531–7.
3. Sharabi Y, Goldstein DS, Bentho O, et al. Sympathoadrenal function in patients with paroxysmal hypertension: pseudopheochromocytoma. J Hypertens 2007; 25(11):2286–95.
4. Hall WD. Resistant hypertension, secondary hypertension, and hypertensive crises. Cardiol Clin 2002;20(2):281–9.
5. Page IH. A syndrome simulating diencephalic stimulation occurring in patients with essential hypertension. Am J Med Sci 1935;190:9–14.
6. Mann SJ. Severe paroxysmal hypertension (pseudopheochromocytoma). Curr Hypertens Rep 2008;10(1):12–8.
7. Mann SJ. Severe paroxysmal hypertension (pseudopheochromocytoma): understanding the cause and treatment. Arch Intern Med 1999;159(7):670–4.
8. Mann SJ. Severe paroxysmal hypertension. An automatic syndrome and its relationship to repressed emotions. Psychosomatics 1996;37(5):444–50.
9. Weinberger DA, Schwartz GE, Davidson RJ. Low-anxious, high-anxious, and repressive coping styles: psychometric patterns and behavioral and physiological responses to stress. J Abnorm Psychol 1979;88(4):369–80.
10. Hoy LJ, Emery M, Wedzicha JA, et al. Obstructive sleep apnea presenting as pseudopheochromocytoma: a case report. J Clin Endocrinol Metab 2004;89(5): 2033–8.
11. Zornitzki T, Knobler H, Schattner A. Reboxetine treatment and pseudopheochromocytoma. QJM 2007;100(1):61–2.
12. Mackenzie IS, Brown MJ. Pseudopheochromocytoma. J Hypertens 2007;25(11): 2204–6.
13. Bravo EL, Tarazi RC, Fouad FM, et al. Blood pressure regulation in pheochromocytoma. Hypertension 1982;4(3 Pt 2):193–9.
14. Goldenberg M, Serlin I, Edwards T, et al. Chemical screening methods for the diagnosis of pheochromocytoma. I. Nor-epinephrine and epinephrine in human urine. Am J Med 1954;16(3):310–27.

15. Widimsky J Jr. Recent advances in the diagnosis and treatment of pheochromocytoma. Kidney Blood Press Res 2006;29(5):321–6.
16. Lenders JW, Duh QY, Eisenhofer G, et al. Pheochromocytoma and paraganglioma: an endocrine society clinical practice guideline. J Clin Endocrinol Metab 2014;99(6):1915–42.
17. Lenders JW, Pacak K, Walther MM, et al. Biochemical diagnosis of pheochromocytoma: which test is best? JAMA 2002;287(11):1427–34.
18. Lenders JW, Eisenhofer G, Mannelli M, et al. Phaeochromocytoma. Lancet 2005; 366(9486):665–75.
19. Eisenhofer G, Lenders JW, Pacak K. Biochemical diagnosis of pheochromocytoma. Front Horm Res 2004;31:76–106.
20. Bravo EL, Tarazi RC, Fouad FM, et al. Clonidine-suppression test: a useful aid in the diagnosis of pheochromocytoma. N Engl J Med 1981;305(11):623–6.
21. Lenz T, Ross A, Schumm-Draeger P, et al. Clonidine suppression test revisited. Blood Press 1998;7(3):153–9.
22. Eisenhofer G, Goldstein DS, Walther MM, et al. Biochemical diagnosis of pheochromocytoma: how to distinguish true- from false-positive test results. J Clin Endocrinol Metab 2003;88(6):2656–66.
23. Eisenhofer G, Sharabi Y, Pacak K. Unexplained symptomatic paroxysmal hypertension in pseudopheochromocytoma: a stress response disorder? Ann N Y Acad Sci 2008;1148:469–78.
24. Balon R, Ortiz A, Pohl R, et al. Heart rate and blood pressure during placebo-associated panic attacks. Psychosom Med 1988;50(4):434–8.
25. Wilkinson DJ, Thompson JM, Lambert GW, et al. Sympathetic activity in patients with panic disorder at rest, under laboratory mental stress, and during panic attacks. Arch Gen Psychiatry 1998;55(6):511–20.
26. Villacres EC, Hollifield M, Katon WJ, et al. Sympathetic nervous system activity in panic disorder. Psychiatry Res 1987;21(4):313–21.
27. Esler M, Lambert E, Alvarenga M, et al. Increased brain serotonin turnover in panic disorder patients in the absence of a panic attack: reduction by a selective serotonin reuptake inhibitor. Stress 2007;10(3):295–304.
28. Garcha AS, Cohen DL. Catecholamine excess: pseudopheochromocytoma and beyond. Adv Chronic Kidney Dis 2015;22(3):218–23.
29. Mann SJ. Labile and paroxysmal hypertension: common clinical dilemmas in need of treatment studies. Curr Cardiol Rep 2015;17(11):99.
30. Mann SJ. The clinical spectrum of labile hypertension: a management dilemma. J Clin Hypertens (Greenwich) 2009;11(9):491–7.
31. Jorge RE. Posttraumatic stress disorder. Continuum (Minneap Minn) 2015;21(3 Behavioral Neurology and Neuropsychiatry):789–805.
32. Kosten TR, Mason JW, Giller EL, et al. Sustained urinary norepinephrine and epinephrine elevation in post-traumatic stress disorder. Psychoneuroendocrinology 1987;12(1):13–20.
33. Zar T, Peixoto AJ. Paroxysmal hypertension due to baroreflex failure. Kidney Int 2008;74(1):126–31.
34. Robertson D, Hollister AS, Biaggioni I, et al. The diagnosis and treatment of baroreflex failure. N Engl J Med 1993;329(20):1449–55.
35. Pickering TG, Clemow L. Paroxysmal hypertension: the role of stress and psychological factors. J Clin Hypertens (Greenwich) 2008;10(7):575–81.
36. Aronow WS. Treatment of hypertensive emergencies. Ann Transl Med 2017; 5(Suppl 1):S5.

37. Mann S. Paroxysmal hypertension (pseudopheochromocytoma). In: Bakris G, ed. UpToDate. Waltham (MA): UpToDate, .Available at: https://www.uptodate.com/contents/paroxysmal-hypertension-pseudopheochromocytoma Accessed March 27, 2019.
38. McNeil JJ, Anderson AE, Louis WJ, et al. Pharmacokinetics and pharmacodynamic studies of labetalol in hypertensive subjects. Br J Clin Pharmacol 1979; 8(Suppl 2):157S–61S.
39. Mann SJ. Neurogenic essential hypertension revisited: the case for increased clinical and research attention. Am J Hypertens 2003;16(10):881–8.
40. Hunt J, Lin J. Paroxysmal hypertension in a 48-year-old woman. Kidney Int 2008; 74(4):532–5.
41. Vaclavik J, Krenkova A, Kocianova E, et al. Effect of sertraline in paroxysmal hypertension. Biomed Pap Med Fac Univ Palacky Olomouc Czech Repub 2018; 162(2):116–20.
42. Muscatello MR, Spina E, Bandelow B, et al. Clinically relevant drug interactions in anxiety disorders. Hum Psychopharmacol 2012;27(3):239–53.

Renovascular Hypertension

Sandra M. Herrmann, MD*, Stephen C. Textor, MD

KEYWORDS

- Renovascular disease • Renal artery stenosis • Ischemic nephropathy
- Hypertension • Renin and angiotensin

KEY POINTS

- Renovascular disease is a major cause of secondary hypertension and may present with a range of clinical manifestations from asymptomatic hypertension to renal insufficiency and pulmonary congestion.
- Distinction among types, degrees, and clinical manifestations of renal artery stenosis should be made in order to define the best management for individual patients.
- Results of prospective trials of optimal medical therapy indicate no additional benefits from renal artery stenting over the course of the trials for individuals with moderate renovascular disease.
- Comprehensive medical therapy, including use of agents that block the renin-angiotensin system and lipid control, should be the cornerstone for management of atherosclerotic renovascular disease.
- Clinicians need to recognize renovascular hypertension progressing to high-risk clinical presentations that should undergo renal revascularization to achieve better renal and cardiovascular outcomes.

INTRODUCTION

Renovascular disease (RVD) is caused by progressive occlusive renal artery disease presenting with a myriad of symptoms ranging from renovascular hypertension to ischemic nephropathy. Renovascular hypertension (RVH) is one of the most common causes of secondary hypertension and has been widely studied as the prototype of angiotensin-dependent hypertension.[1] Most cases are caused by atherosclerotic lesions followed by fibromuscular dysplasia, but a variety of causes, such renal artery

The content is solely the responsibility of the authors and does not necessarily represent the official views of the National Institute for Diabetes, Digestive and Kidney Diseases (NIDDK) or the National Institutes of Health (NIH). Support: This work was partially supported by grant R01 DK100081 and K08 DK118120 from the NIDDK and NIH/National Center for Research Resources.
Division of Nephrology and Hypertension, Mayo Clinic, 200 First Street Southwest, Rochester, MN 55902, USA
* Corresponding author.
E-mail address: herrmann.sandra@mayo.edu

Endocrinol Metab Clin N Am 48 (2019) 765–778
https://doi.org/10.1016/j.ecl.2019.08.007
endo.theclinics.com

dissection or embolic disease, can produce the same symptoms. However, they are much less common.

Seminal studies performed by Goldblatt and colleagues[2] using a 2-kidney, 1-clip (2K1C) model in the early twentieth century established the role of hemodynamic hypoperfusion as a major cause of hypertension. Those studies were later corroborated by Page and Braun-Menendez,[3] identifying the vasoactive peptide angiotensin and its role of renin-angiotensin-aldosterone system (RAAS) axis activation in RVD.[4] These findings identified a potentially reversible cause of systemic increased blood pressure. This finding was translated into clinical practice creating a potential therapy by surgical removal of the pressor kidney when renal artery occlusive disease was identified.[5] This intervention allowed a possible cure, or better control, of hypertension in an era when medical therapy for hypertension was not available. However, surgical nephrectomy was often not successful in treating hypertension and was later discouraged. Intensive development of antihypertensive drugs led to the discovery of multiple therapeutic classes, including RAAS blockers in the 1980s, which coincided with the expansion of endovascular dilatation and stenting procedures.

Although moderate renal artery stenosis (RAS) may be asymptomatic, hypertension eventually develops as RAS progresses. A commonly used criterion to identify hemodynamically significant stenosis is a decrease of at least 60% of the luminal diameter of the renal artery, which is associated with a peak systolic velocity greater than 200 to 300 cm/s per Doppler ultrasonography.[6,7] Nonetheless, studies have shown that the stenotic kidney is able to adapt to moderate flow reduction allowing fairly safe long-term use of antihypertensive drug therapy to control blood pressure.[8] Over time, some renovascular occlusions progress and medical therapy alone fails to treat refractory hypertension. In these cases, RVH can progress with the development of high-risk syndromes, including hypertensive emergency associated with flash pulmonary edema and progressive decline of kidney function.[9] At such a point, the combination of medical therapy plus revascularization of RAS may be required. This article describes the epidemiology, types of RVD, pathophysiology, clinical features, diagnosis, and treatment recommendations for clinicians caring for complex patients in the current era.

EPIDEMIOLOGY AND CAUSES OF RENOVASCULAR HYPERTENSION

RVD is a major cause of hypertension that accounts for 1% to 5% of all cases of hypertension in the general population and 5.4% of secondary hypertension cases in young adults.[10–12] RVD is more prevalent in the older population, greater than 65 years of age, in which the incidence of significant RAS (>60% occlusion by Doppler ultrasonography) may be nearly 7%.[13] However, the incidence and prevalence vary because of the variability of RAS definition and the type of populations being studied. The prevalence may reach 40% in highly selected referral populations.[14,15] In 90% of cases, RVD is caused by atherosclerotic renal artery stenosis (ARAS) (**Fig. 1**) followed by fibromuscular dysplasia (9%). The remainder have miscellaneous causes, as described in **Box 1**.[16,17]

ATHEROSCLEROTIC RENAL ARTERY STENOSIS

ARAS is most common and is predominantly seen in older patients in the context of systemic atherosclerosis. Many of those plaques are extensions of aortic plaque into the renal artery. Hence, the location of atherosclerotic disease is usually near the origin of the artery, although it can be observed anywhere in the renal vessel. It can affect 1 or both renal arteries. Patients often have other associated risk factors,

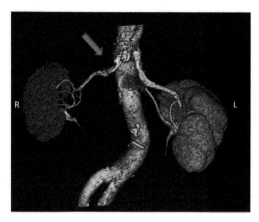

Fig. 1. Computed tomography angiography depicting moderate atherosclerotic RVD affecting the right kidney (*arrow*). L, left; R, right.

Box 1
Causes of renovascular disease

Unilateral renal artery disease

Unilateral atherosclerotic renal artery stenosis

Unilateral fibromuscular dysplasias

Renal artery aneurism

Arterial embolus

Arteriovenous fistula (eg, congenital, traumatic)

Segmental arterial occlusion (eg, posttraumatic, radiation, thrombi)

Extrinsic compression of renal artery (eg, tumor)

Bilateral renal artery disease or solitary functional kidney

Renal artery stenosis to a solitary kidney

Bilateral renal artery stenosis

Aortic coarctation

Atheroembolic disease

Systemic vasculitis (eg, polyarteritis nodosa, Takayasu arteritis)

Vascular occlusion caused by endovascular stent graft

Data from Hirsch AT, Haskal ZJ, Hertzer NR, et al. ACC/AHA 2005 Practice Guidelines for the management of patients with peripheral arterial disease (lower extremity, renal, mesenteric, and abdominal aortic): a collaborative report from the American Association for Vascular Surgery/Society for Vascular Surgery, Society for Cardiovascular Angiography and Interventions, Society for Vascular Medicine and Biology, Society of Interventional Radiology, and the ACC/AHA Task Force on Practice Guidelines (Writing Committee to Develop Guidelines for the Management of Patients With Peripheral Arterial Disease): endorsed by the American Association of Cardiovascular and Pulmonary Rehabilitation; National Heart, Lung, and Blood Institute; Society for Vascular Nursing; TransAtlantic Inter-Society Consensus; and Vascular Disease Foundation. Circulation 2006;113:e463-654.)

such as diabetes, hypertension, smoking history, peripheral vascular disease, and coronary artery disease. It can vary from asymptomatic disease, discovered incidentally during imaging studies or other interventional procedures, to clinical syndromes that present with active cardiovascular symptoms, including refractory hypertension, recurrent flash pulmonary edema, and progressive decline of renal function.[9,18,19]

Atherosclerotic RVD of some degree is found in 12% to 45% of patients undergoing vascular studies for peripheral vascular disease and 14% to 40% of patients undergoing coronary angiography.[14,20,21]

FIBROMUSCULAR DYSPLASIA

Fibromuscular dysplasia (FMD) is a heterogeneous group of nonatherosclerotic and noninflammatory diseases affecting intima or fibrous layers of the vascular wall. FMD commonly affects the renal and cerebral arteries (65%–70%) but can affect other vascular beds as well.[22,23] It can result in arterial stenosis, aneurysm formation, with dissection and/or occlusion of medium-sized arteries. There are 2 subtypes: multifocal FMD, which has the appearance of a string of beads and is the more common form; and focal FMD, which appears as a circumferential or tubular stenosis. FMD lesions are typically located away from the origin of the renal artery, often in the midportion of the vessel or at the first arterial bifurcation. It predominately affects women and is most commonly diagnosed in middle age. Interventional studies have suggested that, among patients referred for renal revascularization for hypertension, FMD accounts for 16% or less.[24] Hypertension is the most common presenting symptom, but other symptoms, such as pulsatile tinnitus, stroke, or chest pain, may result from other affected vascular beds.[25] Reports from arteriograms obtained from renal organ donors have shown the presence of mild FMD in 3% to 5% of those individuals without affecting renal blood flow or arterial pressure.[18] Furthermore, a study using the US FMD Registry showed that patients 65 years of age or older at the time of diagnosis of multifocal FMD were more likely to be asymptomatic and may have a more benign phenotype and fewer symptoms.[26]

In the prospective ARCADIA (Assessment of Renal and Cervical Artery Dysplasia) registry, symptomatic patients with FMD underwent tomographic or magnetic resonance angiography from the aortic arch to the intracranial arteries, and those with cervical FMD from the diaphragm to the pelvis. Among patients with a cerebrovascular presentation, the prevalence of renal artery lesions was higher in patients with hypertension than in those without. Among patients with a renal presentation, the prevalence of cervical lesions was higher in patients with bilateral RAS than in those with unilateral renal artery lesions. These studies characterize FMD as a systemic arterial disease.[27]

PATHOPHYSIOLOGY OF RENOVASCULAR HYPERTENSION

Renovascular hypertension is caused by reduction of blood flow perfusion to the kidney. Incidental RVD can be found in patients undergoing vascular imaging for other causes, but minor hemodynamic stenosis may not be of clinical significance.[20,28] Studies using latex casts to characterize luminal occlusion fail to detect measurable pressure or flow changes at levels of RAS less than 60% and suggest that the threshold for hemodynamic effects develops between 75% and 85% of luminal occlusion.[29] Clinical studies show that occlusion using an expanded balloon causes renin release only after the pressure distal to the balloon decreases by 10% to 20% less than the pressure proximal to the lesion.[30] These measurements correspond with a translesional peak systolic gradient of at least 20 to 25 mm Hg and luminal stenosis

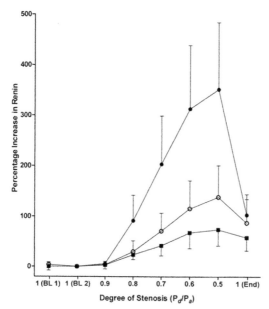

Fig. 2. Studies from human subjects with translesional pressure gradients indicate that an aortic-renal pressure gradient of 10% to 20% is necessary to detect renin release. BL 1, baseline before stenting; BL 2, baseline after stenting; Pd, mean aortic pressure; Pa, mean pressure distal to the RAS. (*From* De Bruyne B, Manoharan G, Pijls NHJ, et al. Assessment of renal artery stenosis severity by pressure gradient measurements. J Am Coll Cardiol. 2006;48:1851-1855.)

of at least 70%.[6] Hence, many lesions identified with clinical imaging tools are hemodynamically insignificant. As RAS progresses, the pressure and flow decrease steeply (**Fig. 2**).[30] The development of hypertension in experimental RVD is directly related to renin release, which increases systemic and distal renal pressures to maintain renal perfusion. The increase in blood pressure can be acute in experimental models using clip stenosis, or more gradual, which is more typical of human RVD. This state of hypoperfusion triggers additional pathways that tend to restore kidney perfusion. It is well established from renovascular experimental models and in humans that activation of RAAS and sodium retention play a major role in RVH.[31,32]

Renovascular occlusive disease results in release of renin from renal juxtaglomerular cells, which acts on its substrate angiotensinogen to produce angiotensin I. Angiotensin I is transformed by angiotensin-converting enzyme (ACE) into angiotensin II in the pulmonary capillary bed. Angiotensin II is a potent vasoconstrictor and promotes the release of aldosterone from the adrenal cortex and retention of salt and water.[33,34] The requirement for angiotensin in RVH was confirmed in a genetically modified angiotensin II subtype 1A receptor knockout (AT1A−/−) mouse model of 2K1C Goldblatt hypertension, which did not develop hypertension. This study indicates the critical role of angiotensin II subtype 1A receptor in blood pressure control.[35]

It is important to point out that the role of the RAAS axis in RVD depends, in part, on whether or not a contralateral nonstenotic kidney is present. Unilateral RVH in humans corresponds to the animal model of the 2K1C Goldblatt model, also called renin-dependent hypertension, characterized by increased peripheral resistance. The increase in blood pressure stimulates pressure natriuresis by the intact contralateral kidney, which prevents volume expansion and sodium retention. Hence the nonstenotic kidney tends to counter the increase of systemic blood pressure, which maintains reduced perfusion of the stenotic kidney and leads to continuous renin release. Although RVD remains a prototype of angiotensin-dependent hypertension, these hormonal responses are usually transient. As the occlusion progresses, or if there is absence of a contralateral perfused kidney, the mechanisms of sustained hypertension differ. As intravascular volume increases because of impaired sodium and water excretion by an ineffective contralateral kidney, there is progressive decrease of renin secretion over time. This phase is referred to as volume-dependent hypertension.[36] Renin activity can be normal or low in this phase.

Glomerular filtration pressure is maintained distal to the stenosis by angiotensin II–mediated vasoconstriction preferentially acting on the efferent arterioles. This action can reach a critical stage at which glomerular filtration rate (GFR) requires angiotensin II as a result of reduced perfusion. Removal of the angiotensin II effect with blockade of the RAAS can dramatically decrease GFR. Clinical examples for this include RAAS blockade with bilateral RAS or significant stenosis in a solitary functioning kidney. Administration of antihypertensive medications, such as ACE inhibitors and angiotensin-receptor blockers (ARBs), in patients with bilateral stenosis or solitary stenotic kidney must be done cautiously because of the potential worsening of renal function caused by this mechanism.[37]

The pathophysiology of RVD has served as the basis for the use of radionuclide studies using captopril renography as well as renal vein renin measurements for the diagnosis and treatment of RAS. The RAAS axis has widespread effects beyond vasoconstriction and sodium retention. Angiotensin II has complex cellular interactions that lead to activation of inflammatory and fibrogenic mechanisms. These mechanisms lead to vascular remodeling and tissue fibrosis within the stenotic kidney and left ventricular hypertrophy.[38–40] Furthermore, ARAS typically occurs in the context of systemic atherosclerosis and the inflammatory milieu that accompanies this disease. Increased sympathetic activation, endothelial dysfunction, and increased oxidative stress have been also shown in clinical studies. All these factors contribute to RVH in this population.[41–43]

The exact degree of vascular occlusion that threatens kidney function is still a matter of debate. The kidney is a highly perfused organ and capable of maintaining autoregulation even with reduced arterial diameters. However, at some point reduced renal perfusion beyond critical stenosis (75%–80%) leads to tissue hypoxia as measured by blood oxygen level–dependent (BOLD) imaging (**Fig. 3**).[8] The possibility cannot be excluded that atherosclerotic RVD represents a gradual process of repeated acute ischemic injury in the setting of an inflammatory milieu, leading to hypoxia and eventual loss of viable kidney function, designated ischemic nephropathy. Identification of this population with decreased renal perfusion before this process becomes irreversible is an important clinical priority.

CLINICAL FEATURES

As discussed earlier, RVH can develop in the setting of any cause of decreased blood flow to the affected kidney. FMD lesions most commonly affect the midportion of the renal artery, leading to early-onset hypertension and affecting women preferentially between 15 and 55 years of age. It rarely causes major renal functional loss, although some progression may be seen in patients who develop vascular injury, such as dissection, but it preferentially affects patients who are smokers.[44] This type of renal artery lesion tends to respond well to percutaneous angioplasty.

BOLD-MRI in Renovascular Disease

Stenotic Kidney   **Contralateral Kidney**

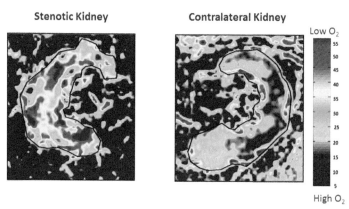

Fig. 3. Oxygenation is threatened lower in the poststenotic kidney compared with the nonstenotic contralateral kidney: representative coronal BOLD images. The R2* map (reflecting the level of deoxyhemoglobin) of the stenotic kidney shows a hypoxic cortical zone and widespread areas of increased deoxyhemoglobin level in the medullary segments (*red*). The unaffected contralateral kidney depicts the R2* map with a lower (*blue*) cortical zone and more gradual development of deeper medullary areas of hypoxia, and it is close to the appearance of a normal nonatherosclerotic RAS kidney. (*From* Herrmann SM, Saad A, Eirin A,et al. Differences in GFR and Tissue Oxygenation, and Interactions between Stenotic and Contralateral Kidneys in Unilateral Atherosclerotic Renovascular Disease. Clin J Am Soc Nephrol. 2016 Mar 7;11(3):458-69.)

Spectrum of Renovascular Disease
Manifestations

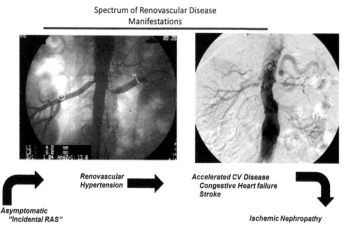

Fig. 4. Spectrum of atherosclerotic RVD. (*Left*) Aortogram obtained during coronary angiography showing moderate incidental stenosis of both renal arteries in a 67-year-old man with symptomatic coronary disease. (*Right*) More severe occlusive disease observed in a 68-year-old woman presenting with severe hypertension and episodes of flash pulmonary edema. Different clinical manifestations depending on severity of vascular occlusion, from asymptomatic hypertension to ischemic nephropathy. As occlusion progresses, this leads to accelerated hypertension, circulatory congestion, and ultimately threatens viability of the kidney. CV, cardiovascular. (*From* Herrmann SM, Saad A, Textor SC. Management of Atherosclerotic Renovascular Disease after Cardiovascular Outcomes in Renal Atherosclerotic Lesions (CORAL). Nephrol Dial Transplant. 2015 Mar;30(3):366-75.)

ARAS is associated with more widespread deleterious effects, often involves both kidneys, and is a multiorgan disease process with a range of manifestations generally related to the severity of the vascular occlusion (**Fig. 4**). ARAS is commonly encountered in the elderly population with other cardiovascular diseases and associated comorbidities. Overall, these individuals have higher mortality compared with normal age-adjusted populations.[45] A thorough physical examination, including auscultation of abdominal/flank area in order to identify the presence of an abdominal bruit, should be performed in all patients evaluated for hypertension. This examination may provide helpful hints to identify hypertensive patients with possible RAS. If such a bruit is found, it should serve as added impetus for further imaging studies.

The diagnosis of RAS often occurs during imaging studies or procedures for other indications, such as coronary catheterization, magnetic resonance (MR), or computed tomography angiography. The diagnosis of RVH in association with RAS is defined by a clinical syndrome with progressive increase of blood pressure, often leading to resistant or refractory hypertension with or without findings of chronic renal disease (**Box 2**). Clinical manifestations include progressive, sometimes rapid, increase in arterial pressure, which often occurs in elderly individuals with preexisting hypertension already treated with antihypertensive drugs. Therefore, clinicians should maintain a high suspicion for superimposed secondary causes of hypertension in patients with progressive increase of antihypertensive drug requirements, especially in the setting of high risk for atherosclerotic disease. This suspicion is particularly important in individuals with a history of smoking, which has a strong association with deleterious cardiorenal outcomes in patients with renovascular hypertension.[46]

Activation of the RAAS axis in this population increases blood pressure fluctuations, especially if the patient is not on optimal medical therapy. Additional reabsorption of salt and water in the setting of increased RAAS activity commonly leads to volume overload and pulmonary congestion. The combination of volume excess and increased RAAS activation can accelerate target organ manifestations, including

---

Box 2
Clinical findings associated with renovascular disease

Onset of hypertension before age of 30 years

Accelerated, resistant, malignant hypertension

Deterioration of renal function in response to ACE inhibitors or angiotensin-receptor blocker

New onset of hypertension after 50 years of age (suggestive of ARAS)

Asymmetric kidneys with more than 1.5 cm of difference in the size and otherwise unexplained loss of kidney function

Sudden unexplained pulmonary edema

Data from Hirsch AT, Haskal ZJ, Hertzer NR, et al. ACC/AHA 2005 Practice Guidelines for the management of patients with peripheral arterial disease (lower extremity, renal, mesenteric, and abdominal aortic): a collaborative report from the American Association for Vascular Surgery/Society for Vascular Surgery, Society for Cardiovascular Angiography and Interventions, Society for Vascular Medicine and Biology, Society of Interventional Radiology, and the ACC/AHA Task Force on Practice Guidelines (Writing Committee to Develop Guidelines for the Management of Patients With Peripheral Arterial Disease): endorsed by the American Association of Cardiovascular and Pulmonary Rehabilitation; National Heart, Lung, and Blood Institute; Society for Vascular Nursing; TransAtlantic Inter-Society Consensus; and Vascular Disease Foundation. Circulation 2006;113:e463-654.

direct vascular injury, left ventricular hypertrophy, and renal dysfunction. These manifestations are seen more commonly in RVD than in patients with essential hypertension, compared with an age-matched population with the same degree of blood pressure control.[47]

RVH in the setting of RVD can accelerate cardiovascular disease. When severe, the increase of blood pressure can be associated with volume retention and precipitate circulatory congestion associated with left ventricular dysfunction. This series of events has been designated flash pulmonary edema and represents a cardiorenal syndrome commonly associated with worsening renal function.[48] Pulmonary edema associated with RVD leads to increased hospitalizations and increased morbidity and mortality in patients with congestive heart failure.[49] Ultimately, progressive occlusive renal artery disease produces overt hypoxia within the kidney and irreversible worsening of kidney function designated ischemic nephropathy, especially in the context of other risk factors such as diabetes, hypertension, and smoking.[50]

IMAGING AND LABORATORY STUDIES

Presence of clinical manifestations that raise suspicion for RVD should prompt consideration of diagnostic imaging. However, before undertaking potentially costly and/or hazardous imaging procedures, clinicians should first establish the goals for the imaging study. Will this study change current medical management? Is the patient presenting with clinical features that warrant consideration for vascular intervention? Will the results of these studies lead to changes in medication, renal revascularization, or even nephrectomy? The choice of imaging is likely to depend on the patient's clinical manifestations in the setting of current medical therapy. Advances in noninvasive imaging techniques have allowed greater diagnostic sensitivity and accuracy than ever before. Computed tomography angiography, MR angiography, and Doppler ultrasonography are noninvasive imaging modalities commonly used to evaluate vasculature. However, none of these tests is perfect, and they are most informative for clinical purposes when the results are positive in a population at high risk for disease.[51,52] Duplex ultrasonography is often the first and least expensive study. There are no issues with intravenous contrast exposure. The limitations of this technique hinge on its dependence on operator skills and patient body habitus. If clinical suspicion for severe RVD is high and noninvasive tests remain inconclusive, catheter angiography may be performed. This procedure is usually reserved for patients considered candidates for endovascular intervention in the same session. Clinicians can also consider the use of functional tests of RVD using radionuclide renography with captopril when there is a need to evaluate the relative function of each kidney before a therapeutic nephrectomy.[7,53] Mercaptoacetyltriglycine is the most commonly used radionuclide because it is more reliable in renal insufficiency. However, functional tests still have limited reliability in renal insufficiency, particularly in the setting of bilateral RVD. Hematologic and electrolytes tests are normal or consistent with the degree of renal insufficiency. If creatinine level progressively increases, this should warrant further evaluation, including renal artery duplex ultrasonography. Urinalysis is generally bland with minimal proteinuria. The presence of significant proteinuria or more active urinary sediment should raise concern for other renal parenchymal diseases.

Plasma renin activity levels alone are of limited value because they vary depending on the sodium and fluid retention status.[54] The plasma aldosterone/renin ratio may be consistent with secondary aldosterone excess, which may lead in some cases to hypokalemia. Measurement of renal vein renin levels has been used for identification of overt lateralization of renin levels in the poststenotic kidney and these levels are reduced in the contralateral kidney. These tests have been limited by the effects of medications and volume status. Because RVH is less commonly the primary indication to consider renal revascularization, as opposed to salvage and/or protection of renal function, these tests are rarely performed. They are most commonly used when contemplating therapeutic nephrectomy for blood pressure control.

MANAGEMENT STRATEGIES FOR RENOVASCULAR DISEASE

The treatment of RVH depends on the type of RVD and clinical manifestations. In patients with FMD, the renal artery may have multiple webs that are amenable to balloon angioplasty. Technical success rates may reach 90%.[55] Approximately 10% to 15% of these cases develop restenosis, although repeat angioplasty can be performed.[56] Despite successful technical outcomes, cure of hypertension with removal of all antihypertensive therapy happens in less than one-third of cases. The likelihood of cure depends on factors such as the age of the patient, and duration and severity of hypertension.[57] In general, clinicians should consider renovascular intervention in patients with FMD, especially for young patients, with the goal of withdrawal or reducing the number of antihypertensive medications.[58]

The treatment of patients with ARAS differs from that of patients with FMD, because angioplasty alone commonly fails to maintain patency for proximal or ostial atherosclerotic lesions. Extensive calcified plaques at the vessel origin tend to recoil, leading to high rates of restenosis.[59] After introduction of endovascular stents, rates of restenosis decreased, leading to technical success in nearly 100%. Nonetheless, restenosis still develops in up to 20% of cases for stents placed in vessels less than 5 mm in diameter.[60]

Results of several randomized controlled trials comparing medical therapy with renal revascularization have failed to show definitive benefits of endovascular stent therapy in addition to medical therapy alone regarding improvement of blood pressure control, renal outcomes, or cardiovascular outcomes.[61–63] It can be argued that contemporary therapies with multitargeted medical management of atherosclerosis, hypertension, and risk factors including smoking and diabetes control may have changed the natural history and clinical outcomes for many patients with atherosclerotic RVD. However, a major limitation of these studies reflects the fact that the population with high-risk clinical presentations were underrepresented in these studies (ie, rapidly progressive renal insufficiency, acute kidney injury during initiation of ACE/ARB therapy, intractable hypertension, and/or flash pulmonary edema). These patients are likely to benefit from restoration of renal artery patency. Multiple observational studies indicate that such patients have major clinical benefits when renal circulation can be restored. The challenge for clinicians is to identify this subgroup of individuals with viable kidneys and intervene appropriately.

A clinical algorithm has been proposed for management of RVH and ischemic nephropathy (**Fig. 5**). As with other vascular occlusive disease, identified patients with RVH should be followed to ensure controlled hypertension and stable renal function. During follow-up of 3 to 5 years with medical therapy in the trial populations, there was no evident advantage of revascularization, although individuals with normal urinary protein levels had evident cardiovascular and mortality benefits in a post hoc analysis.[64] Atherosclerotic disease commonly progresses over longer time period, and some individuals with other comorbidities develop further

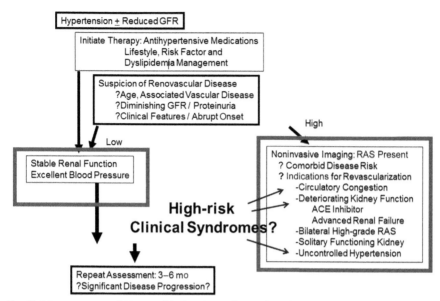

Fig. 5. Management of RVH and ischemic nephropathy. The goal is to reduce morbidity associated with hypertension by controlling blood pressure and preserving kidney function. If medical therapy fails or RVD progresses, revascularization of renal artery should be considered. (*From* Herrmann SM, Saad A, Textor SC. Management of atherosclerotic renovascular disease after Cardiovascular Outcomes in Renal Atherosclerotic Lesions (CORAL). Nephrol Dial Transplant. 2015 Mar;30(3):366-75.)

manifestations of high-grade stenosis and high-risk features. For such individuals, clinicians need to periodically reevaluate risks versus benefits of revascularization of a potential salvageable kidney in order to prevent complete occlusion and/or irreversible injury.

REFERENCES

1. Herrmann SM, Textor SC. Current concepts in the treatment of renovascular hypertension. Am J Hypertens 2018;31:139–49.
2. Goldblatt H, Lynch J, Hanzal RF, et al. Studies on experimental hypertension: I. The production of persistent elevation of systolic blood pressure by means of renal ischemia. J Exp Med 1934;59:347–79.
3. Frohlich ED. Sixtieth anniversary of Angiotensin. Hypertension 2001;38(6):1245.
4. Basso N, Terragno NA. History about the discovery of the renin-angiotensin system. Hypertension 2001;38:1246–9.
5. Stanley JC, David M. Hume memorial lecture. Surgical treatment of renovascular hypertension. Am J Surg 1997;174:102–10.
6. Drieghe B, Madaric J, Sarno G, et al. Assessment of renal artery stenosis: side-by-side comparison of angiography and duplex ultrasound with pressure gradient measurements. Eur Heart J 2008;29:517–24.
7. Hirsch AT, Haskal ZJ, Hertzer NR, et al. ACC/AHA 2005 Practice Guidelines for the management of patients with peripheral arterial disease (lower extremity, renal, mesenteric, and abdominal aortic): a collaborative report from the American Association for Vascular Surgery/Society for Vascular Surgery, Society for

Cardiovascular Angiography and Interventions, Society for Vascular Medicine and Biology, Society of Interventional Radiology, and the ACC/AHA Task Force on Practice Guidelines (Writing Committee to Develop Guidelines for the Management of Patients With Peripheral Arterial Disease): endorsed by the American Association of Cardiovascular and Pulmonary Rehabilitation; National Heart, Lung, and Blood Institute; Society for Vascular Nursing; TransAtlantic Inter-Society Consensus; and Vascular Disease Foundation. Circulation 2006;113: e463–654.

8. Gloviczki ML, Glockner JF, Crane JA, et al. Blood oxygen level-dependent magnetic resonance imaging identifies cortical hypoxia in severe renovascular disease. Hypertension 2011;58:1066–72.

9. Ritchie J, Green D, Chrysochou C, et al. High-risk clinical presentations in atherosclerotic renovascular disease: prognosis and response to renal artery revascularization. Am J Kidney Dis 2014;63:186–97.

10. Olin JW, Piedmonte MR, Young JR, et al. The utility of duplex ultrasound scanning of the renal arteries for diagnosing significant renal artery stenosis. Ann Intern Med 1995;122:833–8.

11. Chrysochou C, Kalra PA. Epidemiology and natural history of atherosclerotic renovascular disease. Prog Cardiovasc Dis 2009;52:184–95.

12. Noilhan C, Barigou M, Bieler L, et al. Causes of secondary hypertension in the young population: a monocentric study. Ann Cardiol Angeiol (Paris) 2016;65: 159–64.

13. Hansen KJ, Edwards MS, Craven TE, et al. Prevalence of renovascular disease in the elderly: a population-based study. J Vasc Surg 2002;36:443–51.

14. de Mast Q, Beutler JJ. The prevalence of atherosclerotic renal artery stenosis in risk groups: a systematic literature review. J Hypertens 2009;27:1333–40.

15. Piecha G, Wiecek A, Januszewicz A. Epidemiology and optimal management in patients with renal artery stenosis. J Nephrol 2012;25:872–8.

16. Safian RD, Textor SC. Renal-artery stenosis. N Engl J Med 2001;344:431–42.

17. Lao D, Parasher PS, Cho KC, et al. Atherosclerotic renal artery stenosis–diagnosis and treatment. Mayo Clin Proc 2011;86:649–57.

18. Lorenz EC, Vrtiska TJ, Lieske JC, et al. Prevalence of renal artery and kidney abnormalities by computed tomography among healthy adults. Clin J Am Soc Nephrol 2010;5:431–8.

19. Rihal CS, Textor SC, Breen JF, et al. Incidental renal artery stenosis among a prospective cohort of hypertensive patients undergoing coronary angiography. Mayo Clin Proc 2002;77:309–16.

20. Conlon PJ, O'Riordan E, Kalra PA. New insights into the epidemiologic and clinical manifestations of atherosclerotic renovascular disease. Am J Kidney Dis 2000;35:573–87.

21. Buller CE, Nogareda JG, Ramanathan K, et al. The profile of cardiac patients with renal artery stenosis. J Am Coll Cardiol 2004;43:1606–13.

22. Sanidas EA, Seferou M, Papadopoulos DP, et al. Renal fibromuscular dysplasia: a not so common entity of secondary hypertension. J Clin Hypertens 2016;18: 240–6.

23. Olin JW, Gornik HL, Bacharach JM, et al. Fibromuscular dysplasia: state of the science and critical unanswered questions: a scientific statement from the American Heart Association. Circulation 2014;129:1048–78.

24. Krijnen P, van Jaarsveld BC, Steyerberg EW, et al. A clinical prediction rule for renal artery stenosis. Ann Intern Med 1998;129:705–11.

25. Olin JW, Froehlich J, Gu X, et al. The United States registry for fibromuscular dysplasia: results in the first 447 patients. Circulation 2012;125:3182–90.
26. Bagh I, Olin JW, Froehlich JB, et al. Association of multifocal fibromuscular dysplasia in elderly patients with a more benign clinical phenotype: data from the US registry for fibromuscular dysplasia. JAMA Cardiol 2018;3:756–60.
27. Plouin PF, Baguet JP, Thony F, et al. High prevalence of multiple arterial bed lesions in patients with fibromuscular dysplasia: the ARCADIA registry (assessment of renal and cervical artery dysplasia). Hypertension 2017;70:652–8.
28. Garovic VD, Textor SC. Renovascular hypertension and ischemic nephropathy. Circulation 2005;112:1362–74.
29. May AG, De Weese JA, Rob CG. Hemodynamic effects of arterial stenosis. Surgery 1963;53:513–24.
30. De Bruyne B, Manoharan G, Pijls NH, et al. Assessment of renal artery stenosis severity by pressure gradient measurements. J Am Coll Cardiol 2006;48:1851–5.
31. Mueller CB, Surtshin A, Carlin MR, et al. Glomerular and tubular influences on sodium and water excretion. Am J Physiol 1951;165:411–22.
32. Dustan HP. Physiologic consequences of renal arterial stenosis. N Engl J Med 1969;281:1348–54.
33. Treadway KK, Slater EE. Renovascular hypertension. Annu Rev Med 1984;35:665–92.
34. Sparks MA, Crowley SD, Gurley SB, et al. Classical renin-angiotensin system in kidney physiology. Compr Physiol 2014;4:1201–28.
35. Cervenka L, Horacek V, Vaneckova I, et al. Essential role of AT1A receptor in the development of 2K1C hypertension. Hypertension 2002;40:735–41.
36. Gavras H, Brunner HR, Thurston H, et al. Reciprocation of renin dependency with sodium volume dependency in renal hypertension. Science 1975;188:1316–7.
37. Pickering TG. Renovascular hypertension: etiology and pathophysiology. Semin Nucl Med 1989;19:79–88.
38. Eirin A, Lerman LO. Darkness at the end of the tunnel: poststenotic kidney injury. Physiology (Bethesda) 2013;28:245–53.
39. Gloviczki ML, Keddis MT, Garovic VD, et al. TGF expression and macrophage accumulation in atherosclerotic renal artery stenosis. Clin J Am Soc Nephrol 2013;8:546–53.
40. Khangura KK, Eirin A, Kane GC, et al. Cardiac function in renovascular hypertensive patients with and without renal dysfunction. Am J Hypertens 2014;27:445–53.
41. Johansson M, Elam M, Rundqvist B, et al. Increased sympathetic nerve activity in renovascular hypertension. Circulation 1999;99:2537–42.
42. Lerman LO, Nath KA, Rodriguez-Porcel M, et al. Increased oxidative stress in experimental renovascular hypertension. Hypertension 2001;37:541–6.
43. Textor SC, Lerman LO. Paradigm shifts in atherosclerotic renovascular disease: where are we now? J Am Soc Nephrol 2015;26:2074–80.
44. O'Connor S, Gornik HL, Froehlich JB, et al. Smoking and adverse outcomes in fibromuscular dysplasia: U.S. registry report. J Am Coll Cardiol 2016;67:1750–1.
45. Vassallo D, Kalra PA. Progress in the treatment of atherosclerotic renovascular disease: the conceptual journey and the unanswered questions. Nephrol Dial Transplant 2016;31:1595–605.
46. Drummond CA, Brewster PS, He W, et al. Cigarette smoking and cardio-renal events in patients with atherosclerotic renal artery stenosis. PLoS One 2017;12:e0173562.

47. Losito A, Fagugli RM, Zampi I, et al. Comparison of target organ damage in renovascular and essential hypertension. Am J Hypertens 1996;9:1062–7.
48. Messerli FH, Bangalore S, Makani H, et al. Flash pulmonary oedema and bilateral renal artery stenosis: the Pickering Syndrome. Eur Heart J 2011;32:2231–5.
49. Kane GC, Xu N, Mistrik E, et al. Renal artery revascularization improves heart failure control in patients with atherosclerotic renal artery stenosis. Nephrol Dial Transplant 2010;25:813–20.
50. Textor SC, Lerman L. Renovascular hypertension and ischemic nephropathy. Am J Hypertens 2010;23:1159–69.
51. Herrmann SM, Textor SC. Diagnostic criteria for renovascular disease: where are we now? Nephrol Dial Transplant 2012;27:2657–63.
52. Textor SC. Pitfalls in imaging for renal artery stenosis. Ann Intern Med 2004;141:730–1.
53. Fommei E, Ghione S, Hilson AJ, et al. Captopril radionuclide test in renovascular hypertension: a European multicentre study. European Multicentre Study Group. Eur J Nucl Med 1993;20:617–23.
54. Wilcox CS. Use of angiotensin-converting-enzyme inhibitors for diagnosing renovascular hypertension. Kidney Int 1993;44:1379–90.
55. Tegtmeyer CJ, Selby JB, Hartwell GD, et al. Results and complications of angioplasty in fibromuscular disease. Circulation 1991;83:I155–61.
56. Surowiec SM, Sivamurthy N, Rhodes JM, et al. Percutaneous therapy for renal artery fibromuscular dysplasia. Ann Vasc Surg 2003;17:650–5.
57. Bonelli FS, McKusick MA, Textor SC, et al. Renal artery angioplasty: technical results and clinical outcome in 320 patients. Mayo Clin Proc 1995;70:1041–52.
58. Davidson RA, Barri Y, Wilcox CS. Predictors of cure of hypertension in fibromuscular renovascular disease. Am J Kidney Dis 1996;28:334–8.
59. van de Ven PJ, Kaatee R, Beutler JJ, et al. Arterial stenting and balloon angioplasty in ostial atherosclerotic renovascular disease: a randomised trial. Lancet 1999;353:282–6.
60. Textor SC, Misra S, Oderich GS. Percutaneous revascularization for ischemic nephropathy: the past, present, and future. Kidney Int 2013;83:28–40.
61. Bax L, Woittiez AJ, Kouwenberg HJ, et al. Stent placement in patients with atherosclerotic renal artery stenosis and impaired renal function: a randomized trial. Ann Intern Med 2009;150:840–8, w150-1.
62. Wheatley K, Ives N, Gray R, et al. Revascularization versus medical therapy for renal-artery stenosis. N Engl J Med 2009;361:1953–62.
63. Cooper CJ, Murphy TP, Cutlip DE, et al. Stenting and medical therapy for atherosclerotic renal-artery stenosis. N Engl J Med 2014;370:13–22.
64. Murphy TP, Cooper CJ, Pencina KM, et al. Relationship of albuminuria and renal artery stent outcomes: results from the CORAL randomized clinical trial (cardiovascular outcomes with renal artery lesions). Hypertension 2016;68:1145–52.

Hypertension and Acromegaly

Soraya Puglisi, MD, Massimo Terzolo, MD*

KEYWORDS

- Blood pressure • Cardiovascular risk • Antihypertensive treatment
- Cardiovascular complication • Mortality • Prevalence • Pathogenesis • Sleep apnea

KEY POINTS

- Hypertension is one of the most important and common complications in acromegaly, for to increased cardiovascular risk, higher rate of hospitalization, and greater costs for the disease management.
- The pathogenesis has not yet been fully elucidated and likely includes multiple factors.
- A comprehensive, patient-centered approach, focusing not only on the biochemical control of acromegaly but also on an early diagnosis of hypertension and a prompt antihypertensive treatment, is required for optimal patient care.

INTRODUCTION

Acromegaly is a rare, chronic disease whose clinical manifestations are the consequence of growth hormone (GH) and insulinlike growth factor (IGF) 1 excess that is usually caused by a GH-secreting pituitary adenoma.[1] The disease is associated with a significant number of complications and comorbid conditions, mainly affecting the cardiovascular (CV) system.[2] Arterial hypertension is among the most frequent CV complications of acromegaly; however, its role as a prognostic factor is not definitely established,[3–7] despite the negative impact of hypertension on the acromegalic cardiomiopathy.[8,9] The classic view, that CV disease is the main culprit for the excess mortality in acromegalic patients,[2,4] has been revisited in more recent studies.[6,10,11] Nevertheless, CV disease is associated with an important disease burden, and significantly increases the rate of hospitalization and the health care costs.[12]

PREVALENCE AND CHARACTERISTICS

The frequency of hypertension in acromegaly varies from 11% to 54.7%, averaging 33.6%, as reported in **Table 1**, which includes the main studies published in the last

Conflicts of interest: S. Puglisi has no conflicts of interest in connection with this article. M. Terzolo has received research grants from Novartis.
Internal Medicine 1, Department of Clinical and Biological Sciences, University of Turin, San Luigi Gonzaga Hospital, Regione Gonzole 10, Orbassano 10043, Italy
* Corresponding author.
E-mail address: terzolo@usa.net

Endocrinol Metab Clin N Am 48 (2019) 779–793
https://doi.org/10.1016/j.ecl.2019.08.008
0889-8529/19/© 2019 Elsevier Inc. All rights reserved.

endo.theclinics.com

Table 1
Frequency of hypertension in acromegaly in studies published over the last 15 years (national or local registries of acromegalic patients)

Country	Patients (N)[a]	Patients with HTN (N)	Patients with HTN (%)[b]	Mean Age (y)	Study Period	References, Year of Publication
Spain	1036	405	39.1	45.0	1997–2003	Mestron et al,[3] 2004
New Zealand	126	69	54.7	42.0	1964–2000	Holdaway et al,[4] 2004
Belgium	409	161	39.4	44.0	2000–2004	Bex et al,[13] 2007
Greece	84	—	46.0	47.0	1980–2009	Anagnostis et al,[14] 2011
Italy	1512	—	33.0	45.0	1980–2002	Arosio et al,[6] 2012
Malta	47	22	46.8	43.4	1979–2008	Mercieca et al,[15] 2012
Canada	537	198	36.9	45.0	1980–2010	Vallette et al,[16] 2013
Iceland	52	25	48.1	44.5	1955–2013	Hoskuldsdottir et al,[17] 2015
Denmark	405	44	11.0	48.7	1991–2010	Dal et al,[18] 2016
Mexico	2057	—	27.0	41.0	2009–present	Portocarrero-Ortiz et al,[19] 2016
United States	120	57	47.5	55.4	1985–2013	Carmichael et al,[20] 2017
Sweden	358	142	39.7	50.0	2005–2013	Lesén et al,[21] 2017
Germany	479	186	45.5	45.7	Up to 2016	Schofl et al,[22] 2017
France	947	—	33.0	46.0	1999–2012	Maione et al,[23] 2017
Weighted mean	—	—	33.6	—		
Range	—	—	11.0–54.7	—		—

Abbreviation: HTN, hypertension.
[a] If specified, only patients with known information about hypertension.
[b] If specified, data at diagnosis.

15 years.[3,4,6,13–23] The variability found in the prevalence of hypertension could be attributed to the different diagnostic criteria adopted over different periods of recruitment, and to population-related risk factors (genetic and racial differences; prevalence of obesity; unhealthy life style, such as smoking and excessive sodium or alcohol intake). Note that all these studies were retrospective and reported only on office measurements of blood pressure (BP), likely overestimating the frequency of hypertension compared with ambulatory BP monitoring (ABPM).

This caveat was first shown by Minniti and colleagues,[24] who reported a frequency of hypertension of 42.5% in acromegalic patients with office BP measurements versus a frequency of 17.5% with ABPM. Similar findings were recently found by Costenaro and colleagues,[25] who showed a rate of 23% hypertension with ABPM versus 32% with clinical measurements. They reported that BP levels recorded by ABPM were correlated with GH and IGF-1 concentrations.

The correlation between severity of hypertension and GH or IGF-1 levels has been investigated in several studies, but findings are discordant.[6,26,27] A recent article tried to dissect the problem, showing a positive correlation between BP levels and IGF-1 concentrations when the latter were above the upper limit of normalcy, with an inverse relationship when IGF-1 levels were within the normal range.[28] The analysis included several studies, most of which have been performed in nonacromegalic patients, and supports a direct relationship in states characterized by overtly increased IGF-1 levels, such as uncontrolled acromegaly. In addition, it is plausible that other variables are important determinants of hypertension in acromegaly, such as the duration of disease,[27,29] patient age, and body mass index, whereas family history of hypertension or gender have more controversial roles.[19,27,30]

Hypertension in acromegalic patients is generally regarded as a mild disease that can be easily managed with standard antihypertensive drugs.[31] A peculiar pattern of acromegaly-associated hypertension may be found in higher diastolic BP and lower systolic BP levels compared with nonacromegalic hypertensive patients.[27,32] Furthermore, studies using ABPM found a higher prevalence of nondippers (almost 50%) in acromegalic hypertensive patients compared with patients with primary hypertension.[32,33] The nondipping pattern is shared with other types of secondary hypertension and is associated with increased CV morbidity and mortality.

PATHOGENESIS

The pathogenesis of hypertension in acromegaly has not yet been fully clarified, but a multifactorial origin is the most convincing explanation (**Fig. 1**). The development of hypertension may be attributable to a combined effect of a chronic GH/IGF-1 excess on different systems that eventually causes expansion of extracellular fluid volume, increase of peripheral vascular resistance, and development of the sleep apnea syndrome.

Expansion of Extracellular Fluid Volume

The increase of total extracellular fluid volume is secondary to sodium and water retention by the kidney, caused by direct and indirect effects of GH/IGF-1.[34]

Direct growth hormone antinatriuretic effects

The hypothesis of a GH direct effect fits well with the demonstration of GH receptors in human adrenal cortex.[35] In rat models of acromegaly, GH had an aldosterone-independent antinatriuretic effect, mediated through the epithelial Na^+ channels (ENaC) of collecting ducts.[36] The rats received furosemide, an antidiuretic drug able to inhibit the sodium reabsorption Na-K-2Cl symporter (NCCK2) channels in the

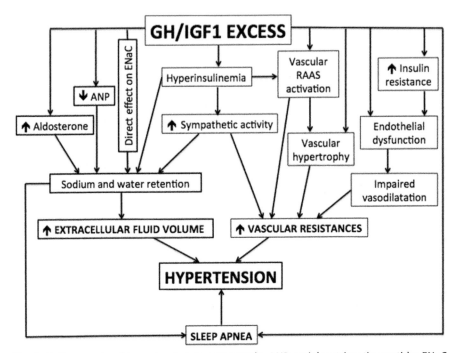

Fig. 1. Pathogenesis of hypertension in acromegaly. ANP, atrial natriuretic peptide; ENaC, epithelial Na+ channels; RAAS, renin-angiotensin-aldosterone system.

loop of Henle, and amiloride, which blocks the ENaC in the collecting ducts. In acromegalic rats, the furosemide-induced natriuresis was lower compared with controls, whereas the amiloride-induced natriuresis was higher, confirming the hypothesis that GH stimulates sodium transport in the distal nephron via ENaC. The increased activity of ENaC in acromegaly was also shown in humans, using a similar model of pharmacologic challenge with amiloride and furosemide.[37]

Effects of growth hormone on the renin-angiotensin-aldosterone system

The relationship between the renin-angiotensin-aldosterone system (RAAS) and GH/IGF-1 excess has been carefully evaluated in the last decades, but remains controversial. The leading hypothesis is that increased aldosterone levels, directly stimulated by GH excess, contribute to hypertension in acromegaly without stimulation of plasma renin activity (PRA).[38] However, no change has been found in RAAS activity during IGF-1 administration,[39] and low levels of PRA have been consistently detected in acromegalic patients.[40,41]

A significant direct correlation between GH and aldosterone values in acromegalic patients has been observed, and serum aldosterone concentration significantly decreased after normalization of GH secretion caused by surgical cure, whereas renin concentrations remained unaffected. In animal models, the association of chronic GH excess with increased aldosterone level was independent of renin, IGF-1, or adrenal aldosterone synthase expression.[38] In contrast, a study concerning the polymorphisms of genes involved in the RAAS has underlined the role of aldosterone synthase (cytochrome P [CYP] 11B2), showing that acromegalic patients with the CYP11B2-344CC genotype were affected by hypertension more frequently than patients with the CT/TT genotypes, with a significant increase of systolic BP.[42] In contrast, no significant effect of polymorphisms in other genes, such as angiotensino-gen or angiotensin-converting enzyme (ACE), was reported, in agreement with the findings of a more recent study.[43]

Insulinlike growth factor 1–mediated inhibition of atrial natriuretic peptide

Some studies showed a reduction of atrial natriuretic peptide (ANP) secretion in acro-megalic patients. McKnight and colleagues[44] compared plasma ANP levels of patients with active acromegaly with those of healthy subjects, before and after a 4-hour intra-venous infusion of normal saline. ANP levels increased significantly in the control group, whereas in acromegalic patients they did not respond to saline stimulation. Although the basal ANP values were similar between the two groups, the 4-hou ANP levels were significantly higher in the group of healthy subjects than in the acro-megalic group. A few years later, Moller and colleagues[39] showed that the inhibition of ANP-induced natriuresis is mediated by IGF-1.

Insulin-mediated effect

It is well known that acromegaly is often associated with insulin resistance and hyper-insulinemia. The antinatriuretic effect of insulin has long been debated, but an action on renal sodium absorption has confirmed it.[45] Although experimental studies in acro-megalic patients are not available, the pathophysiologic role of insulin-mediated changes in sodium balance fits well with the finding of higher insulin levels after oral glucose tolerance load in hypertensive compared with normotensive acromegalic pa-tients,[46] and higher BP levels in hyperinsulinemic acromegalic patients.[47] In contrast, other studies did not find a difference in fasting or postload plasma insulin values be-tween hypertensive and normotensive acromegalic patients,[48,49] suggesting that other factors could be involved in the pathogenesis, such as the insulin-mediated activation of the sympathetic nervous system.[50,51]

Sympathetic nervous system–mediated effect

The influence of the sympathetic nervous system on tubular processing of sodium is well known.[51] In contrast, controversial data on the role of an impaired sympathetic tone in acromegaly have been reported in the last decades.[50] In this area of debate, the assessment of the 24-hour profiles of plasma catecholamine levels and BP in 14 acromegalic patients (before and after pituitary surgery) and 8 healthy controls showed a flattened 24-hour profile of norepinephrine and BP in acromegalic patients, whereas the circadian norepinephrine rhythm was restored after surgery with normal-ization/reduction of GH/IGF-1 levels.[52]

Increase of Peripheral Vascular Resistances

The effect of chronic GH and IGF-1 excess on vascular resistance could explain the more apparent increase of diastolic versus systolic BP in acromegalic patients.[27,32] Recently, a study used renal ultrasonography to assess 57 acromegalic patients and showed that the Renal Resistive Index (RRI) was higher in 16 hypertensive acro-megalic patients compared with 49 normotensive patients.[53] Moreover, the RRI value was independently related to the presence of hypertension and correlated with IGF-1 levels, supporting the hypothesis of a link between the severity of acromegaly and hypertension.

Stimulation of vascular renin-angiotensin-aldosterone system and vascular hypertrophy

It has been shown in vitro that both IGF-1 and insulin are able to stimulate angiotensi-nogen production in cultures of vascular smooth muscle cells.[54] The same study showed the role of the two hormones in the development of vascular hypertrophy, through activation of the vascular RAAS. It is conceivable that the same mechanism could play a role in the pathogenesis of hypertension in acromegaly, according to studies that showed an association between hyperinsulinemia and hypertension in this group of patients.[46,47] This hypothesis sits well with evidence of a hypertrophic remodeling of subcutaneous small resistance arteries in acromegalic patients compared with the eutrophic remodeling in patients with essential hypertension.[55] The assessment of the structure of small arteries in biopsies of subcutaneous fat and of the calculated media-to-lumen ratio and growth indices showed the effect of growth factors in the development of vascular morphologic alterations. A weak but statistically significant correlation between the media-to-lumen ratio and IGF-1 values was also found in this small group of 9 acromegalic patients. Similar findings on vascular hypertrophy in acromegaly, and a positive association between wall thickness and IGF-1 levels, were shown in a subsequent study including a larger sample of 41 patients.[56]

Endothelial dysfunction

The comparison of the cutaneous vasoreactivity responses of 10 normotensive acromegalic patients with 10 healthy controls showed in the former group an impaired endothelium-dependent vasodilatation, which is mediated by nitric oxide (NO).[57] The NO pathway was subsequently evaluated, also taking into consideration its effects on vascular resistance, platelet aggregation, and inhibition of smooth muscle cell proliferation. A few years later, a decrease of NO concentrations was shown in acromegalic patients, caused by a reduced endothelial NO synthase expression, and an inverse correlation between NO and GH/IGF-1 levels, and duration of acromegaly.[58] Several recent studies confirmed the impairment of flow-mediated vasodilation[59,60] and the role of reduced NO levels in acromegaly,[56,61] which may contribute to both hypertension and erectile dysfunction in male acromegalic patients.[62] In addition, the association between endothelial dysfunction and insulin resistance deserves to be mentioned[63] as a further possible mechanism in this complex scenario.

Sympathetic activation

The evidence of an over-reactivity to sympathetic stimulation in acromegaly has been provided using a cold pressor test to study sympathetic vasoreactivity.[57] The study showed a significantly more pronounced increase in systolic BP, and a trend to a greater decrease in skin perfusion, in acromegalic patients compared with healthy controls, with a greater, although not statistically significant, vasoconstriction in acromegaly. In contrast, there are few and contradictory data on catecholamine levels, without any clear evidence of increased sympathetic tone in acromegalic patients.[50] A study comparing acromegalic patients and hypertensive controls reported a 24-hour catecholamine secretion that was quantitatively similar, but without any circadian rhythm, and a normal decrease during the night in acromegalic patients.[52] This report is in agreement with other findings indicating a reduced nocturnal decrease in BP in both normotensive and hypertensive acromegalic patients, with a prevalence of the nondipper profile (mean nocturnal BP $\leq 10\%$ of the average daytime BP).[32,64]

Sleep Apnea

Sleep apnea syndrome (SAS) is common in acromegaly, mainly caused by anatomic changes in the respiratory system.[29] In particular, alterations of the bone and soft tissues in the craniofacial region (mandibular prognathism caused by the growth effect of GH/IGF-1, macroglossia, pharyngeal and laryngeal swelling caused by sodium and water retention) reduce the airflow during sleep, causing repeated hypoxic and hypercapnic episodes.[65] Therefore, the prevalence of SAS in active acromegaly is 45% to 80% of patients, according to different studies.[66] As in the general population, SAS is independently associated with hypertension and cardiovascular disease,[67,68] and the role of SAS in the pathogenesis of hypertension in acromegaly should not be overlooked because of its contribution to the flattening of the nocturnal BP decrease.

DIAGNOSIS AND MANAGEMENT

A recent consensus on the diagnosis and treatment of acromegaly complications[31] recommended an early diagnosis and aggressive treatment of high BP levels, regardless of the specific treatment of acromegaly. Therefore, BP measurement is always recommended at diagnosis of acromegaly, but it must be reassessed during the long-term follow-up (every 6 months, or when acromegaly treatment is changed, if hypertensive).[31] It could be argued that the sole use of office measurements can lead to an overestimation of the frequency of hypertension,[24,25] but this risk could be minimized using a self-measurement pressure diary or AMBP.

The choice of the antihypertensive agents, mainly ACE inhibitors (ACEi), angiotensin II receptor blockers (ARBs), thiazide-type diuretics, and calcium channel blockers, does not significantly differ from the choice in nonacromegalic patients and there is no recommendation on a preferential class of drugs,[31] although recent research has suggested that amiloride is a potentially interesting option.[36,37] Moreover, a recent study including a small number of acromegalic patients has shown, with cardiac magnetic resonance, that cardiac indices were improved in hypertensive patients on ACEi or ARBs compared with other antihypertensive drugs.[69] Given that sleep apnea exacerbates hypertension,[68] its effective management is mandatory to improve BP control.

EFFECT OF ACROMEGALY CONTROL

The effect of attaining control of GH and IGF-1 excess on BP levels is heterogeneous across studies. In 2008, a study showed significantly lower systolic and diastolic BP levels in 76 acromegalic patients achieving disease control after 36 months, compared with the remaining 29 uncontrolled patients. Moreover, increased doses, and/or greater number of antihypertensive drugs, were needed in patients with uncontrolled disease.[70] In addition, the biochemical control of acromegaly also seems to have beneficial effects on BP levels in nonhypertensive patients, preventing the progression toward hypertension.[33] A recent study, including 121 acromegalic patients (of whom 79 achieved biochemical control during follow-up), confirmed that hypertension was more frequent in uncontrolled acromegaly.[20]

However, some recently published articles downplayed the role of acromegaly control on BP levels. A study including 552 acromegalic patients, stratified according to disease activity at the last visit, showed that the prevalence of hypertension was not modified by the successful treatment of acromegaly.[71] Previously, a study including 200 acromegalic patients did not show at multivariate analysis that the lack of biochemical control was a predictor of hypertension, although the univariate analysis showed a 6-fold higher risk of hypertension in uncontrolled patients compared with patients in remission after surgery.[30] Although the question is still open, the authors reviewed a selection of articles addressing this issue and classified them according to the treatment approach (**Table 2**).

Table 2
Effects of different treatments of acromegaly on hypertension

Treatment	Effect on HTN	References
Surgery	Amelioration of HTN with conflicting data on a more prominent effect on SBP vs DBP	73–78
Somatostatin analogues	Possible amelioration of HTN with long-term control of acromegaly	81–84
Pegvisomant	Amelioration of HTN with long-term control of acromegaly	90–95
Cabergoline	NA	—
Radiotherapy	NA	—

Abbreviations: DBP, diastolic BP; NA, not available; SBP, systolic BP.

Surgery

The surgical removal of a GH-secreting adenoma, in most cases using a transsphenoidal approach, still represents the mainstay of treatment and a potentially rapid curative option.[72] Several studies have investigated the impact of neurosurgery on BP levels and reported contrasting findings, probably caused by different sample sizes, type of measurements (clinical measurements vs ABPM), BP cutoffs used, and timing of assessment after surgery. Studies showed a significant decrease of both clinical systolic and diastolic BP at 3[73] and 6 months after surgery.[74] The first study used only office BP measurement, whereas ABPM was also performed in the second study, showing a significant postoperative decrease of the 24-hour diurnal and nocturnal systolic BP profile with no change in the diastolic profile. Moreover, a circadian rhythm of BP was restored in most of the patients with a blunted preoperative BP profile. Similarly, Minniti and colleagues,[75] using both clinical measurement and ABPM before and 6 months after surgery, showed a significant decrease of the clinical and 24-hour systolic BP in 15 well-controlled patients after surgery, in contrast with no change in 15 poorly controlled acromegalic subjects. In the first group, a normal BP circadian rhythm was restored in almost all patients, whereas no changes occurred in the second group. The reduction in systolic BP, but not diastolic BP, 6 months after surgery was confirmed by Reyes-Vidal and colleagues[76]; in addition, a decreased diastolic BP was found 1 year after surgery. Colao and colleagues,[77] comparing 56 acromegalic patients controlled with somatostatin analogue (SSA) and 33 cured with surgery, reported at 1 year a significant decrease of diastolic (but not systolic) BP in both groups. The long-term effect of remission on diastolic BP was confirmed by a study reporting that, after a mean period from surgery of 12.7 years, diastolic (but not systolic) BP was significantly lower in patients in remission than in patients with active acromegaly.[78]

Somatostatin Analogues

Although surgery is the treatment of choice, SSA (octreotide and lanreotide and the second-generation multireceptor-targeted pasireotide) is the first-line medical therapy, with a proven efficacy in more than 50% of patients, and he ability to significantly improve acromegalic comorbidities.[79,80] A retrospective study comparing 36 acromegalics treated with SSA and 33 sex-matched, age-matched, and body mass index–matched patients cured after surgery, did not find any significant difference in diastolic and systolic BP between the two groups.[81] Previously, a prospective study showed a significant reduction of systolic and diastolic BP in 36 acromegalic patients treated for 12 to 24 months with depot long-acting octreotide.[82] However, in 2007, a metanalysis showed that SSA therapy did not lead to a clear decrease in BP, suggesting a pressure-independent effect of SSA on heart.[83] In 2009, a study evaluated the efficacy of 5 years of depot SSA as first-line therapy in acromegaly and showed a reduction in BP and a reduction in the rate of hypertension.[84]

Pegvisomant

The second-line medical therapy consists of pegvisomant (PEG), an antagonist of the GH receptor able to normalize IGF-1 levels in 60% to 90% of patients[85–88] and recently indicated as potentially responsible for permanent remission in selected patients with SSA-resistant acromegaly.[89] However, data on its impact on BP levels are limited to small studies and are conflicting.

A prospective study including 16 patients with SSA-resistant acromegaly treated with PEG showed no change in systolic and diastolic BP overall; however, a significant decrease of diastolic BP was apparent in the 4 hypertensive patients evaluated separately.[90] Although 6 months of therapy with PEG in 17 acromegalic patients did not significantly change systolic and diastolic BP,[91] 18 months of therapy with PEG in 10 acromegalic patients significantly decreased systolic BP in the entire group, as well as in the group of hypertensive patients, but decreased diastolic BP only in the hypertensive patients.[92] A recent prospective study of the same group, including 50 acromegalic patients assessed at baseline, after long-term treatment with SSA and after 12 and 60 months of combined treatment with SSA and PEG, showed only a slight and nonsignificant improvement of systolic and diastolic BP after combined treatment compared with long-term SSA therapy.[93] In 2010, Berg and colleagues[94] assessed BP levels at baseline and after 12 months of PEG therapy in 62 acromegalic patients, of whom 42 had normalized IGF-1 levels (controlled patients) and 20 had reduced, but not normalized, IGF-1 levels (partially controlled patients). Systolic BP was significantly lower in the former than in the latter group, and decreased significantly during treatment only in controlled patients, but not in partially controlled patients. Diastolic BP was significantly lower in controlled than in partially controlled patients, but without significant changes in each group compared with baseline.[94] More recently, a retrospective study including 96 patients treated with different modalities (surgery, SSA, or PEG) reported a significant reduction, among the 11 patients who were hypertensive at diagnosis and whose antihypertensive treatment was not modified, in systolic BP after surgery but not after PEG treatment, regardless of IGF-1 changes.[95]

Cabergoline

Cabergoline is a dopamine agonist, used in acromegaly as an adjuvant treatment as monotherapy in patients with mild disease or in combination with SSA.[72] To date, no prospective randomized trial evaluating its efficacy in acromegaly is available and no study reporting its effect on hypertension in acromegalic patients has been performed.

Radiotherapy

Radiotherapy is currently considered a third-line option in acromegalic patients uncontrolled after surgery and medical therapy, or in cases of aggressive GH-secreting tumors.[72] To our knowledge, no data focusing on the effect of radiotherapy on hypertension in acromegalic patients have been reported.

SUMMARY

Hypertension is one of the most important and common complications in acromegaly. Its pathogenesis has not yet been fully elucidated, and likely includes multiple factors. A comprehensive, patient-centered approach, focusing not only on the biochemical control of acromegaly but also on an early diagnosis of hypertension and prompt antihypertensive treatment, is required for optimal patient care. However, there is an urgent need for prospective, large-scale studies focusing on hypertension, and its response to treatment of acromegaly, to solve the conundrum whether control of GH–IGF-1 excess ameliorates BP levels.

REFERENCES

1. Melmed S. Acromegaly. N Engl J Med 1990;322:966–77.
2. Colao A, Ferone D, Marzullo P, et al. Systemic complications of acromegaly: epidemiology, pathogenesis, and management. Endocr Rev 2004;25:102–52.
3. Mestron A, Webb SM, Astorga R, et al. Epidemiology, clinical characteristics, outcome, morbidity and mortality in acromegaly based on the Spanish Acromegaly Registry (Registro Espanol de Acromegalia, REA). Eur J Endocrinol 2004;151:439–46.
4. Holdaway IM, Rajasoorya RC, Gamble GD. Factors influencing mortality in acromegaly. J Clin Endocrinol Metab 2004;89:667–74.
5. Holdaway IM, Bolland MJ, Gamble GD. A meta-analysis of the effect of lowering serum levels of GH and IGF-1 on mortality in acromegaly. Eur J Endocrinol 2008; 159:89–95.
6. Arosio M, Reimondo G, Malchiodi E, et al. Predictors of morbidity and mortality in acromegaly: an Italian survey. Eur J Endocrinol 2012;167:189–98.
7. Ragonese M, Alibrandi A, Di Bella G, et al. Cardiovascular events in acromegaly: distinct role of Agatston and Framingham score in the 5-year prediction. Endocrine 2014;47:206–12.
8. López-Velasco R, Escobar-Morreale HF, Vega B, et al. Cardiac involvement in acromegaly: specific myocardiopathy or consequence of systemic hypertension? J Clin Endocrinol Metab 1997;82:1047–53.
9. Colao A, Baldelli R, Marzullo P, et al. Systemic hypertension and impaired glucose tolerance are independently correlated to the severity of the acromegalic cardiomyopathy. J Clin Endocrinol Metab 2000;85:193–9.
10. Mercado M, Gonzalez B, Vargas G, et al. Successful mortality reduction and control of comorbidities in patients with acromegaly followed at a highly specialized multidisciplinary clinic. J Clin Endocrinol Metab 2014;99:4438–46.
11. Ritvonen E, Löyttyniemi E, Jaatinen P, et al. Mortality in acromegaly: a 20-year follow-up study. Endocr Relat Cancer 2015;23:469–80.
12. Broder MS, Neary MP, Chang E, et al. Treatments, complications, and healthcare utilization associated with acromegaly: a study in two large United States databases. Pituitary 2014;17:333–41.
13. Bex M, Abs R, T'Sjoen G, et al. AcroBel the Belgian registry on acromegaly: a survey of the 'real-life' outcome in 418 acromegalic subjects. Eur J Endocrinol 2007; 157:399–409.
14. Anagnostis P, Efstathiadou ZA, Polyzos SA, et al. Acromegaly: presentation, morbidity and treatment outcomes at a single centre. Int J Clin Pract 2011;65: 896–902.
15. Mercieca C, Gruppetta M, Vassallo J. Epidemiology, treatment trends and outcomes of acromegaly. Eur J Intern Med 2012;23:e206–7.

16. Vallette S, Ezzat S, Chik C, et al. Emerging trends in the diagnosis and treatment of acromegaly in Canada. Clin Endocrinol (Oxf) 2013;79:79–85.
17. Hoskuldsdottir GT, Fjalldal SB, Sigurjonsdottir HA. The incidence and prevalence of acromegaly, a nationwide study from 1955 through 2013. Pituitary 2015;18: 803–7.
18. Dal J, Feldt-Rasmussen U, Andersen M, et al. Acromegaly incidence, prevalence, complications and long-term prognosis: a nationwide cohort study. Eur J Endocrinol 2016;175:181–90.
19. Portocarrero-Ortiz LA, Vergara-Lopez A, Vidrio-Velazquez M, et al. The Mexican acromegaly registry: clinical and biochemical characteristics at diagnosis and therapeutic outcomes. J Clin Endocrinol Metab 2016;101:3997–4004.
20. Carmichael JD, Broder MS, Cherepanov D, et al. Long-term treatment outcomes of acromegaly patients presenting biochemically-uncontrolled at a tertiary pituitary center. BMC Endocr Disord 2017;17:49.
21. Lesén E, Granfeldt D, Houchard A, et al. Comorbidities, treatment patterns and cost-of-illness of acromegaly in Sweden: a register-linkage population-based study. Eur J Endocrinol 2017;176:203–12.
22. Schofl C, Petroff D, Tonjes A, et al. Incidence of myocardial infarction and stroke in acromegaly patients: results from the German Acromegaly Registry. Pituitary 2017;20:635–42.
23. Maione L, Brue T, Beckers A, et al. Changes in the management and comorbidities of acromegaly over three decades: the French Acromegaly Registry. Eur J Endocrinol 2017;176:645–55.
24. Minniti G, Moroni C, Jaffrain-Rea ML, et al. Prevalence of hypertension in acromegalic patients: clinical measurement versus 24-hour ambulatory blood pressure monitoring. Clin Endocrinol (Oxf) 1998;48:149–52.
25. Costenaro F, Martin A, Horn RF, et al. Role of ambulatory blood pressure monitoring in patients with acromegaly. J Hypertens 2016;34:1357–63.
26. Ohtsuka H, Komiya I, Aizawa T, et al. Hypertension in acromegaly: hereditary hypertensive factor produces hypertension by enhancing IGF-I production. Endocr J 1995;42:781–7.
27. Vitale G, Pivonello R, Auriemma RS, et al. Hypertension in acromegaly and in the normal population: prevalence and determinants. Clin Endocrinol (Oxf) 2005;63: 470–6.
28. Schutte AE, Volpe M, Tocci G, et al. Revisiting the relationship between blood pressure and insulin-like growth factor-1. Hypertension 2014;63:1070–7.
29. Powlson AS, Gurnell M. Cardiovascular disease and sleep disordered breathing in acromegaly. Neuroendocrinology 2016;103:75–85.
30. Sardella C, Cappellani D, Urbani C, et al. Disease activity and lifestyle influence comorbidities and cardiovascular events in patients with acromegaly. Eur J Endocrinol 2016;175(5):443–53.
31. Melmed S, Casanueva FF, Klibanski A, et al. A consensus on the diagnosis and treatment of acromegaly complications. Pituitary 2013;16:294–302.
32. Terzolo M, Matrella C, Boccuzzi A, et al. Twenty-four hour profile of blood pressure in patients with acromegaly. Correlation with demographic, clinical and hormonal features. J Endocrinol Invest 1999;22:48–54.
33. Sardella C, Urbani C, Lombardi M, et al. The beneficial effect of acromegaly control on blood pressure values in normotensive patients. Clin Endocrinol 2014;81: 573–81.
34. Feld S, Hirschgerg R. Growth Hormone, the insulin-like growth factor system, and the kidney. J Clin Endocrinol Metab 1996;5:423–80.

35. Lin CJ, Mendonca BB, Lucon AM, et al. Growth hormone receptor messenger ribonucleic acid in normal and pathologic human adrenocortical tissues—An analysis by quantitative polymerase chain reaction technique. J Clin Endocrinol Metab 1997;82:2671–6.

36. Kamenicky P, Viengchareun S, Blanchard A, et al. Epithelial sodium channel is a key mediator of growth hormone induced sodium retention in acromegaly. Endocrinology 2008;149:3294–305.

37. Kamenicky P, Blanchard A, Frank M, et al. Body fluid expansion in acromegaly is related to enhanced epithelial sodium channel (ENaC) activity. J Clin Endocrinol Metab 2011;96:2127–35.

38. Bielohuby M, Roemmler J, Manolopoulou J, et al. Chronic growth hormone excess is associated with increased aldosterone: a study in patients with acromegaly and in growth hormone transgenic mice. Exp Biol Med (Maywood) 2009;234:1002–9.

39. Moller J, Jorgensen JO, Marqversen J, et al. Insulin-like growth factor I administration induces fluid and sodium retention in healthy adults: Possible involvement of renin and atrial natriuretic factor. Clin Endocrinol (Oxf) 2000;52:181–6.

40. Kraatz C, Benker G, Weber F, et al. Acromegaly and hypertension: Prevalence and relationship to the renin-angiotensin-aldosterone system. Klin Wochenschr 1990;68:583–7.

41. Zacharieva S, Andreeva M, Andonova K. Effect of sodium depletion on the renin-angiotensin-aldosterone system and renal prostaglandins in acromegalic patients. Exp Clin Endocrinol 1990;96:213–8.

42. Mulatero P, Veglio F, Maffei P, et al. CYP11B2-344T/C Gene Polymorphism and Blood Pressure in Patients with Acromegaly. J Clin Endocrinol Metab 2006;91:5008–12.

43. Erbas T, Cinar N, Dagdelen S, et al. Association between ACE and AGT polymorphism and cardiovascular risk in acromegalic patients. Pituitary 2017;20:569–77.

44. McKnight JA, McCance DR, Hadden DR, et al. Basal and saline-stimulated levels of plasma atrial natriuretic factor in acromegaly. Clin Endocrinol 1989;31:431–8.

45. Brands MW, Manhiani MM. Sodium-retaining effect of insulin in diabetes. Am J Physiol Regul Integr Comp Physiol 2012;303:R1101–9.

46. Slowinska-Srzednicka J, Zgliczynski S, Soszynski P, et al. High blood pressure and hyperinsulinaemia in acromegaly and in obesity. Clin Exp Hypertens 1989;A11:407–25.

47. Ikeda T, Terasawa H, Ishimura M, et al. Correlation between blood pressure and plasma insulin in acromegaly. J Intern Med 1993;234:61–3.

48. Ezzat S, Forster MJ, Berchtold P, et al. Acromegaly. Clinical and biochemical features in 500 patients. Medicine (Baltimore) 1994;73:233–40.

49. Jaffrain-Rea ML, Moroni C, Baldelli R, et al. Relationship between blood pressure and glucose tolerance in acromegaly. Clin Endocrinol (Oxf) 2001;54:189–95.

50. Bondanelli M, Ambrosio MR, degli Uberti EC. Pathogenesis and prevalence of hypertension in acromegaly. Pituitary 2001;4:239–49.

51. Grassi G, Mark A, Esler M. The sympathetic nervous system alterations in human hypertension. Circ Res 2015;116:976–90.

52. Bondanelli M, Ambrosio MR, Franceschetti P, et al. Diurnal rhythm of plasma catecholamines in acromegaly. J Clin Endocrinol Metab 1999;84:2458–67.

53. Sumbul HE, Koc AS. Hypertension is Common in Patients with Newly Diagnosed Acromegaly and is Independently Associated with Renal Resistive Index. High Blood Press Cardiovasc Prev 2019;26:69–75.

54. Kamide K, Hori MT, Zhu JH, et al. Insulin and insulin-like growth factor-I promotes angiotensinogen production and growth in vascular smooth muscle cells. J Hypertens 2000;18:1051–6.
55. Rizzoni D, Porteri E, Giustina A, et al. Acromegalic patients show the presence of hypertrophic remodeling of subcutaneous small resistance arteries. Hypertension 2004;43:561–5.
56. Paisley AN, Izzard AS, Gemmell I, et al. Small vessel remodeling and impaired endothelial-dependent dilatation in subcutaneous resistance arteries from patients with acromegaly. J Clin Endocrinol Metab 2009;94:1111–7.
57. Maison P, Démolis P, Young J, et al. Vascular reactivity in acromegalic patients: preliminary evidence for regional endothelial dysfunction and increased sympathetic vasoconstriction. Clin Endocrinol (Oxf) 2000;53:445–51.
58. Ronconi V, Giacchetti G, Mariniello B, et al. Reduced nitric oxide levels in acromegaly: cardiovascular implications. Blood Press 2005;14:227–32.
59. Baykan M, Erem C, Gedikli O, et al. Impairment in flow-mediated vasodilatation of the brachial artery in acromegaly. Med Princ Pract 2009;18:228–32.
60. Yaron M, Izkhakov E, Sack J, et al. Arterial properties in acromegaly: relation to disease activity and associated cardiovascular risk factors. Pituitary 2016;19: 322–31.
61. Anagnostis P, Efstathiadou ZA, Gougoura S, et al. Oxidative stress and reduced antioxidative status, along with endothelial dysfunction in acromegaly. Horm Metab Res 2013;45:314–8.
62. Chen Z, Yu Y, He M, et al. Higher growth hormone levels are associated with erectile dysfunction in male patients with acromegaly. Endocr Pract 2019;25(6): 562–71.
63. Cersosimo E, DeFronzo RA. Insulin resistance and endothelial dysfunction: the road map to cardiovascular diseases. Diabetes Metab Res Rev 2006;22:423–36.
64. Pietrobelli DJ, Akopian M, Olivieri AO, et al. Altered circadian blood pressure profile in patients with active acromegaly. Relationship with left ventricular mass and hormonal values. J Hum Hypertens 2001;15:601–5.
65. Attal P, Chanson P. Endocrine aspects of obstructive sleep apnea. J Clin Endocrinol Metab 2010;95:483–95.
66. Davì MV, Giustina A. Sleep apnea in acromegaly: a review on prevalence, pathogenetic aspects and treatment. Expert Rev Endocrinol Metab 2012;7:55–62.
67. Lavie P, Herer P, Hoffstein V. Obstructive sleep apnoea syndrome as a risk factor for hypertension: Population study. BMJ 2000;320:479–82.
68. Bradley TD, Floras JS. Obstructive sleep apnoea and its cardiovascular consequences. Lancet 2009;373:82–93.
69. Thomas JDJ, Dattani A, Zemrak F, et al. Renin-angiotensin system blockade improves cardiac indices in acromegaly patients. Exp Clin Endocrinol Diabetes 2017;125:365–7.
70. Colao A, Terzolo M, Bondanelli M, et al. GH and IGF-I excess control contributes to blood pressure control: results of an observational, retrospective, multicentre study in 105 hypertensive acromegalic patients on hypertensive treatment. Clin Endocrinol (Oxf) 2008;69:613–20.
71. González B, Vargas G, de Los Monteros ALE, et al. Persistence of diabetes and hypertension after multimodal treatment of acromegaly. J Clin Endocrinol Metab 2018;103:2369–75.
72. Katznelson L, Laws ER Jr, Melmed S, et al, Endocrine Society. Acromegaly: an endocrine society clinical practice guideline. J Clin Endocrinol Metab 2014;99: 3933–51.

73. Yonenaga M, Fujio S, Habu M, et al. Postoperative changes in metabolic parameters of patients with surgically controlled acromegaly: assessment of new stringent cure criteria. Neurol Med Chir (Tokyo) 2018;58:147–55.

74. Jaffrain-Rea ML, Minniti G, Moroni C, et al. Impact of successful transsphenoidal surgery on cardiovascular risk factors in acromegaly. Eur J Endocrinol 2003;148: 193–201.

75. Minniti G, Moroni C, Jaffrain-Rea ML, et al. Marked improvement in cardiovascular function after successful transsphenoidal surgery in acromegalic patients. Clin Endocrinol (Oxf) 2001;55:307–13.

76. Reyes-Vidal C, Fernandez JC, Bruce JN, et al. Prospective study of surgical treatment of acromegaly: effects on ghrelin, weight, adiposity, and markers of CV risk. J Clin Endocrinol Metab 2014;99:4124–32.

77. Colao A, Pivonello R, Galderisi M, et al. Impact of treating acromegaly first with surgery or somatostatin analogs on cardiomyopathy. J Clin Endocrinol Metab 2008;93:2639–46.

78. Serri O, Beauregard C, Hardy J. Long-term biochemical status and disease-related morbidity in 53 postoperative patients with acromegaly. J Clin Endocrinol Metab 2004;89:658–61.

79. Carmichael JD, Bonert VS, Nuño M, et al. Acromegaly clinical trial methodology impact on reported biochemical efficacy rates of somatostatin receptor ligand treatments: a meta-analysis. J Clin Endocrinol Metab 2014;99:1825–33.

80. Gadelha MR, Bronstein MD, Brue T, et al. Pasireotide versus continued treatment with octreotide or lanreotide in patients with inadequately controlled acromegaly (PAOLA): a randomised, phase 3 trial. Lancet Diabetes Endocrinol 2014;2: 875–84.

81. Ronchi CL, Varca V, Beck-Peccoz P, et al. Comparison between six-year therapy with long-acting somatostatin analogs and successful surgery in acromegaly: effects on cardiovascular risk factors. J Clin Endocrinol Metab 2006;91:121–8.

82. Colao A, Ferone D, Marzullo P, et al. Long-term effects of depot long-acting somatostatin analog octreotide on hormone levels and tumor mass in acromegaly. J Clin Endocrinol Metab 2001;86:2779–86.

83. Maison P, Tropeano AI, Macquin-Mavier I, et al. Impact of somatostatin analogs on the heart in acromegaly: a metaanalysis. J Clin Endocrinol Metab 2007;92: 1743–7.

84. Colao A, Auriemma RS, Galdiero M, et al. Effects of initial therapy for five years with somatostatin analogs for acromegaly on growth hormone and insulin-like growth factor-I levels, tumor shrinkage, and cardiovascular disease: a prospective study. J Clin Endocrinol Metab 2009;94:3746–56.

85. Trainer P, Drake W, Katznelson L, et al. Treatment of acromegaly with the growth hormone-receptor antagonist pegvisomant. N Engl J Med 2000;342:1171–7.

86. van der Lely AJ, Hutson RK, Trainer PJ, et al. Long-term treatment of acromegaly with pegvisomant, a growth hormone receptor antagonist. Lancet 2001;358: 1754–9.

87. Grottoli S, Maffei P, Bogazzi F, et al. ACROSTUDY: the Italian experience. Endocrine 2015;48:334–41.

88. Ragonese M, Grottoli S, Maffei P, et al. How to improve effectiveness of pegvisomant treatment in acromegalic patients. J Endocrinol Invest 2017;41:575–81.

89. Puglisi S, Spagnolo F, Ragonese M, et al. First report on persistent remission of acromegaly after withdrawal of long-term pegvisomant monotherapy. Growth Horm IGF Res 2019;45:17–9.

90. Colao A, Pivonello R, Auriemma RS, et al. Efficacy of 12-month treatment with the GH receptor antagonist pegvisomant in patients with acromegaly resistant to long-term, high-dose somatostatin analog treatment: effect on IGF-I levels, tumor mass, hypertension and glucose tolerance. Eur J Endocrinol 2006;154:467–77.

91. Pivonello R, Galderisi M, Auriemma RS, et al. Treatment with growth hormone receptor antagonist in acromegaly: effect on cardiac structure and performance. J Clin Endocrinol Metab 2007;92:476–82.

92. De Martino MC, Auriemma RS, Brevetti G, et al. The treatment with growth hormone receptor antagonist in acromegaly: effect on vascular structure and function in patients resistant to somatostatin analogues. J Endocrinol Invest 2010; 33:663–70.

93. Auriemma RS, Grasso LF, Galdiero M, et al. Effects of long-term combined treatment with somatostatin analogues and pegvisomant on cardiac structure and performance in acromegaly. Endocrine 2017;55:872–84.

94. Berg C, Petersenn S, Lahner H, et al. Cardiovascular risk factors in patients with uncontrolled and long-term acromegaly: comparison with matched data from the general population and the effect of disease control. J Clin Endocrinol Metab 2010;95:3648–56.

95. Briet C, Ilie MD, Kuhn E, et al. Changes in metabolic parameters and cardiovascular risk factors after therapeutic control of acromegaly vary with the treatment modality. Data from the Bicêtre cohort, and review of the literature. Endocrine 2019;63:348–60.

Monogenic Forms of Hypertension

Filippo Ceccato, MD, PhD*, Franco Mantero, MD

KEYWORDS

- Low-renin hypertension • Hypokalemia • Steroidogenesis
- Congenital adrenal hyperplasia • Liddle syndrome • Gordon syndrome
- Apparent excess of mineralocorticoids

KEY POINTS

- Endocrine secondary hypertension is rare; however, it must be considered in patients with young onset–age, with resistant hypertension, electrolyte imbalance, or ambiguous genitalia.
- Monogenic forms of hypertension are characterized by suppressed renin-aldosterone axis (except familial hyperaldosteronism type I-III) and hypokalemia (except Gordon syndrome).
- Monogenic forms of hypertension may present with severe or mild phenotype, secondary to the degree of enzymatic defect or channel mutation.
- Treatment with glucocorticoids, mineralocorticoid receptor antagonists, or thiazides should be considered after an appropriate diagnostic work-up.

INTRODUCTION

The close relationship between blood pressure (BP) and cardiovascular events is continuous, thus complicating the distinction between normal BP levels and hypertension. Therefore, despite its definition (>140/90 mm Hg is widely accepted), hypertension is a highly prevalent disease in the general population (up to 30%–40% in large epidemiologic studies).[1] The most common is essential hypertension[2]; however, recent acquisition regarding complex genetic alterations in essential hypertension suggests that mechanistically driven personalized treatment is feasible, and this could be the challenge of the next century.[3]

Disclosure of Potential Conflicts of Interest: All authors declare that they have no conflicts of interest that might be perceived as influencing the impartiality of the reported research.
Funding: This study did not receive any specific grant from any funding agency in the public, commercial or not-for-profit sector.
Research involving human participants and patient consent: Informed consent to describe patients' history has been obtained.
Endocrinology Unit, Department of Medicine DIMED, University-Hospital of Padova, Via Ospedale Civile, 105, Padova 35128, Italy
* Corresponding author.
E-mail address: filippo.ceccato@unipd.it

On the contrary, at least 15% to 20% of patients are affected by secondary hypertension (considering endocrine and renovascular forms), characterized by a specific and potentially reversible cause of increased BP levels. All patients with young onset–age (not evidence-based, albeit <40–45 years is widely accepted), with resistant hypertension (defined as the use of three antihypertensive drugs, with at least one diuretic), or electrolyte imbalance should be screened for secondary forms. Pseudoresistance (inadequate cuff size or patient rest before BP measurement) and poor compliance to medical treatment should be investigated before the screening of secondary hypertension.[2,4]

The adrenals produce several hormones from the cortex (mainly cortisol and aldosterone) and from the medulla (catecholamines) that control plasma volume and vascular resistance, therefore an endocrine excess of these hormones is encountered in some of the most common endocrine forms of hypertension, such as primary aldosteronism, Cushing syndrome, and pheochromocytoma.[5,6] Besides these classic forms of adrenal hormones excess (encountering the larger part of secondary endocrine hypertension), some rare mutations characterizing monogenic forms of low-renin hypertension are now identified, and are summarized in this review. Albeit rare, these forms of hypertension are relevant, because they represent models for the physiology or the pathophysiology of the renal control of sodium levels and plasma volume, some of the major players in BP levels. Some rare forms of familial primary aldosteronism (eg, glucocorticoid remediable aldosteronism or familial aldosteronism type 2 and 3) are also monogenic forms of hypertension (discussed elsewhere in this issue).

CONGENITAL ADRENAL HYPERPLASIA CAUSED BY 11β-HYDROXYLASE DEFICIENCY

Steroidogenesis is the complex process by which cholesterol is converted to biologically active steroid hormones, especially in adrenal, gonads, and placenta. Steroidogenic enzymes fall into two groups: cytochrome P-450 enzymes (type 1 in mitochondria or type 2 in endoplasmic reticulum) and hydroxysteroid dehydrogenases (HSD; aldo-keto reductase or short-chain dehydrogenase/reductase families).[7] In humans, the most potent steroids are 11 β-hydroxylated compounds, derived from 11β-hydroxylase (whose expression is directly controlled by corticotropin), and present glucocorticoid (particularly cortisol) or mineralocorticoid activity (especially aldosterone).[8] As depicted in **Fig. 1**, the first two steps of aldosterone and cortisol biosynthesis (from cholesterol to progesterone) are identical and are mediated by the same enzymes in zona fasciculate and glomerulosa.

Congenital adrenal hyperplasia (CAH) is an autosomal-recessive disorder caused by defects in one of the various steroidogenesis enzymes. Patients with CAH have a wide spectrum of clinical presentation depending on the underlying enzymatic deficiency; the most common are 21-hydroxylase deficiency (21-OHD; up to 90% of all CAH), 11β-hydroxylase deficiency (11β-OHD, accounting for 1%–8%), 3β-HSD, and 17α-hydroxylase.[9] The condition was first described in 1865 by De Crecchio on autopsy of a male who died of an adrenal crisis.[10] However, only in 1965 was it proposed that a deficiency of 11β-hydroxylase enzyme could explain CAH and hypertension.[11]

As in 21-OHD, also 11β-OHD may present with a classic (complete, severe) or nonclassic (mild) phenotype, depending on the percentage of enzyme activity.[10,12] In classic 11β-OHD, common signs and symptoms are features of androgen excess, such as virilization of external genitalia in females and precocious puberty in males. Hypertension is present in two-third of the cases with 11β-OHD caused by excess steroid production with mineralocorticoid activity (salt-wasting syndrome and adrenal insufficiency are not key features of 11β-OHD).[10]

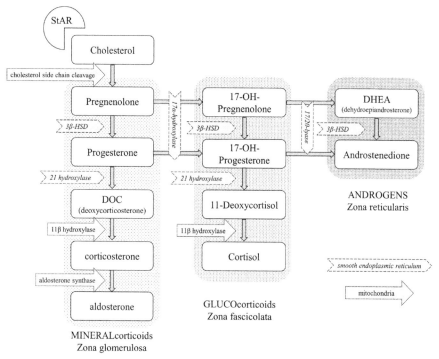

Fig. 1. Adrenal steroidogenesis.

Cortisol is synthesized in zona fasciculata: CYP11B1 (11β-hydroxylase) is responsible for the conversion of 11-deoxycortisol to cortisol, which is the final step in cortisol synthesis, and 11-deoxycorticosterone (DOC) to corticosterone (then only in zona glomerulosa corticosterone is converted to aldosterone with CYP11B2, termed aldosterone synthase). Mutations in the CYP11B1 gene result in a defective 11β-hydroxylase enzyme, with a decreased conversion of 11-deoxycortisol to cortisol. The low cortisol level activates the negative feedback mechanism of pituitary-adrenal axis leading to increased corticotropin production, with consequential adrenal cortex hyperplasia and overproduction of steroid precursors before the block. Therefore, steroidogenesis is shunted toward the androgen pathway (causing virilization in females) and elevated mineralocorticoid precursors (as summarized in **Fig. 2A**), leading to the development of hyporeninemic hypertension.[13]

Features of hyperandrogenism in women may be detected at any age from infancy to early adulthood: female karyotypes present with varying degrees of virilization of external genitalia (caused by androgen secretion during embryonic and fetal development; therefore, surgical reconstruction is required in most virilized girls), with intact functional gonads, Mullerian-derived structures that are independent from androgens.[14] Left untreated, males can develop precocious pubertal development, gynecomastia, Leydig cell hyperplasia, and testicular adrenal rest tumors.[15] Moreover, accelerated somatic growth with premature epiphyseal closure and resultant short adult stature is observed.[10]

Mild to moderate hypertension (which is one of the main clinical differences with CAH caused by 21-OHD) is observed in up to 60% of 11β-OHD cases at the time of diagnosis. The mechanism proposed is not only related to elevated mineralocorticoid

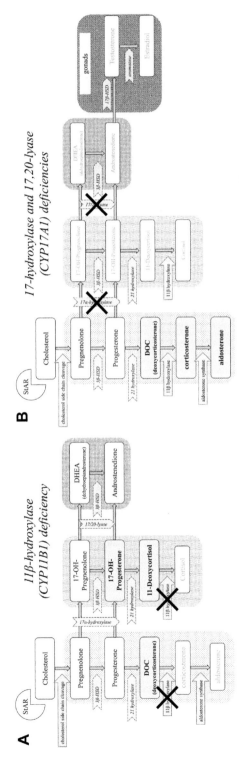

Fig. 2. Aberrant steroidogenesis in 11β-hydroxylase deficiency (*A*) and 17-hydroxylase and 17,20-lyase deficiency (*B*).

precursors (mainly DOC), because they present only weak mineralocorticoid activity and there is no relationship between DOC and BP levels. Moreover, poorly controlled hypertension and glucocorticoid overtreatment can adversely affect the cardiometabolic profile. Therefore, it has been proposed that 18-hydroxylated compounds are the main cause of hypertension in 11β-OHD.[16] On the contrary, hypokalemia is the result of excess mineralocorticoid activity, and is not correlated to hypertension.[17]

The diagnosis of 11β-OHD is based on increased glucocorticoid and mineralocorticoid precursors (11-deoxycortisol and DOC) (**Fig. 3**A) and androgens, and on suppression of aldosterone-renin axis. In mild cases (late-onset, or nonclassic form), measurements of basal and corticotropin-stimulated 11-deoxycortisol and DOC may be helpful. Besides hormonal assessment, genetic profile and functional characterization of mutations is of particular interest to confirm diagnosis.[18] In humans, there are two 11β-hydroxylase isoenzymes in chromosome 8, sharing 95% of homology in coding regions: CYP11B1 gene encoding 11β-hydroxylase is close to the CYP11B2 gene, which codes for aldosterone synthase.[19]

As in CAH, the goals of therapy are to replace deficient cortisol secretion and to reduce excessive androgens and mineralocorticoid secretion. Treatment is short-acting glucocorticoids as hydrocortisone in children (10–20 mg/m²/d) in two to three doses (as in 21-OHD), and long-acting glucocorticoids as prednisolone or dexamethasone (2.5–7.5 mg/d and 0.25–0.5 mg/d, respectively) in adults. Once adequate

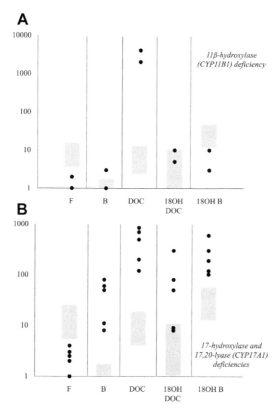

Fig. 3. Levels of cortisol (F, in μg/dL), corticosterone (B, in μg/dL), desossicorticosterone (DOC, in ng/dL), 18-OH DOC (in ng/dL), and 18-OH B (in ng/dL) in 11β-hydroxylase deficiency (*A*) and 17-hydroxylase and 17,20-lyase deficiency (*B*).

glucocorticoid treatment is initiated, DOC and renin levels should normalize, whereas the control of hypertension may require additional antihypertensive drugs.[8,10] An immediate three- to five-fold increased dosage in illness or acute stress is mandatory, to prevent adrenal crisis.[20]

CONGENITAL ADRENAL HYPERPLASIA CAUSED BY 17-HYDROXYLASE AND 17,20-LYASE (CYP17A1) DEFICIENCIES

All vertebrates with different genders require, in adrenal and gonads, the activity of 17,20-lyase (CYP17A1) to synthesize 19-carbon androgens and subsequently 18-carbon estrogen. Based on its location in the steroidogenic pathways, CYP17A1 is fundamental for sex steroid production in gonads (summarized in **Fig. 2**B). Human steroidogenesis is different from mice, in whom corticosterone is the dominant glucocorticoid. Thus, in human adrenal 17-hydroxylase activity is essential to produce cortisol, and complete deficiency of CYP17A1 leads to CAH, with hormone deficiency (mainly cortisol, androgens, and estrogens) and hormone excess (DOC and corticosterone, Kendall's Compound B).[21] Nevertheless, adrenal 17-OHD does not really result in glucocorticoid deficiency because extremely high corticosterone levels adequately supply cortisol deficiency, therefore adrenal crisis are rare, and the critical issue is the low-renin hypertension from DOC excess.

The human CYP17A1 gene is located on chromosome 10, and the enzyme system CYP17A1 and P-450-oxidoreductase (the redox partner) catalyzes the 17-hydroxylase and 17,20-lyase activities.[22] More than 100 mutations in the CYP17A1 gene have been described, with combined degree of 17-hydroxylase/17,20-lyase deficiency,[23,24] up to isolated 17,20-lyase deficiency.[25] Because production of androgens and estrogens requires the 17,20-lyase activity of CYP17A1 and the availability of 17-hydroxysteroid substrates for this reaction, which are exclusive products of CYP17A1, the clinical features are closely related to the enzyme impairment.

The two common clinical presentations of 17-OHD are children with 46,XY karyotype and female or ambiguous genitalia (with inguinal or abdominal testes, characterized by high levels of gonadotropins and low testosterone, thus excluding androgen insensitivity), or the adolescent girl (46,XX karyotype) with primary amenorrhea and absent secondary sexual characteristics (because of absent estrogen production) with hypertension and hypokalemia.[26,27] Individuals with both 46,XX and 46,XY karyotypes have female external genitalia from absent testosterone (and dihydrotestosterone) synthesis in fetal life. Moreover, male 46,XY individuals do not have internal Müllerian structure, because of preservation of anti-Müllerian hormone (which does not depend on steroidogenesis) from the testes. From infancy to adulthood, DOC accumulates, but manifestations of mineralocorticoid excess (hypertension with hypokalemia) tend not to occur in infancy, because the newborn kidney is rather insensitive to mineralocorticoids. Gradually and typically in adolescence, DOC excess causes overt and severe hypertension, with hypokalemia, that respond well to mineralocorticoid receptor (MR) antagonist (MRA) treatment.[27] Intriguingly, aldosterone levels in 17-OHD are low, despite normal enzymes of the mineralocorticoid pathway (see **Fig. 1**) and high amounts of precursors (see **Figs. 2**B and **3**A). It is likely that suppressed renin (caused by increased DOC) leads to low aldosterone levels; low-dose dexamethasone treatment is able to reduce DOC and increase renin and aldosterone.[28]

Glucocorticoid substitutive treatment in patients with 17-OHD is not always necessary; however, a low-dose regiment treatment may be useful to reduce DOC production. Moreover, these patients present an increased sensitivity to glucocorticoids, therefore the risk of overtreatment must be carefully balanced before developing cushingoid features.[28] Amiloride is effective in controlling hypokalemia; however, it is not as potent as spironolactone in controlling BP. In phenotypically female patients, treatment of primary amenorrhea is estrogen replacement during adolescence, combined with progestin only for those with 46,XX karyotype and an intact uterus.[21]

APPARENT MINERALOCORTICOID EXCESS

Apparent mineralocorticoid excess (AME) is a rare autosomal-recessive condition. However, it represents a clear model of bench-to-bedside research, because it demonstrates the physiologic mechanisms underlying selective activation of epithelial MR by aldosterone in mineralocorticoid tissue, protecting them from circulating cortisol. Cortisol is the biologically active glucocorticoid, and is regulated mainly by 11β-HSD isoenzymes and the glucocorticoid receptor (GR). The tissue-specific expression of 11β-HSDs and GR/MR play an important role in regulation of the differential mineralocorticoid and glucocorticoid effects.[29,30] Diagnosis of AME relies on a triad of hypertension, hypokalemia, suppressed aldosterone and renin levels, plus an abnormal urinary cortisol to cortisone ratio, either free steroids or their metabolites.[29]

AME was described for the first time in 1979 in hypertensive patients with hypokalemia, low renin and aldosterone levels, and marked response to MRA (spironolactone), suggesting a decreased rate of cortisol conversion to cortisone.[31] Four years later, it has been reported in the same patients that hydrocortisone treatment was able to increase BP and reduce potassium levels,[32] simulating mineralocorticoid activity. The first cloning of 11β-dehydrogenase by Rusvai was performed in 1993,[33] and the demonstration that 11β-dehydrogenase type 2 (11β-HSD2, which gene is located on chromosome 16) finally confirm its role to protect aldosterone-sensitive tissue from cortisol.[34,35] The kidneys receive 20% to 25% of the cardiac output, and plasma free cortisol levels are 100-fold higher than those of aldosterone, providing a large amount of cortisol in the main mineralocorticoid organ. Moreover, in terms of physiology, aldosterone is not the best ligand for MR, because cortisol is the ligand of MR.[29] 11β-HSD1 is a bidirectional enzyme, with (11-oxo) reductase and dehydrogenase activity dependent on the available cofactor (NADP/H+). The predominant reaction is the former, within the endoplasmic reticulum in liver, lung, gonads, pituitary, brain, adipose, bone, muscle, and stromal tissues, where activation of cortisol from cortisone facilitates cortisol action via the GR. On the contrary, 11β-HSD2 is a dehydrogenase that inactivates cortisol to cortisone, it is expressed predominantly in mineralocorticoid responsive tissues, such as distal nephron, colon, and salivary glands (**Fig. 4**).[36]

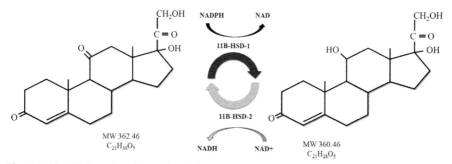

Fig. 4. 11β-HSD type 1 and type 2 activity.

It is now clear that in aldosterone target tissues 11β-HSD2 is coexpressed at high levels with MR: in humans it inactivates cortisol to cortisone, thus allowing aldosterone to activate selectively MR and therefore transepithelial sodium transport.[29] Nevertheless, 11β-HSD2 activity is not only to reduce cortisol levels close to MR, but also to generate NADH: around 90% of the "protected" renal MR are normally occupied by cortisol but not activated, so it is reasonable (albeit not yet demonstrated) that such cortisol-MR complexes are held inactive by the cogenerated NADH.[37] When 11β-HSD2 is deficient or compromised NADH levels fall, allowing cortisol-MR complexes to mimic aldosterone-MR and activate transcription of aldosterone-related genes, thus leading to the syndrome of AME (mainly hypertension and hypokalemia).[29,37]

AME is severe or mild (type 1 and type 2, respectively) (**Fig. 5**; Franco Mantero, MD, personal communication, 1994), depending on absent or residual 11β-HSD2 activity.[38] Severe AME, without enzymatic activity, presents early in life, with the diagnostic triad of hypertension, suppressed renin and aldosterone concentration, and hypokalemia; persistent metabolic alkalosis; and an elevated urinary cortisol to cortisone ratio. Untreated (or inadequately treated) subjects may be afflicted by a wide variety of morbidity (cardiac, renal, retinal, and central nervous system) reflecting their very high BP, expanded vascular volume, and hypokalemia.[29,39]

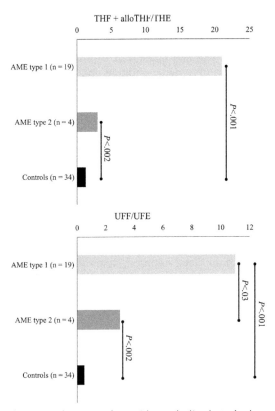

Fig. 5. Comparison between the rates of steroid metabolite (tetrahydrocortisol, tetrahydrocortisone) and urinary free cortisol to urinary free cortisone ratio in AME type 1 and type 2. THE, tetrahydrocortisone; THF, tetrahydrocortisol; UFE, urinary free cortisone; UFF, urinary free cortisol.

Similar to AME, some common conditions are able to induce an AME, such as excessive licorice consumption. The active principles in licorice (glycyrrhetinic acid, glycyrrhizic acid) are potent competitive inhibitors of 11β-HSD2, thus reducing its activity and leading to an acquired AME. Overconsumption of grapefruit has also been reported to affect 11β-HSD2 activity, as have endogenous glycyrrhetinic acid–like factors related to bile acids.[29] Extremely high cortisol levels, as those observed in Cushing syndrome, are able to saturate 11β-HSD2 activity, leading to the mineralocorticoid effect of cortisol also in case of normal enzymatic activity.[40]

The treatment of AME is based on MRA (spironolactone or eplerenone), combined with a low sodium/high potassium diet, plus potassium supplementation if required, in the most severe forms.

LIDDLE SYNDROME

In the early 1960s, Liddle reported on a family in which a young teenager and her adolescent brother presented with severe hypertension, hypokalemia, increased urinary potassium excretion, and metabolic alkalosis. Their mother and grandmother died prematurely, and were both hypertensive. Intriguingly, renin-aldosterone axis was suppressed, and MRA treatment was ineffective; however, triamterene (a pteridine derivative that blocks sodium flow into the cell) and sodium restriction corrected hypertension and hypokalaemia.[41] Thirty years later, an autosomal-dominant inheritance pattern had been described, and the three subunits of the epithelial sodium channel (ENaC; a heteromeric protein) were cloned and characterized,[42] identifying activating mutations of β, γ, and α subunits of ENaC.[43] This gain-of-function of ENaC led to Liddle syndrome (LS), a rare autosomal-dominant form of hypertension: 30 different LS-causing heterozygous mutations have been reported to date, occurring either in familial or in sporadic cases: no more than about 100 familiar or sporadic cases have been reported.[43,44] However, large genetic screening for LS has not been conducted, and it may be largely underdiagnosed, because in some populations its prevalence is close to 1% to 2%.[44,45]

In LS, ENaC is constitutively active, because it is neither ligand- nor voltage-gated, and is highly selective for sodium and lithium ions, which are smaller than potassium (selectivity ratio between 100 and 1000, the selectivity filter is formed by nine amino acids, three for each subunit), and is blocked by amiloride and triamterene, which share a common binding site proximal to transmembrane domain 2, and competitively interact with sodium.[46]

In the kidney, ENaC is expressed in the luminal membrane of the principal cells of the distal nephron, mediating the rate-limiting step in sodium absorption: ENaC is the final sodium transporter along the nephron, and it may reabsorb up to 100% of the sodium entering the distal nephron (**Fig. 6**). Aldosterone (through MR) is the main regulator of ENaC, by inducing its genetic transcription and the redistribution of channel subunits from intracellular sites to the apical membrane, in the collecting duct, whereas ENaC activity in the most proximal parts (distal convolute tubule and connecting tubule) is partly aldosterone independent.[43]

In LS, increased ENaC activity in the apical surface of distal nephron leads to a greater sodium reabsorption, increased plasmatic volume (thus leading to low aldosterone and renin levels), high BP, increased potassium extraction (explaining hypokalemia), and metabolic alkalosis. In addition, the increased sodium reabsorption through ENaC generates a transepithelial lumen-negative voltage that drives potassium secretion across ROMK channels in the apical membrane of the principal cells and facilitates the proton secretion by the proton pump in the intercalated cells of

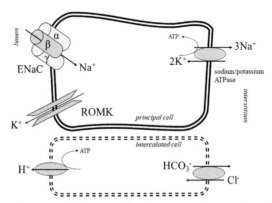

Fig. 6. In Liddle syndrome, ENaC allows sodium transport from the lumen into the cell. Reabsorbed sodium is shunted from the principal cell into the interstitium through sodium/potassium ATPase pump. Sodium flow (thorough ENaC and the ATPase pump) generates a negative transepithelial voltage, which leads to potassium diffusion through potassium channels (ROMK) from the cell to the lumen and facilitates the active H+ secretion into the lumen.

Aldosterone-Sensitive Distal Nephron, resulting in the hypokalemic metabolic alkalosis. Moreover, sodium retention and vascular dysfunction (through increased peripheral resistance) are required for the development of salt-sensitive hypertension, and recent functional studies reported that abnormalities in vascular function, resulting from increased expression of ENaC in the brain and in the vessels, are involved in the initiation and stabilization of hypertension in LS.[47] Finally, ENaC is expressed in the taste bud cells of the anterior tongue, thus explaining novel features of sodium attraction and increased dietary sodium intake in LS,[48] which is not merely a tubulopathy.

LS is associated with an increased risk of cardiovascular events (premature stroke, myocardial infarction, sudden death), related not only to misdiagnosed and undertreated hypertension, but also to endothelial dysfunction. Therefore, LS should be considered in all patients with early onset hypertension, regardless of potassium concentration, even in the absence of a familial history, because de novo mutations may occur.[43,45]

The diagnosis of LS is based on clinical suspicion, considering the signs and symptoms described; however, a good response to 4-week treatment of either triamterene (100 mg/d) or amiloride (10 mg/d) to correct hypokalemia and hypertension is a cornerstone. Direct sequencing of the involved genes and the finding of a known mutation is the most accurate tool to identify LS, because the discovery of a novel ENaC mutation does not necessarily imply its causal role and needs to be confirmed with the injection of the mutant and the wild ENaC cRNA in oocytes, followed by the electrophysiologic measurement of the amiloride-sensitive sodium current (available only in a few research laboratories).

Mild forms of familial AME may be indistinguishable from LS. However, the inheritance pattern (autosomal recessive) and the response to MRA treatment are characteristic of AME.

GORDON SYNDROME

Gordon syndrome (GS) is a rare familial monogenic form of hypertension with autosomal-dominant trait (although recently has been described with recessive inheritance); it is characterized mainly by the hallmark severe hyperkalemia (reaching 8–9 mmol/L), which distinguishes GS from all other rare syndromic monogenic forms of low-renin hypertension. Patients with GS respond to aggressive diet salt-restriction or small doses of thiazide diuretics, which suggests activation of the thiazide-sensitive Na/Cl cotransporter (NCC) in the distal nephron.[49] Gordon and Hodsman[50] in 1964 reported a case of hypertension and severe hyperkalemia, with an inheritable characteristic phenotype, metabolic acidosis, symptoms of periodic paralysis (because of increased potassium levels), and with preserved renal function.

There is a clear phenotype-genotype correlation, and some families or sporadic cases presented with milder symptoms. In the past, GS and Gitelman syndrome (a form of hypotension with electrolyte disorder) were considered as mirror images of each other, with NCC involvement. However, the coding sequence of NCC is not mutated in patients with GS, and GS is related to the independent action of two serine-threonine kinases (With No Lysine Kinase 1 and 4 [WNK1 and WNK4]), suppressing sodium flux by a marked inhibition of NCC expression at the cell membrane, through early lysosomal degradation.[51,52] Furthermore, the WNK1 and WNK4 do not phosphorylate NCC directly, because they act to STE20 serine/threonine kinases that are involved in the increased transporter (NCC) activity in association with insertion of the transporter into the apical surface membrane (**Fig. 7**).[49,53] In some patients WNK4 gene variants are related to osteoporosis, without evidence of hypertension.[54]

Also hyperkalemia in GS arises from different mechanisms. The effect of NCC activation is to extract more sodium from the DCT, leading to reduced electrogenic recovery of sodium in the collecting ducts and thereby a reduction in the lumen (negative) potential required for potassium secretion through the secretory K-channel in the collecting ducts (ROMK).[49] Recent papers reported WNK1 and WNK4 activity to reduce cell-surface expression of ROMK, accelerating the endocytosis of ROMK through a

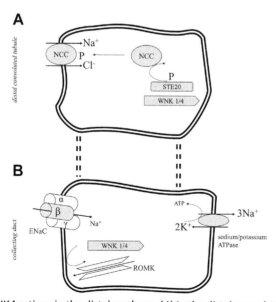

Fig. 7. WNK1/WNK4 actions in the distal nephron. (*A*) In the distal convoluted tubule WNK1/4 phosphorylates the STE20/SPS1-related proline/alanine-rich kinase (SPAK) and activates the thiazide-sensitive NCC. (*B*) In the collecting duct WNK1/4 accelerates internalization of the secretory ROMK channel.

clathrin-coated pit pathway.[55,56] Further genes have emerged through whole-genome sequencing, regulating the ubiquitination and proteasomal degradation of WNK kinases; these proteins are Cullin-3 (CUL3, coding for a scaffold protein in an ubiquitin–E3 ligase) and Kelch3 (KLHL3, coding for an adaptor protein respectively).[49,57] Mutations in CUL3 invariably cause onset of the GS phenotype in very early childhood and the most profound electrolyte disturbances, with severe hyperkalemia, and it was discovered in the Gordon index case.[57]

Considering aldosterone-renin axis, patients with GS usually have suppressed renin (because of their constitutive salt-loaded state) and low aldosterone levels. Both conditions are reversed by dietary salt-restriction (20 mmol/d) and thiazide treatment.[49,50,58]

As in LS, also in GS the hypertension is not entirely explained by salt-retention through NCC activation, but also a vascular endothelial function must be considered, because vasoconstriction by an increased vascular smooth muscle is described in GS with CUL3 deletion.[59]

ACTIVATING MINERALOCORTICOID RECEPTOR MUTATION IN HYPERTENSION EXACERBATED BY PREGNANCY (GELLER SYNDROME)

In 2000, Geller described a rare form of hypertension caused by constitutive MR activity, exacerbated during pregnancy, where high levels of progesterone are characterized by mineralocorticoid effect. He described an adolescent boy (and then several relatives, of whom three died of heart failure <50 years) with severe hypertension, suppressed renin-aldosterone axis, hypokalemia with urinary potassium excretion, and no other underlying cause of hypertension. They discovered a missense mutation, resulting in substitution of leucine for serine, altering the hormone-binding domain of the MR. MR-aldosterone complex activity was similar among wild-type and mutated; however, mutated MR was active also without the natural ligand. Moreover, 21-carbon steroids (eg, progesterone, normally an MR antagonists) were potent activators of mutated MR, and likewise also spironolactone act as an agonist in mutated MR. Two females of this family presented severe hypertension during pregnancy, and were carriers of the mutated MR.[60]

Recently, it has been shown that cortisone, the principal metabolite of cortisol produced in the distal nephron by 11β-HSD2, binds to and activates mutated MR,[61] suggesting that cortisone could be the agonist responsible for hypertension in male and nonpregnant patients with GS.

SUMMARY

All these low-renin monogenic forms of hypertension are rare (or extremely rare) diseases, or at least are considered rare, because evidence-based large population studies have never been conducted. Their relevance lies in representing models that, starting from a phenotype that is easy to identify, such as arterial hypertension with low renin (and often hypokalemia), have led to the discovery of genes involved in the regulation of sodium metabolism and plasma volume, and therefore of BP.

Although their role in essential arterial hypertension has not been clearly defined, it must be recognized that these models of monogenic hypertension, if nothing else, have a high scientific interest. Furthermore, as often happens when studying a model, it is expected to identify forms with a phenotype less "extreme," caused by mild genetic variants or polymorphisms, probably closer to the phenotype of essential hypertension and susceptible to personalized and targeted drug treatment.[3,62]

REFERENCES

1. Mancia G, Fagard R, Narkiewicz K, et al. 2013 ESH/ESC guidelines for the management of arterial hypertension: the Task Force for the management of arterial hypertension of the European Society of Hypertension (ESH) and of the European Society of Cardiology (ESC). Eur Heart J 2013;34(28):2159–219.
2. Rimoldi SF, Scherrer U, Messerli FH. Secondary arterial hypertension: when, who, and how to screen? Eur Heart J 2014;35(19):1245–54.
3. Manosroi W, Williams GH. Genetics of human primary hypertension: focus on hormonal mechanisms. Endocr Rev 2019;40(3):825–56.
4. Calhoun DA, Jones D, Textor S, et al. Resistant hypertension: diagnosis, evaluation, and treatment: a scientific statement from the American Heart Association Professional Education Committee of the Council for High Blood Pressure Research. Circulation 2008;117(25):e510–26.
5. Grasso M, Boscaro M, Scaroni C, et al. Secondary arterial hypertension: from routine clinical practice to evidence in patients with adrenal tumor. High Blood Press Cardiovasc Prev 2018;25(4):345–54.
6. Barbot M, Ceccato F, Scaroni C. The pathophysiology and treatment of hypertension in patients with Cushing's syndrome. Front Endocrinol (Lausanne) 2019; 10:321.
7. Miller WL, Auchus RJ. The molecular biology, biochemistry, and physiology of human steroidogenesis and its disorders. Endocr Rev 2011;32(1):81–151.
8. Peter M. Congenital adrenal hyperplasia: 11β-hydroxylase deficiency. Semin Reprod Med 2002;20(3):249–54.
9. Merke DP. Approach to the adult with congenital adrenal hyperplasia due to 21-hydroxylase deficiency. J Clin Endocrinol Metab 2008;93(3):653–60.
10. Bulsari K, Falhammar H. Clinical perspectives in congenital adrenal hyperplasia due to 11β-hydroxylase deficiency. Endocrine 2017;55(1):19–36.
11. Bongiovanni AM, Eberlein WR. Plasma and urinary corticosteroids in the hypertensive form of congenital adrenal hyperplasia. J Biol Chem 1956;223(1): 85–94. Available at: http://www.ncbi.nlm.nih.gov/pubmed/13376579.
12. Valadares LP, Pfeilsticker ACV, de Brito Sousa SM, et al. Insights on the phenotypic heterogeneity of 11β-hydroxylase deficiency: clinical and genetic studies in two novel families. Endocrine 2018. https://doi.org/10.1007/s12020-018-1691-4.
13. Nimkarn S, New MI. Steroid 11β- hydroxylase deficiency congenital adrenal hyperplasia. Trends Endocrinol Metab 2008;19(3):96–9.
14. Nordenskjöld A, Holmdahl G, Frisén L, et al. Type of mutation and surgical procedure affect long-term quality of life for women with congenital adrenal hyperplasia. J Clin Endocrinol Metab 2008;93(2):380–6.
15. Breil T, Yakovenko V, Inta I, et al. Typical characteristics of children with congenital adrenal hyperplasia due to 11β-hydroxylase deficiency: a single-centre experience and review of the literature. J Pediatr Endocrinol Metab 2019;32(3): 259–67.
16. Zachmann M, Tassinari D, Prader A. Clinical and biochemical variability of congenital adrenal hyperplasia due to 11 beta-hydroxylase deficiency. A study of 25 patients. J Clin Endocrinol Metab 1983;56(2):222–9.
17. Rösler A, Leiberman E, Sack J, et al. Clinical variability of congenital adrenal hyperplasia due to 11 beta-hydroxylase deficiency. Horm Res 1982;16(3):133–41. Available at: http://www.ncbi.nlm.nih.gov/pubmed/7049883.

18. Khattab A, Haider S, Kumar A, et al. Clinical, genetic, and structural basis of congenital adrenal hyperplasia due to 11β-hydroxylase deficiency. Proc Natl Acad Sci U S A 2017;114(10):E1933–40.

19. Curnow KM, Slutsker L, Vitek J, et al. Mutations in the CYP11B1 gene causing congenital adrenal hyperplasia and hypertension cluster in exons 6, 7, and 8. Proc Natl Acad Sci U S A 1993;90(10):4552–6.

20. Bornstein SR, Allolio B, Arlt W, et al. Diagnosis and treatment of primary adrenal insufficiency: an endocrine society clinical practice guideline. J Clin Endocrinol Metab 2016;101(2):364–89.

21. Auchus RJ. Steroid 17-hydroxylase and 17,20-lyase deficiencies, genetic and pharmacologic. J Steroid Biochem Mol Biol 2017;165:71–8.

22. Zuber MX, Simpson ER, Waterman MR. Expression of bovine 17 alpha-hydroxylase cytochrome P-450 cDNA in nonsteroidogenic (COS 1) cells. Science 1986;234(4781):1258–61.

23. Biason A, Mantero F, Scaroni C, et al. Deletion within the CYP17 gene together with insertion of foreign DNA is the cause of combined complete 17 alpha-hydroxylase/17,20-lyase deficiency in an Italian patient. Mol Endocrinol 1991; 5(12):2037–45.

24. Biason-Lauber A, Boscaro M, Mantero F, et al. Defects of steroidogenesis. J Endocrinol Invest 2010;33(10):756–66.

25. Sherbet DP, Tiosano D, Kwist KM, et al. CYP17 mutation E305G causes isolated 17,20-lyase deficiency by selectively altering substrate binding. J Biol Chem 2003;278(49):48563–9.

26. Mantero F, Busnardo B, Riondel A, et al. Arterial hypertension, hypokalemic alkalosis and male pseudohermaphroditism caused by 17 alpha-hydroxylase deficiency. Schweiz Med Wochenschr 1971;101(2):38–43 [in French]. Available at: http://www.ncbi.nlm.nih.gov/pubmed/5101501.

27. Biglieri EG, Kater CE. 17 alpha-hydroxylation deficiency. Endocrinol Metab Clin North Am 1991;20(2):257–68. Available at: http://www.ncbi.nlm.nih.gov/pubmed/1879398.

28. Mantero F, Opocher G, Rocco S, et al. Long-term treatment of mineralocorticoid excess syndromes. Steroids 1995;60(1):81–6. Available at: http://www.ncbi.nlm.nih.gov/pubmed/7792822.

29. Funder JW. Apparent mineralocorticoid excess. J Steroid Biochem Mol Biol 2017; 165:151–3.

30. Limumpornpetch P, Stewart PM. Apparent mineralocorticoid excess. In: Encyclopedia of endocrine diseases, vol. 3. Elsevier; 2019. p. 638–43. https://doi.org/10.1016/B978-0-12-801238-3.64338-6.

31. Ulick S, Kodama T, Gunczier P, et al. A syndrome of apparent mineralocorticoid excess associated with defects in the peripheral metabolism of cortisol. J Clin Endocrinol Metab 1979;49(5):757–64.

32. Oberfield SE, Levine LS, Carey RM, et al. Metabolic and blood pressure responses to hydrocortisone in the syndrome of apparent mineralocorticoid excess. J Clin Endocrinol Metab 1983;56(2):332–9.

33. Rusvai E, Náray-Fejes-Tóth A. A new isoform of 11 beta-hydroxysteroid dehydrogenase in aldosterone target cells. J Biol Chem 1993;268(15):10717–20. Available at: http://www.ncbi.nlm.nih.gov/pubmed/8496139.

34. Wilson RC, Krozowski ZS, Li K, et al. A mutation in the HSD11B2 gene in a family with apparent mineralocorticoid excess. J Clin Endocrinol Metab 1995;80(7):2263–6.

35. Obeyesekere VR, Ferrari P, Andrews RK, et al. The R337C mutation generates a high Km 11 beta-hydroxysteroid dehydrogenase type II enzyme in a family with apparent mineralocorticoid excess. J Clin Endocrinol Metab 1995;80(11):3381–3.

36. Chapman K, Holmes M, Seckl J. 11β-hydroxysteroid dehydrogenases: intracellular gate-keepers of tissue glucocorticoid action. Physiol Rev 2013;93(3): 1139–206.

37. Fjeld CC, Birdsong WT, Goodman RH. Differential binding of NAD+ and NADH allows the transcriptional corepressor carboxyl-terminal binding protein to serve as a metabolic sensor. Proc Natl Acad Sci U S A 2003;100(16):9202–7.

38. Mantero F, Palermo M, Petrelli MD, et al. Apparent mineralocorticoid excess: type I and type II. Steroids 1996;61(4):193–6. Available at: http://www.ncbi.nlm.nih.gov/pubmed/8732999.

39. New MI, Geller DS, Fallo F, et al. Monogenic low renin hypertension. Trends Endocrinol Metab 2005;16(3):92–7.

40. Ceccato F, Trementino L, Barbot M, et al. Diagnostic accuracy of increased urinary cortisol/cortisone ratio to differentiate ACTH-dependent Cushing's syndrome. Clin Endocrinol (Oxf) 2017;87(5). https://doi.org/10.1111/cen.13391.

41. Liddle GW, Bledsoe T, Coppage WS Jr. A familial renal disorder simulating primary aldosteronism but with negligible aldosterone secretion. Trans Assoc Am Physicians 1963;76:199–213.

42. Canessa CM, Schild L, Buell G, et al. Amiloride-sensitive epithelial Na+ channel is made of three homologous subunits. Nature 1994;367(6462):463–7.

43. Rossi E, Rossi GM. Liddle syndrome. In: Encyclopedia of endocrine diseases, vol. 3. Elsevier; 2019. p. 652–63. https://doi.org/10.1016/B978-0-12-801238-3.65187-5.

44. Pagani L, Diekmann Y, Sazzini M, et al. Three reportedly unrelated families with Liddle syndrome inherited from a common ancestor. Hypertension 2018;71(2): 273–9.

45. Cui Y, Tong A, Jiang J, et al. Liddle syndrome: clinical and genetic profiles. J Clin Hypertens 2017;19(5):524–9.

46. Hanukoglu I. ASIC and ENaC type sodium channels: conformational states and the structures of the ion selectivity filters. FEBS J 2017;284(4):525–45.

47. Kurtz TW, Dominiczak AF, DiCarlo SE, et al. Molecular-based mechanisms of mendelian forms of salt-dependent hypertension. Hypertension 2015;65(5): 932–41.

48. Chandrashekar J, Kuhn C, Oka Y, et al. The cells and peripheral representation of sodium taste in mice. Nature 2010;464(7286):297–301.

49. O'Shaughnessy KM. Gordon syndrome: a continuing story. Pediatr Nephrol 2015; 30(11):1903–8.

50. Gordon RD, Hodsman GP. The syndrome of hypertension and hyperkalaemia without renal failure: long term correction by thiazide diuretic. Scott Med J 1986;31(1):43–4.

51. Zhou B, Zhuang J, Gu D, et al. WNK4 enhances the degradation of NCC through a sortilin-mediated lysosomal pathway. J Am Soc Nephrol 2010;21(1):82–92.

52. Sakoh T, Sekine A, Mori T, et al. A familial case of pseudohypoaldosteronism type II (PHA2) with a novel mutation (D564N) in the acidic motif in WNK4. Mol Genet Genomic Med 2019;7(6):e705.

53. Glover M, Mercier Zuber A, Figg N, et al. The activity of the thiazide-sensitive Na + –Cl – cotransporter is regulated by protein phosphatase PP4. Can J Physiol Pharmacol 2010;88(10):986–95.

54. Mendes AI, Mascarenhas MR, Matos S, et al. A WNK4 gene variant relates to osteoporosis and not to hypertension in the Portuguese population. Mol Genet Metab 2011;102(4):465–9.

55. Lazrak A, Liu Z, Huang C-L. Antagonistic regulation of ROMK by long and kidney-specific WNK1 isoforms. Proc Natl Acad Sci U S A 2006;103(5):1615–20.

56. Vidal-Petiot E, Elvira-Matelot E, Mutig K, et al. WNK1-related familial hyperkalemic hypertension results from an increased expression of L-WNK1 specifically in the distal nephron. Proc Natl Acad Sci U S A 2013;110(35):14366–71.

57. Glover M, Ware JS, Henry A, et al. Detection of mutations in KLHL3 and CUL3 in families with FHHt (familial hyperkalaemic hypertension or Gordon's syndrome). Clin Sci 2014;126(10):721–6.

58. Mayan H, Vered I, Mouallem M, et al. Pseudohypoaldosteronism type II: marked sensitivity to thiazides, hypercalciuria, normomagnesemia, and low bone mineral density. J Clin Endocrinol Metab 2002;87(7):3248–54.

59. Pelham CJ, Ketsawatsomkron P, Groh S, et al. Cullin-3 regulates vascular smooth muscle function and arterial blood pressure via PPARγ and RhoA/Rho-kinase. Cell Metab 2012;16(4):462–72.

60. Geller DS. Activating mineralocorticoid receptor mutation in hypertension exacerbated by pregnancy. Science 2000;289(5476):119–23.

61. Rafestin-Oblin M-E, Souque A, Bocchi B, et al. The severe form of hypertension caused by the activating S810L mutation in the mineralocorticoid receptor is cortisone related. Endocrinology 2003;144(2):528–33.

62. Mariniello B, Ronconi V, Sardu C, et al. Analysis of the 11β-hydroxysteroid dehydrogenase type 2 gene (HSD11B2) in human essential hypertension. Am J Hypertens 2005;18(8):1091–8.

Resistant Hypertension
A Clinical Perspective

Fady Hannah-Shmouni, MD, FRCPC[a],*,
Sriram Gubbi, MD[b],
J. David Spence, MD, FRCPC[c],
Constantine A. Stratakis, MD, D(Med)Sci[a],
Christian A. Koch, MD, PhD[d]

KEYWORDS

- Hypertension • Resistant hypertension • Primary aldosteronism • Renin
- Aldosterone • Liddle syndrome • Amiloride

KEY POINTS

- True resistant hypertension is defined as suboptimal blood pressure response to a well-constructed antihypertensive therapy.
- Secondary forms of hypertension should be excluded in all cases.
- A renin/aldosterone-based approach for diagnosis and treatment is encouraged.

INTRODUCTION

Hypertension is an important contributor to cardiovascular morbidity and mortality in humans. The prevalence of hypertension is estimated between 34% and 53%, as observed in large-scale randomized controlled trials, including ALLHAT

Disclosure Statement: F. Hannah-Shmouni is a member of the Endocrine Hypertension Subcommittee of the Canadian Hypertension Guidelines (Hypertension Canada) and has no relevant disclosures to report. C.A. Koch is receiving royalties from Springer for the book "Endocrine Hypertension." All other authors have no relevant disclosures to report.
Source of support: This research was supported in part by the Intramural Research Program of *Eunice Kennedy Shriver* National Institute of Child Health and Human Development, National Institutes of Health, protocol 00-CH-0160 (Clinical and Molecular Analysis of ACTH-Independent Steroid Hormone Production in Adrenocortical Tissue).
[a] Internal Medicine-Endocrinology, Hypertension and Metabolic Genetics, Section on Endocrinology and Genetics, *Eunice Kennedy Shriver* National Institute of Child Health and Human Development, National Institutes of Health, 10 Center Drive, MSC 1109, Bethesda, MD 20892, USA; [b] Diabetes, Endocrinology, and Obesity Branch, National Institute of Diabetes and Digestive and Kidney diseases, National Institutes of Health, 10 Center Drive, Bethesda, MD 20892, USA; [c] Stroke Prevention and Atherosclerosis Research Centre, Robarts Research Institute, Western University, 1400 Western Road, London, ON N6G 2V4, Canada; [d] The University of Tennessee Health Science Center, 910 Madison Avenue, Memphis, TN 38163, USA
* Corresponding author.
E-mail address: fady.hannah-shmouni@nih.gov

(Antihypertensive and Lipid-Lowering Treatment to Prevent Heart Attack Trial; 34%), NHANES (National Health and Nutrition Examination Survey; 53%), and the Framingham Heart Study (48%).[1] These prevalence numbers certainly depend on the definition of hypertension. Using a threshold of 140/90 mm Hg, approximately 32% of adults of the United States are hypertensive, whereas the prevalence would increase to 46% with a lower threshold of 130/80 mm Hg.[2] Hypertension is the leading cause of cardiovascular disease in the United States, with a major economic burden.[3] Several subtypes of hypertension exist: controlled, uncontrolled, refractory, pseudo-resistant, apparent, and true resistant (**Table 1**).[4] An important and challenging subtype in clinical practice is resistant hypertension, defined as suboptimal blood pressure (BP) response to a well-constructed antihypertensive therapy. This definition identifies patients who are at high risk of having reversible causes of hypertension, such as obstructive sleep apnea, primary aldosteronism, or renal artery stenosis. The definition also includes patients who require ≥3 antihypertensives. A lower cutoff to ascertain the diagnosis of resistant hypertension (130/80 mm Hg) could be used in high-risk patients with diabetes mellitus or kidney disease.[5] Patients with resistant hypertension generally share several comorbidities that increase the relative risk of cardiovascular morbidity and mortality, including obesity, metabolic syndrome, chronic kidney disease, obstructive sleep apnea, sedentary lifestyle, smoking, and high salt intake.[6]

The exact prevalence of resistant hypertension is unknown owing to the difficulty of assessing medication adherence and/or accurate measurement of ambulatory BP in research studies that are mainly observational. Approximately 10% to 15% of treated hypertensive patients meet the definition of true resistant hypertension. In 1 cross-sectional study of more than 470,000 patients, 60,327 had resistant hypertension

Table 1
Hypertension subtypes

Hypertension Subtype	Definition	Reference
Resistant	BP above goal despite full doses of at least 3 well-constructed antihypertensive medications, including a diuretic	Burnier,[4] 2016
Pseudo-resistant	Apparent lack of BP control despite full doses of at least 3 well-constructed antihypertensive medications, including a diuretic	Judd & Calhoun,[7] 2014
Masked	Normal BP in the office, elevated BP out of the office	Papadopoulos & Makris[8] 2007
White-coat	Elevated BP in office, normal BP out of the office	Franklin et al,[9] 2013
Refractory	Uncontrolled BP despite maximal medical therapy after ≥3 visits to a hypertension clinic within a minimum 6-mo follow-up period	Acelajado et al,[10] 2012
Isolated systolic	Elevated systolic BP	Bavishi et al,[11] 2016
Isolated nocturnal	Elevated nocturnal BP	Abdalla et al,[12] 2016
Malignant	Hypertension with multiorgan involvement appearing over a short period of time	Funder et al,[13] 2016
Sustained	BP >150/100 mm Hg on each of 3 measurements obtained on different days without antihypertensive therapy	Funder et al,[13] 2016

(~12.8% of all hypertensives and 15.3% of patients on antihypertensive therapy).[14] Other estimates from patients receiving antihypertensive therapy suggest that resistant hypertension ranges from 9% to 18%.[15] Prevalence of resistant hypertension is higher in older age[16] and in individuals with obstructive sleep apnea and obesity, 3 of its strongest risk factors.[17,18] Given the heightened risk of resistant hypertension on cardiovascular morbidity and mortality, intensive management to target a systolic blood pressure (SBP) $\leq$120 mm Hg should be considered, particularly in individuals older than 50 years. The impact on renal and cerebral function should be taken into account in the individual patient. This recommendation stems from the SPRINT (Systolic Blood Pressure Intervention Trial), a National Heart, Lung, and Blood Institute (NHLBI)–supported randomized controlled trial that randomized 9631 subjects at high risk for cardiovascular disease but without diabetes mellitus or prior stroke, to an SBP less than 120 mm Hg or standard SBP less than 140 mm Hg.[19] The trial was stopped early (ie, after 3.2 years of the planned 5 years of follow-up) after an interim analysis found a significant reduction in cardiovascular events with intensive treatment. BP optimization using multiple strategies, including lifestyle changes, screening for secondary forms of hypertension, such as disorders of the adrenal glands and kidneys, and optimal doses of single-pill combination therapies is encouraged. Therapy should be aimed at reducing cardiovascular events, improving BP control, promoting adherence, and reducing medication side effects. In this review, the authors describe a clinical perspective on the diagnosis and management of resistant hypertension.

DIAGNOSIS OF HYPERTENSION

The diagnostic cutoff for hypertension is a subject of debate and a moving target by various national and international organizations (**Table 2**). For several decades,

Table 2 Selected guidelines for the diagnosis of hypertension	
Guidelines	**Definition, Diagnostic Method, and Targets**
2011 UK National Institute for Health and Clinical Excellence[22]	• $\geq$140/90 mm Hg and ABPM or HBPM
2013 European Society of Hypertension[23]	• $\geq$140/90 mm Hg, office ABPM (gold standard) • Ambulatory or HBPM for resistant hypertension
2014 Joint National Committee 8[20,21]	• Did not define hypertension • Office ABPM favored • Ambulatory BPM is not mentioned
2014 American Society of Hypertension–International Society of Hypertension[24]	• $\geq$140/90 mm Hg on office ABPM (gold standard) • Ambulatory or HBPM for resistant hypertension
2017 Canadian Hypertension Education Program[25]	• Daytime mean $\geq$135/85 mm Hg, 24 h mean 130/80 on ABPM. Home BPM mean $\geq$135/85. Mean office BP >180/110 mm Hg
2017 American College of Cardiology/American Heart Association[2]	• Elevated BP: $\geq$120–129/80 mm Hg • Hypertension: $\geq$130/80 mm Hg • Stage 1 hypertension: $\geq$130–139/80–89 mm Hg • Stage 2 hypertension: $\geq$140/90 mm Hg

Adapted from Hannah-Shmouni F, Melcescu E, Koch CA. Testing for endocrine hypertension. In: Feingold KR, Anawalt B, Boyce A, et al, editors. Endotext. South Dartmouth (MA): MDText.com, Inc; 2000; with permission.

hypertension was classified as a BP ≥140/90 mm Hg. The Joint National Committee 8[20,21] did not address the definition of hypertension. Recently, the American College of Cardiology/American Heart Association Task Force on Clinical Practice Guidelines defined hypertension as a BP ≥130/80 mm Hg,[2] which will lead to a new diagnosis in approximately 14% more Americans and the percentage of US adults considered to have hypertension will increase to 45.6% (103.3 million adults). Elevated BP (previously prehypertension) is now defined as ≥120 to 129/80 mm Hg. Stage 1 hypertension (previously prehypertension) is now ≥130 to 139/80 to 89 mm Hg, and stage 2 hypertension (previously stage 1 hypertension) is anything above that BP target. The suggested "normal" BP target is less than 120/80 mm Hg.

There is consistent evidence that BP is not accurately assessed in routine practice, which is particularly true when BP is measured manually using an auscultatory technique and when standardized methodology is not followed. Studies suggest that BP obtained in clinical practice is, on average, 9/6 mm Hg higher than when standardized measurement tools are used. Inaccuracies in BP measurement can have clinical consequences, such as misclassification of cardiovascular risk. Thus, it is important to correctly use a reliable BP measurement technique. It is encouraged to use a validated electronic digital oscillometric device for accurate BP measurement, and an out-of-office BP measurement should be performed to confirm a diagnosis of hypertension. The advantages of automated office BP (AOBP; the mean calculated and displayed by the device) are that it uses fully automated electronic oscillometric devices without any patient-provider interaction and designed to be used while the patient rests alone in a quiet room or private area. There are several other advantages of AOBP over manual approaches, including eliminating the risk of conversation during readings, facilitating multiple measurements with each clinical encounter, calculating a mean BP, demonstrating consistency of measurements from visit to visit, and eliminating the need for the health care provider to perform sequential electronic measurements.

The best options for out-of-office BP assessment are the ambulatory 24-hour BP measurement (ABPM) and home BP measurement (HBPM). The 24-hour ABPM is the preferred out-of-office BP measurement modality because it assesses BP throughout the day and night. However, if ABPM is not available or if the patient is unable to tolerate it, HBPM is a suitable alternative. Out-of-office measurement can ascertain hypertension and/or identify white-coat hypertension and masked hypertension (see **Table 1**). Masked hypertension describes the situation in which BP appears to be controlled when measured in the office but not at home (see **Table 1**). Their distinction is important because white-coat hypertensives are at somewhat lower relative risk of cardiovascular morbidity, whereas masked hypertensives show more extensive target organ damage than true normotensives.[26,27] Therefore, relying on office-based BP measurement alone may result in missed cases of masked hypertension. However, white-coat hypertension is not benign, and its presence should not be regarded as validating neglect of the condition.[28]

DIAGNOSIS OF RESISTANT HYPERTENSION

True resistant hypertension represents BP above goal despite full doses of at least 3 well-constructed antihypertensive medications, including a diuretic. BP cutoff values for the diagnosis of resistant hypertension include ambulatory BP ≥135/85 mm Hg during the daytime or ≥130/80 mm Hg over 24 hours.[29] The first steps in evaluating a patient with resistant hypertension should ensure medication compliance and appropriate full dosing through an objective assessment (such as measurement of drug levels), and exclusion of secondary forms of hypertension,[29] as detailed later.

Pseudo-resistant hypertension should be assessed in all cases. This clinical entity represents an apparent lack of BP control despite full doses of at least 3 well-constructed antihypertensive medications, including a diuretic.[7] Common factors that may lead to pseudo-resistance include poor adherence to drug treatment, periodic changes in dietary factors (eg, high sodium intake, high alcohol consumption, natural licorice, glycyrrhiza glabra), rapid weight gain, periodic changes in concomitant drugs (nonsteroidal anti-inflammatory agents, selective COX-2 inhibitors, sympathomimetic agents, such as decongestants, and stimulants), weight loss medications, and herbal compounds (eg, arnica, bitter orange, ephedra, ginkgo, and ginseng).[4,30]

In patients with stiff arteries, BP measured by cuff may be falsely elevated; the term "pseudohypertension" was used to describe this situation. Among patients aged greater than 60 years with diastolic blood pressure (DBP) greater than 100 mm Hg but no hypertensive end-organ disease, half had a 30 mm Hg false elevation of the cuff pressure, when compared with simultaneous intraarterial pressure measurement.[31] A better name for this situation is "cuff artefact." In this context, it is important to note that aging promotes atherosclerosis and that at present there is no randomized trial evidence to support starting antihypertensive therapy at SBP less than 150 mm Hg in persons aged 60 years or older.

SECONDARY FORMS OF HYPERTENSION

Secondary forms of hypertension refer to a disorder that is potentially correctable, as listed in **Table 3**. Compelling evidence suggests that 10% to 20% of hypertensives have an underlying secondary form of hypertension.[32] In 1 study, the prevalence of secondary hypertension in hypertensives was estimated at 10.2%.[33] Several clues on physical and biochemical examination may point toward a secondary form of

Table 3
Common and rare causes of secondary hypertension

Common Causes	Rare Causes
• Obstructive sleep apnea	• CAH: 11β-hydroxylase deficiency
• Primary aldosteronism	• CAH: 17α-hydroxylase deficiency
• Renal vascular hypertension	• Familial hyperaldosteronism
• Hypothyroidism	• Apparent mineralocorticoid excess (classic and
• Thyrotoxicosis	nonclassic)
• Nonparathyroid hormone mediated	• Liddle syndrome
hypercalcemia	• Pseudohypoaldosteronism type 1
• Parathyroid hormone-mediated	• Pseudohypoaldosteronism type 2
hypercalcemia	• Glucocorticoid resistance syndrome
• Insulin resistance	• Growth hormone excess: gigantism and
• Obesity	acromegaly
• Pheochromocytoma and paraganglioma	• Neuroendocrine neoplasms (secretory)
• Chronic kidney disease	• Medullary thyroid cancer
• Metabolic syndrome	• Geller syndrome
• Polycystic ovary syndrome	• Adrenocortical cancer
• Hypogonadism	• Cushing syndrome
• Vitamin D deficiency	
• Exogenous steroids	

Adapted from Hannah-Shmouni F, Melcescu E, Koch CA. Testing for endocrine hypertension. In: Feingold KR, Anawalt B, Boyce A, et al, editors. Endotext. South Dartmouth (MA): MDText.com, Inc; 2000; with permission.

hypertension, including flushing and excessive sweating,[34] holosystolic high-pitched renal bruit,[35] young onset (<40 years), worsening BP despite maximum drug therapy (failing triple-drug therapy including a diuretic), controlled BP (<140/90 mm Hg) on ≥4 antihypertensive drugs, spontaneous or diuretic-induced hypokalemia, snoring and apneic spells, atypical skin lesions (such as mucosal neuromas, fibromas, café-au-lait spots, striaes, axillary freckling, angiofibromas, or collagenomas), retinal angiomas, marfanoid body habitus, worsening glycemic control, kidney stones, and personal or family history of rare cancers.[30]

BIOCHEMICAL SCREENING FOR SECONDARY HYPERTENSION

Once confirmed by ABPM and assessment of adherence is completed, patients with resistant hypertension should be evaluated for secondary forms of hypertension (**Fig. 1**). It is important to note that biochemical assays differ widely in their accuracy, variability, precision, and functional limit of detection and should be chosen based on their performance. **Fig. 2** lists the major pathophysiologic mechanisms of resistant hypertension. As shown, these mechanisms are complex and involve an interplay between the central nervous system, kidneys, adrenal glands, heart, and carotid afferent and baroreceptors. Specifically, the intricate interplay involves sympathetic overactivity and the renin-aldosterone-angiotensin system (RAAS), altered renal sodium handling in the kidneys and volume loading, psychosocial factors, and endothelial and adrenocortical dysfunction (see **Fig. 1**). The biochemical phenotype of resistant hypertension could be categorized into 2 major subtypes based on the renin and aldosterone values: low or suppressed renin subtypes (primary aldosteronism type, or hyporeninemic hyperaldosteronism; low renin/high aldosterone); Liddle syndrome type, or hyporeninemic hypoaldosteronism; low renin/low aldosterone); and normal to high renin subtypes (hypereninemic hyperaldosteronism [high renin/high aldosterone]; normoreninemic normoaldosteronism) (see **Fig. 1**).

A renin/aldosterone-based approach should be considered the initial diagnostic strategy for the evaluation of individuals with resistant hypertension (see **Fig. 1**). Renin is a protease that is produced in the juxtaglomerular apparatus of the kidneys and catalyzes the first step in the activation of the RAAS. The secretion of renin is regulated by renal baroreceptors and sodium chloride delivery to the macula densa; thus, circulating plasma renin is influenced by changes in BP and salt balance. Plasma renin tests, either plasma renin activity (PRA) or direct renin concentration (DRC), are available commercially and are useful for screening and management purposes. PRA are within reference range in ~50% of patients with renovascular hypertension, whereas, conversely, increased levels may be found in ≤10% of patients with primary HTN.[36–38]

In renovascular hypertension, the low-pressure flow state within the afferent renal arterioles at the juxtaglomerular cells results in a log-unit (>10-fold) increase in plasma renin. Although no studies to date have evaluated the overall sensitivity and specificity of plasma renin as a diagnostic test in patients with resistant hypertension, the recognition of a plasma renin that is many-fold higher than the normal range (hypereninemic hypertension, as seen in renovascular hypertension), at the lower end of reference range (hyporeninemic hypertension), as seen in the Liddle phenotype (low-renin/low aldosterone) hypertension or hyporeninemic hyperaldosteronism hypertension, as seen in primary aldosteronism/inappropriate secretion of aldosterone, may be useful in guiding the next diagnostic or therapeutic steps (see **Fig. 1**).[37] The threshold set to diagnose a low-renin state is assay specific but generally defined as a PRA <0.65 ng/mL/h or a DRC <15 mU/L.[30,39] Although PRA is convenient for estimating the biological activity of the renin system, it does not necessarily reflect its

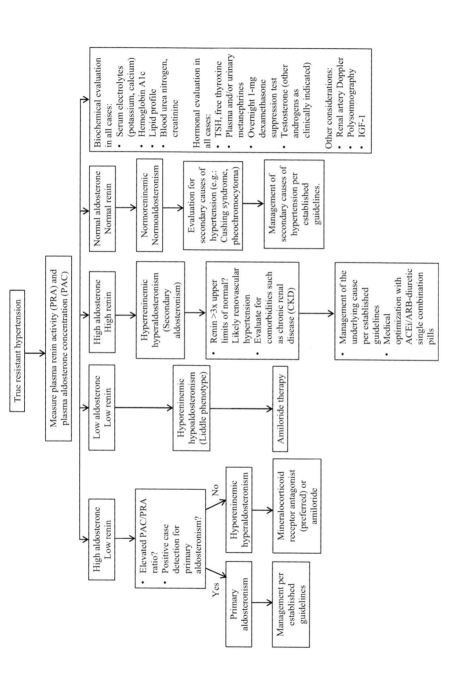

actual concentration. A DRC (conversion factor from PRA to DRC is 12) is an alternative test that can confirm a low-renin state, which could be particularly useful in low-renin hypertension.[39,40] DRC and PRA are poorly correlated in the range where PRA is less than 1 ng/mL/h.

Systematic screening for other endocrinopathies in concert or sequentially is encouraged following a renin/aldosterone-based subtyping of resistant hypertension (see **Fig. 1**). Screening tests could be influenced by several factors, including medications, advanced age, dietary sodium/potassium, and hypokalemia. Primary aldosteronism is screened with the easy, rapid, and inexpensive PAC-to-PRA ratio (ARR).[41] A minimum PAC of 15 ng/dL (410 pmol/L) and PRA of less than 1 ng/mL/h are used as screening criteria, with the most commonly adopted cutoff values for ARR being 30 (in conventional units; 90% sensitivity and 91% specificity).[13] Although hypokalemia is suggestive of primary aldosteronism, most patients are normokalemic,[13,42] and a suppressed renin test does not differentiate between primary aldosteronism and the Liddle phenotype or other forms of secondary hypertension, such as classic or partial apparent mineralocorticoid excess.[43] Recent evidence suggests milder forms of primary aldosteronism that manifest with suppressed renin and aldosterone values below the guidelines cutoffs.[44–46] Other causes of low or suppressed renin include licorice, nonsteroidal anti-inflammatory drugs, excess mineralocorticoids, apparent mineralocorticoid excess, and Liddle syndrome (see **Table 2**).[30,46] For accurate interpretation of the renin/aldosterone phenotypes, it is therefore important that plasma renin and aldosterone be measured in a stimulated condition, while the patient is taking a diuretic and/or angiotensin-converting enzyme inhibitor (ACEi)/angiotensin-receptor blocker (ARB).[47,48] The lower limit of detection varies among different PRA assays and can have a dramatic effect on ARR; because ARR is highly dependent on plasma renin, false positive PRA could be expected when PAC is low. Thus, a high index of suspicion is needed.

Screening for hypercortisolism is confirmed with the late-night cortisol (2 measurements), 1-mg overnight dexamethasone suppression test (DST), 24 hour urine free cortisol (at least 2 measurements), or the longer low-dose DST (2 mg/d for 48 hours).[49] Any concurrent or recent use of glucocorticoid products could lead to false positive testing.[50] The most reliable and specific screening test for the diagnosis of pheochromocytomas and paragangliomas is the plasma free or urinary fractionated metanephrines.[51–54] False positives could arise with certain antidepressive agents, caffeine, smoking, and alcohol intake, which should be withheld for 24 hours before testing.[30,54]

RESISTANT HYPERTENSION IN AFRICAN AMERICANS

African Americans and other people of African descent show a higher incidence of hypertension and its related comorbidities.[3] Moreover, they have higher degrees of BP levels beginning in childhood as well as a higher incidence and prevalence of

---

Fig. 1. Once BP is confirmed by ABPM and assessment of adherence is completed, patients with resistant hypertension should be evaluated for secondary forms of hypertension. A renin/aldosterone-based approach could be considered the initial diagnostic test for the evaluation of individuals with resistant hypertension. Low-renin/high-aldosterone hypertension favors treatment with a mineralocorticoid receptor antagonist; low-renin/low-aldosterone hypertension is best treated with amiloride. Normal to high renin favors screening of other secondary forms of hypertension and treatment with ACEi/ARB-diuretic single-pill combination. IGF1, insulin-like growth factor 1. (*Courtesy of* S. Gubbi, MD, Bethesda, MD.)

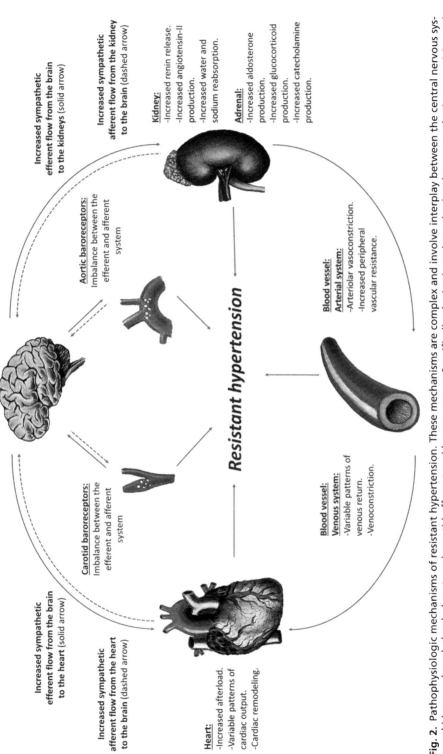

Fig. 2. Pathophysiologic mechanisms of resistant hypertension. These mechanisms are complex and involve interplay between the central nervous system, kidneys, adrenal glands, heart, and carotid afferent and baroreceptors. Specifically, the intricate interplay involves sympathetic overactivity and the RAAS, altered renal sodium handling in the kidneys and volume loading, psychosocial factors, endothelial and adrenocortical dysfunction. (*Courtesy of* S. Gubbi, MD, Bethesda, MD.)

hypertension across the lifespan.[55-60] Major predictors of hypertension in African Americans exist when compared with other ethnicities, including greater impairment of arterial elasticity,[61-63] increased aldosterone sensitivity (magnitude of the association between PAC and BP),[64] poor BP control and resistance,[65] and hypertensive diagnostic inertia, defined as a failure to investigate the underlying cause of hypertension.[66,67] Moreover, African Americans excrete a sodium load more slowly and less completely than whites,[68] leading to RAAS suppression from volume loading that typically begins in childhood,[69-72] and the ensuing low-renin hypertension.[30,73,74] One study demonstrated lower levels of PRA and PAC in normotensive African Americans across all ages, with BP positively correlating with PAC, an effect that increased as PRA decreased.[71] Thus, a typical biochemical profile in an African American person with hypertension is a low- or high-aldosterone test, a low or suppressed renin test, and suppressed angiotensin I and II,[75-78] leading to 2 possible renin subtypes: primary aldosteronism type, or hyporeninemic hyperaldosteronism, and hyporeninemic hypoaldosteronism or Liddle phenotype.[79]

Several genes implicated in the regulation of sodium reabsorption in the kidneys were likely selected as an adaptation to hot environments, particularly in people from sub-Saharan Africa.[65,80] These genes include genes in the 2 different streams of low-renin hypertension. Sodium retention owing to overactivity of the renal tubular epithelial sodium channel (ENaC) can be due to variants of ENaC itself (SCNN1B), or variants of at least 5 other genes affecting ENaC function: GRK, NEDD4L, CYP4A11, NPPA, and UMOD.[39,48,65,81] For this reason, the Liddle phenotype is much more common than true Liddle syndrome because of variants of SCNN1B. The other stream is genes affecting increased aldosterone production from the adrenal cortex, due to CYP11B2, KCNJ5, ATP1A1, ATP2B3, CACNA1D, and armadillo repeat containing 5 (ARMC5).[39,82,83] Adrenocortical hyperplasia is likely more prevalent in African Americans,[39,83,84] suggesting the possibility of aldosterone and/or cortisol excess (or their precursors) as an important contributor to the pathogenesis of hypertension and in particular the primary aldosteronism phenotype (see **Fig. 2**). Collectively, these genetic factors might have played an important physiologic adaptation ("natural selection") to the low sodium environments and survival of African Americans during their passage from Africa to America,[65,80] where they experienced extreme conditions, including severe heat, hyperhidrosis, and fluid loss through vomiting and diarrhea. Indeed, this selection process might have contributed to the increased prevalence of salt and water retention, and therefore, hypertension in this population.[85,86] That hypothesis is supported by the observation that hypertension is nearly twice as prevalent in US-born than in foreign-born African Americans.[87,88] Spence[48] hypothesized that some patients may have variants that predispose both to inappropriate aldosterone secretion and to overactivity of ENaC.

MEDICAL MANAGEMENT OF RESISTANT HYPERTENSION

Some patients with severe renovascular hypertension may require revascularization, and some patients with pheochromocytoma or primary aldosteronism may require adrenalectomy, even with bilateral adrenonodular hyperplasia,[84] but it is important to recognize that primary aldosteronism is commonly (even usually) due to bilateral adrenocortical hyperplasia (**Fig. 3**).[89-91] Most patients with resistant hypertension are therefore best managed medically. However, the key to controlling resistant hypertension is to identify the physiologic drivers of the hypertension.[65]

Patients with true resistant hypertension are on effective doses of ≥3 different classes of antihypertensives, including a diuretic. Some patients remain uncontrolled with

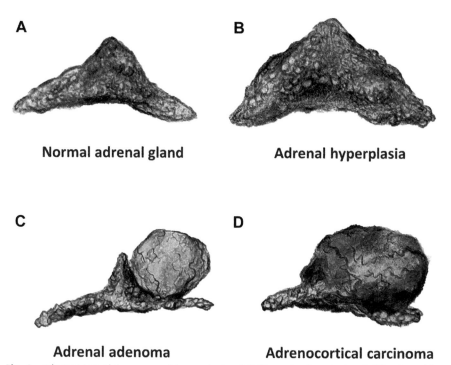

A   Normal adrenal gland

B   Adrenal hyperplasia

C   Adrenal adenoma

D   Adrenocortical carcinoma

Fig. 3. Adrenocortical tumors and hyperplasias. (*A*) Normal adrenal gland; (*B*) adrenal hyperplasia; (*C*) adrenal adenoma; (*D*) adrenal cancer. Adrenal hyperplasia is likely more prevalent in individuals of African descent, suggesting the possibility of aldosterone and/or cortisol excess as an important contributor to the pathogenesis of hypertension and the primary aldosteronism phenotype. Adrenal hyperplasia and ensuing hyperaldosteronism could have emerged as an important physiologic adaptation ("natural selection") to the low sodium environments and survival of African Americans during their passage from Africa to America. (*Courtesy of* S. Gubbi, MD, Bethesda, MD.)

$\geq$5 different antihypertensives, including a long-acting thiazide-like diuretic, such as chlorthalidone, and/or a mineralocorticoid receptor antagonist. This subtype of hypertension is referred to as refractory (see **Table 1**). One cross-sectional study (REGARDS cohort) found 78 of 14,809 patients being treated for hypertension as having refractory hypertension and were more likely to be of African American descent (strongest predictor, prevalence ratio of 4.88, 95% confidence interval, 2.79–8.72), male sex, and higher body mass index.[92]

Important management approaches to the treatment of true resistant hypertension include medication adherence and reinforcement, regular exercise, weight loss, reduction of salt intake, behavioral interventions, and management of risk factors, such as obesity, obstructive sleep apnea, hyperglycemia, and insulin resistance.[29] Medical therapy is optimized and tailored based on the renin/aldosterone phenotype, and single-pill combination therapy with the highest tolerable doses, including the use of a thiazide-like diuretic, and a mineralocorticoid receptor antagonist, particularly in the setting of low-renin hypertension or hyperaldosteronism, suggestive of mineralocorticoid receptor activation with heightened cardiovascular risk. Moreover, mineralocorticoid receptor antagonists are also effective throughout the distribution of baseline renin tests,[93] making it an important first-line therapy. Conversely, amiloride, a renal tubular ENaC antagonist, is an alternative therapy to mineralocorticoid receptor antagonists,[94] particularly in individuals with adverse effects to mineralocorticoid receptor antagonists, such as hyperkalemia, gynecomastia in men, breast tenderness and engorgement in women (very rare), or pregnancy (category B). Amiloride is particularly useful in individuals with hypertension and variants affecting ENaC function. Spironolactone is commonly used in resistant hypertension, but amiloride should be used more widely. Although in the PATHWAYS 2 trial[93] amiloride and spironolactone were equally effective overall in resistant hypertension, spironolactone was more effective in patients with inappropriate aldosterone secretion,[93] and it is important to recognize that amiloride will be more effective in patients with the Liddle phenotype, as shown by Laffer and colleagues[95,96] in patients with a variant of the CYP4A11 gene. The importance of ENaC in sodium retention and low renin hypertension has been reviewed elsewhere.[65]

In the high-renin/high-aldosterone phenotype, an ACEi/ARB-diuretic single-combination pill, with/without calcium channel antagonist and mineralocorticoid receptor antagonist is favored. Serial BP checks with ABPM are encouraged in 2- to 3-week intervals until BP control is achieved.[29] In low or suppressed renin hypertension, the dose of medication should be optimized to increase plasm renin substantially, suggesting sufficient mineralocorticoid receptor antagonism to mitigate the heightened cardiovascular risk.[46] Thus, measuring renin serially has an added value in tailoring and optimizing therapy in these clinical scenarios, until other biochemical measures of RAAS are commercially available for tailoring therapy.

Egan and colleagues[97] conducted a randomized trial of renin-based management of resistant hypertension, and although BPs were somewhat lower with less medication, there was not a significant increase in BP control. The problem with using only plasma renin to guide therapy is that there are 2 categories of low-renin hypertension: primary aldosteronism/inappropriate aldosterone secretion, with a low-renin/high-aldosterone phenotype, and those owing to overactivity of ENaC, with a low-renin/low-aldosterone phenotype. In a trial in Africa, BP control was significantly better controlled with physiologically individualized therapy based on renin/aldosterone phenotyping (PhysRx) than with usual care.[98] At the Nigerian site, where patients were randomized, and where amiloride was available, SBP was controlled in 15% of usual care versus 85% of PhysRx, DBP was controlled in 45 versus 75%, and both SBP and DBP were controlled in 15 versus 75% (P<.0001), even though the renal function of patients was poorer at that site.[98] The biggest difference in medication was that at the end of the study, only 2.8% of usual care patients were receiving amiloride versus 19% of PhysRx.[98] This suggests that the Liddle phenotype is much more common than previously thought and highlights the importance of considering amiloride and renin/aldosterone phenotyping in the management of resistant hypertension.[96]

SUMMARY

Hypertension is the leading cause of cardiovascular disease, and resistant hypertension represents an important subtype particularly in African Americans. Suboptimal BP response to a well-constructed antihypertensive therapy, including a diuretic, contributes to this increased risk. Some individuals with resistant hypertension have a reversible cause, such as obstructive sleep apnea, primary aldosteronism, or renal artery stenosis. Thus, all patients with resistant hypertension should undergo a systematic and sequential biochemical screening for secondary forms of hypertension. A renin/aldosterone-based diagnostic and treatment strategy is encouraged to attain optimal selection of therapy, adherence, and BP response.

REFERENCES

1. Calhoun DA, Jones D, Textor S, et al. Resistant hypertension: diagnosis, evaluation, and treatment. A scientific statement from the American Heart Association Professional Education Committee of the Council for High Blood Pressure Research. Hypertension 2008;51(6):1403–19.
2. Whelton PK, Carey RM, Aronow WS, et al. 2017 ACC/AHA/AAPA/ABC/ACPM/ AGS/APhA/ASH/ASPC/NMA/PCNA guideline for the prevention, detection, evaluation, and management of high blood pressure in adults: executive summary: a report of the American College of Cardiology/American Heart Association Task Force on clinical practice guidelines. Circulation 2018;138(17):e426–83.
3. Mozaffarian D, Benjamin EJ, Go AS, et al. Heart disease and stroke statistics– 2015 update: a report from the American Heart Association. Circulation 2015; 131(4):e29–322.
4. Burnier M. Resistant hypertension: is the number of drugs a reliable marker of resistance? Hypertension 2016;68(6):1346–8.
5. Moser M, Setaro JF. Clinical practice. Resistant or difficult-to-control hypertension. N Engl J Med 2006;355(4):385–92.
6. Daugherty SL, Powers JD, Magid DJ, et al. Incidence and prognosis of resistant hypertension in hypertensive patients. Circulation 2012;125(13):1635–42.
7. Judd E, Calhoun DA. Apparent and true resistant hypertension: definition, prevalence and outcomes. J Hum Hypertens 2014;28(8):463–8.
8. Papadopoulos DP, Makris TK. Masked hypertension definition, impact, outcomes: a critical review. J Clin Hypertens 2007;9(12):956–63.
9. Franklin SS, Thijs L, Hansen TW, et al. White-coat hypertension: new insights from recent studies. Hypertension 2013;62(6):982–7.
10. Acelajado MC, Pisoni R, Dudenbostel T, et al. Refractory hypertension: definition, prevalence, and patient characteristics. J Clin Hypertens 2012;14(1):7–12.
11. Bavishi C, Goel S, Messerli FH. Isolated systolic hypertension: an update after SPRINT. Am J Med 2016;129(12):1251–8.
12. Abdalla M, Goldsmith J, Muntner P, et al. Is isolated nocturnal hypertension a reproducible phenotype? Am J Hypertens 2016;29(1):33–8.
13. Funder JW, Carey RM, Mantero F, et al. The management of primary aldosteronism: case detection, diagnosis, and treatment: an Endocrine Society Clinical Practice guideline. J Clin Endocrinol Metab 2016;101(5):1889–916.
14. Sim JJ, Bhandari SK, Shi J, et al. Characteristics of resistant hypertension in a large, ethnically diverse hypertension population of an integrated health system. Mayo Clin Proc 2013;88(10):1099–107.
15. Achelrod D, Wenzel U, Frey S. Systematic review and meta-analysis of the prevalence of resistant hypertension in treated hypertensive populations. Am J Hypertens 2015;28(3):355–61.
16. Sinnott SJ, Smeeth L, Williamson E, et al. Trends for prevalence and incidence of resistant hypertension: population based cohort study in the UK 1995-2015. BMJ 2017;358:j3984.
17. de Abreu-Silva EO, Beltrami-Moreira M. Sleep apnea: an underestimated cause of resistant hypertension. Curr Hypertens Rev 2014;10(1):2–7.
18. Goodfriend TL, Calhoun DA. Resistant hypertension, obesity, sleep apnea, and aldosterone: theory and therapy. Hypertension 2004;43(3):518–24.
19. Group SR, Wright JT Jr, Williamson JD, et al. A randomized trial of intensive versus standard blood-pressure control. N Engl J Med 2015;373(22):2103–16.

20. James PA, Oparil S, Carter BL, et al. 2014 evidence-based guideline for the management of high blood pressure in adults: report from the panel members appointed to the Eighth Joint National Committee (JNC 8). JAMA 2014;311(5): 507–20.

21. Reisin E, Harris RC, Rahman M. Commentary on the 2014 BP guidelines from the panel appointed to the Eighth Joint National Committee (JNC 8). J Am Soc Nephrol 2014;25(11):2419–24.

22. National Clinical Guideline Centre (UK). Hypertension: the clinical management of primary hypertension in adults: update of clinical guidelines 18 and 34 [Internet]. London: Royal College of Physicians (UK); 2011.

23. Mancia G, Fagard R, Narkiewicz K, et al. 2013 ESH/ESC guidelines for the management of arterial hypertension: the Task Force for the management of arterial hypertension of the European Society of Hypertension (ESH) and of the European Society of Cardiology (ESC). J Hypertens 2013;31(7):1281–357.

24. Weber MA, Schiffrin EL, White WB, et al. Clinical practice guidelines for the management of hypertension in the community: a statement by the American Society of Hypertension and the International Society of Hypertension. J Clin Hypertens 2014;16(1):14–26.

25. Daskalopoulou SS, Rabi DM, Zarnke KB, et al. The 2015 Canadian Hypertension Education Program recommendations for blood pressure measurement, diagnosis, assessment of risk, prevention, and treatment of hypertension. Can J Cardiol 2015;31(5):549–68.

26. Pickering TG, Davidson K, Gerin W, et al. Masked hypertension. Hypertension 2002;40(6):795–6.

27. Ohkubo T, Kikuya M, Metoki H, et al. Prognosis of "masked" hypertension and "white-coat" hypertension detected by 24-h ambulatory blood pressure monitoring 10-year follow-up from the Ohasama study. J Am Coll Cardiol 2005; 46(3):508–15.

28. Spence JD. Dilemmas in diagnosing and managing hypertension: is white coat hypertension benign? Can J Cardiol 2015;31(5):580–2.

29. Wei FF, Zhang ZY, Huang QF, et al. Diagnosis and management of resistant hypertension: state of the art. Nat Rev Nephrol 2018;14(7):428–41.

30. Hannah-Shmouni F, Melcescu E, Koch CA. Testing for endocrine hypertension. In: Feingold KR, Anawalt B, Boyce A, et al, editors. Endotext. South Dartmouth (MA): MDText.com, Inc; 2000. Available at: https://www.ncbi.nlm.nih.gov/books/NBK278965/.

31. Spence JD, Sibbald WJ, Cape RD. Pseudohypertension in the elderly. Clin Sci Mol Med Suppl 1978;4:399s–402s.

32. Funder JW. Primary aldosteronism: seismic shifts. J Clin Endocrinol Metab 2015; 100(8):2853–5.

33. Anderson GH Jr, Blakeman N, Streeten DH. The effect of age on prevalence of secondary forms of hypertension in 4429 consecutively referred patients. J Hypertens 1994;12(5):609–15.

34. Hannah-Shmouni F, Stratakis CA, Koch CA. Flushing in (neuro)endocrinology. In: Reviews in endocrine & metabolic disorders. 2016.

35. Turnbull JM. The rational clinical examination. Is listening for abdominal bruits useful in the evaluation of hypertension? JAMA 1995;274(16):1299–301.

36. Derkx FH, Schalekamp MA. Renal artery stenosis and hypertension. Lancet 1994; 344(8917):237–9.

37. Petruzzelli M, Taylor KP, Koo B, et al. Telling tails: very high plasma renin levels prompt the diagnosis of renal artery stenosis, despite initial negative imaging. Hypertension 2016;68(1):11–6.

38. Brown MJ. Clinical value of plasma renin estimation in the management of hypertension. Am J Hypertens 2014;27(8):1013–6.

39. Zilbermint M, Hannah-Shmouni F, Stratakis CA. Genetics of hypertension in African Americans and others of African descent. Int J Mol Sci 2019;20(5) [pii: E1081].

40. Campbell DJ, Nussberger J, Stowasser M, et al. Activity assays and immunoassays for plasma renin and prorenin: information provided and precautions necessary for accurate measurement. Clin Chem 2009;55(5):867–77.

41. Schwartz GL, Turner ST. Screening for primary aldosteronism in essential hypertension: diagnostic accuracy of the ratio of plasma aldosterone concentration to plasma renin activity. Clin Chem 2005;51(2):386–94.

42. Rossi E, Regolisti G, Negro A, et al. High prevalence of primary aldosteronism using postcaptopril plasma aldosterone to renin ratio as a screening test among Italian hypertensives. Am J Hypertens 2002;15(10 Pt 1):896–902.

43. Tapia-Castillo A, Baudrand R, Vaidya A, et al. Clinical, biochemical, and genetic characteristics of "nonclassic" apparent mineralocorticoid excess syndrome. J Clin Endocrinol Metab 2019;104(2):595–603.

44. Brown JM, Robinson-Cohen C, Luque-Fernandez MA, et al. The spectrum of subclinical primary aldosteronism and incident hypertension: a cohort study. Ann Intern Med 2017;167(9):630–41.

45. Vaidya A, Mulatero P, Baudrand R, et al. The expanding spectrum of primary aldosteronism: implications for diagnosis, pathogenesis, and treatment. Endocr Rev 2018;39(6):1057–88.

46. Baudrand R, Vaidya A. The low-renin hypertension phenotype: genetics and the role of the mineralocorticoid receptor. Int J Mol Sci 2018;19(2) [pii:E546].

47. Wallach L, Nyarai I, Dawson KG. Stimulated renin: a screening test for hypertension. Ann Intern Med 1975;82(1):27–34.

48. Spence JD. Hypertension in Africa. Eur J Prev Cardiol 2019;26(5):455–7.

49. Nieman LK, Biller BM, Findling JW, et al. The diagnosis of Cushing's syndrome: an Endocrine Society Clinical Practice Guideline. J Clin Endocrinol Metab 2008;93(5):1526–40.

50. Hannah-Shmouni F, Demidowich A, Stratakis CA. Cortisol in the evaluation of adrenal insufficiency. JAMA 2016;316(5):535–6.

51. Eisenhofer G, Peitzsch M. Laboratory evaluation of pheochromocytoma and paraganglioma. Clin Chem 2014;60(12):1486–99.

52. Peaston RT, Graham KS, Chambers E, et al. Performance of plasma free metanephrines measured by liquid chromatography-tandem mass spectrometry in the diagnosis of pheochromocytoma. Clin Chim Acta 2010;411(7–8):546–52.

53. Lenders JW, Pacak K, Walther MM, et al. Biochemical diagnosis of pheochromocytoma: which test is best? JAMA 2002;287(11):1427–34.

54. Hannah-Shmouni F, Pacak K, Stratakis CA. Metanephrines for evaluating palpitations and flushing. JAMA 2017;318(4):385–6.

55. Writing Group M, Mozaffarian D, Benjamin EJ, et al. Heart disease and stroke statistics–2016 update: a report from the American Heart Association. Circulation 2016;133(4):e38–360.

56. Berenson GS, Wattigney WA, Webber LS. Epidemiology of hypertension from childhood to young adulthood in black, white, and Hispanic population samples. Public Health Rep 1996;111(Suppl 2):3–6.

57. Bao W, Threefoot SA, Srinivasan SR, et al. Essential hypertension predicted by tracking of elevated blood pressure from childhood to adulthood: the Bogalusa Heart Study. Am J Hypertens 1995;8(7):657–65.

58. Carson AP, Howard G, Burke GL, et al. Ethnic differences in hypertension incidence among middle-aged and older adults: the multi-ethnic study of atherosclerosis. Hypertension 2011;57(6):1101–7.

59. Calhoun DA, Nishizaka MK, Zaman MA, et al. Hyperaldosteronism among black and white subjects with resistant hypertension. Hypertension 2002;40(6):892–6.

60. Chor D, Pinho Ribeiro AL, Sa Carvalho M, et al. Prevalence, awareness, treatment and influence of socioeconomic variables on control of high blood pressure: results of the ELSA-Brasil study. PLoS One 2015;10(6):e0127382.

61. Ge D, Young TW, Wang X, et al. Heritability of arterial stiffness in black and white American youth and young adults. Am J Hypertens 2007;20(10):1065–72.

62. Sherva R, Miller MB, Lynch AI, et al. A whole genome scan for pulse pressure/stroke volume ratio in African Americans: the HyperGEN study. Am J Hypertens 2007;20(4):398–402.

63. Chen W, Srinivasan SR, Boerwinkle E, et al. Beta-adrenergic receptor genes are associated with arterial stiffness in black and white adults: the Bogalusa Heart Study. Am J Hypertens 2007;20(12):1251–7.

64. Tu W, Li R, Bhalla V, et al. Age-related blood pressure sensitivity to aldosterone in blacks and whites. Hypertension 2018;72(1):247–52.

65. Spence JD, Rayner BL. Hypertension in blacks: individualized therapy based on renin/aldosterone phenotyping. Hypertension 2018;72(2):263–9.

66. Spence JD, Rayner BL. J curve and cuff artefact, and diagnostic inertia in resistant hypertension. Hypertension 2016;67(1):32–3.

67. Spence JD. Blood pressure control in Canada: the view from a stroke prevention clinic. Can J Cardiol 2015;31(5):593–5.

68. Brier ME, Luft FC. Sodium kinetics in white and black normotensive subjects: possible relevance to salt-sensitive hypertension. Am J Med Sci 1994;307(Suppl 1):S38–42.

69. Helmer OM, Judson WE. Metabolic studies on hypertensive patients with suppressed plasma renin activity not due to hyperaldosternosm. Circulation 1968;38(5):965–76.

70. Wilson DK, Bayer L, Krishnamoorthy JS, et al. The prevalence of salt sensitivity in an African-American adolescent population. Ethn Dis 1999;9(3):350–8.

71. Tu W, Eckert GJ, Hannon TS, et al. Racial differences in sensitivity of blood pressure to aldosterone. Hypertension 2014;63(6):1212–8.

72. Li R, Richey PA, DiSessa TG, et al. Blood aldosterone-to-renin ratio, ambulatory blood pressure, and left ventricular mass in children. J Pediatr 2009;155(2):170–5.

73. Gillum RF. Pathophysiology of hypertension in blacks and whites. A review of the basis of racial blood pressure differences. Hypertension 1979;1(5):468–75.

74. Monticone S, Losano I, Tetti M, et al. Diagnostic approach to low-renin hypertension. Clin Endocrinol (Oxf) 2018;89(4):385–96.

75. Rayner BL, Myers JE, Opie LH, et al. Screening for primary aldosteronism–normal ranges for aldosterone and renin in three South African population groups. S Afr Med J 2001;91(7):594–9.

76. Gafane LF, Schutte R, Van Rooyen JM, et al. Plasma renin and cardiovascular responses to the cold pressor test differ in black and white populations: The SABPA study. J Hum Hypertens 2016;30(5):346–51.

77. van Rooyen JM, Poglitsch M, Huisman HW, et al. Quantification of systemic renin-angiotensin system peptides of hypertensive black and white African men established from the RAS-Fingerprint(R). J Renin Angiotensin Aldosterone Syst 2016; 17(4) [pii:1470320316669880].

78. Rayner BL, Owen EP, King JA, et al. A new mutation, R563Q, of the beta subunit of the epithelial sodium channel associated with low-renin, low-aldosterone hypertension. J Hypertens 2003;21(5):921–6.

79. Tetti M, Monticone S, Burrello J, et al. Liddle syndrome: review of the literature and description of a new case. Int J Mol Sci 2018;19(3) [pii:E812].

80. Grim CE, Robinson M. Salt, slavery and survival- hypertension in the African diaspora. Epidemiology 2003;14(1):120–2 [discussion: 124–6].

81. Jones ES, Spence JD, McIntyre AD, et al. High frequency of variants of candidate genes in black Africans with low renin-resistant hypertension. Am J Hypertens 2017;30(5):478–83.

82. Nanba K, Omata K, Gomez-Sanchez CE, et al. Genetic characteristics of aldosterone-producing adenomas in blacks. Hypertension 2019;73(4):885–92.

83. Zilbermint M, Xekouki P, Faucz FR, et al. Primary aldosteronism and ARMC5 variants. J Clin Endocrinol Metab 2015;100(6):E900–9.

84. Spence JD. Physiologic tailoring of therapy for resistant hypertension: 20 years' experience with stimulated renin profiling. Am J Hypertens 1999;12(11 Pt 1): 1077–83.

85. Wilson TW, Grim CE. Biohistory of slavery and blood pressure differences in blacks today. A hypothesis. Hypertension 1991;17(1 Suppl):I122–8.

86. Tishkoff SA, Reed FA, Friedlaender FR, et al. The genetic structure and history of Africans and African Americans. Science 2009;324(5930):1035–44.

87. Brown AGM, Houser RF, Mattei J, et al. Hypertension among US-born and foreign-born non-Hispanic blacks: National Health and Nutrition Examination Survey 2003-2014 data. J Hypertens 2017;35(12):2380–7.

88. Spence JD. Hypertension in US-born vs. foreign-born African-Americans. J Hypertens 2017;35(12):2369–71.

89. Biglieri EG, Kater CE, Arteaga EE. Primary aldosteronism is comprised of primary adrenal hyperplasia and adenoma. J Hypertens Suppl 1984;2(3):S259–61.

90. Banks WA, Kastin AJ, Biglieri EG, et al. Primary adrenal hyperplasia: a new subset of primary hyperaldosteronism. J Clin Endocrinol Metab 1984;58(5):783–5.

91. Spence JD. The current epidemic of primary aldosteronism: causes and consequences. J Hypertens 2004;22(10):2038–9 [author reply: 2039].

92. Calhoun DA, Booth JN 3rd, Oparil S, et al. Refractory hypertension: determination of prevalence, risk factors, and comorbidities in a large, population-based cohort. Hypertension 2014;63(3):451–8.

93. Williams B, MacDonald TM, Morant S, et al. Spironolactone versus placebo, bisoprolol, and doxazosin to determine the optimal treatment for drug-resistant hypertension (PATHWAY-2): a randomised, double-blind, crossover trial. Lancet 2015; 386(10008):2059–68.

94. Saha C, Eckert GJ, Ambrosius WT, et al. Improvement in blood pressure with inhibition of the epithelial sodium channel in blacks with hypertension. Hypertension 2005;46(3):481–7.

95. Laffer CL, Elijovich F, Eckert GJ, et al. Genetic variation in CYP4A11 and blood pressure response to mineralocorticoid receptor antagonism or ENaC inhibition: an exploratory pilot study in African Americans. J Am Soc Hypertens 2014;8(7): 475–80.

96. Tapolyai M, Uysal A, Dossabhoy NR, et al. High prevalence of liddle syndrome phenotype among hypertensive US Veterans in Northwest Louisiana. J Clin Hypertens (Greenwich) 2010;12(11):856–60.

97. Egan BM, Basile JN, Rehman SU, et al. Plasma renin test-guided drug treatment algorithm for correcting patients with treated but uncontrolled hypertension: a randomized controlled trial. Am J Hypertens 2009;22(7):792–801.

98. Akintunde A, Nondi J, Gogo K, et al. Physiological phenotyping for personalized therapy of uncontrolled hypertension in Africa. Am J Hypertens 2017;30(9): 923–30.

Evaluation and Management of Endocrine Hypertension During Pregnancy

Salvatore M. Corsello, MD, Rosa Maria Paragliola, MD, PhD*

KEYWORDS

- Hypertension • Pheochromocytoma • Hyperaldosteronism • Cushing syndrome
- Pregnancy

KEY POINTS

- The diagnosis of endocrine hypertension in pregancy based on clinical suspicion often can be difficult. In many cases, symptoms in pregnant patients can be similar to those detected in preeclampsia. Differential diagnosis is mandatory.
- The biochemical diagnosis of endocrine hypertension in pregnancy can be challenging. Physiologic changes of renin-angiotensin-aldosterone system and physiologic hypercortisolism make the diagnosis more difficult.
- The medical management of secondary hypertension in pregnancy is the most crucial challenge. The choice of the more suitable medical therapy is related to a careful evaluation of the risks and benefits. In particular, it is mandatory to consider the possible teratogenic effects of several drugs usually used in nonpregnant patients affected by Cushing syndrome and primary hyperaldosteronism.
- Surgery often is considered the therapy of choice, in particular for pheochromocytoma and Cushing syndrome.

INTRODUCTION

Hypertension is a common clinical problem in pregnancy and represents a possible short-term and long-term risk of complications for both mothers and babies. Hypertension can affect approximately 6% to 8% of all pregnant women. A large observational study about chronic hypertension in pregnancy, reported that approximately 46% of patients with mild gestational hypertension develop preeclampsia, with progression to severe disease in 9.6%.[1]

In a majority of cases (88%), hypertension is essential, whereas secondary causes are more rare and affect less than 1% of pregnancies.[2] Secondary hypertension can

Endocrinology, Fondazione Policlinico Universitario Agostino Gemelli, IRCCS - Università Cattolica del Sacro Cuore, Largo Agostino Gemelli 8, I-00168, Rome, Italy
* Corresponding author.
E-mail address: rosamariaparagliola@gmail.com

Endocrinol Metab Clin N Am 48 (2019) 829–842
https://doi.org/10.1016/j.ecl.2019.08.011
0889-8529/19/© 2019 Elsevier Inc. All rights reserved.

be the result of various endocrine and renal disorders. A prompt and correct diagnosis is mandatory, to avoid the increased risk of adverse outcome.

In this review, the most important causes of endocrine hypertension in pregnancy are discussed, focusing on the importance of a prompt diagnosis and adequate treatment.

ENDOCRINE HYPERTENSION DURING PREGNANCY

The most important causes of endocrine hypertension in pregnancy are

- Primary hyperaldosteronism (PA)
- Pheochromocytoma (PCC)/paraganglioma (PG)
- Cushing syndrome (CS)

Primary Hyperaldosteronism

Causes and epidemiology of primary hyperaldosteronism

In the general population, PA represents the most common cause of endocrine hypertension. Reported for the first time in 1954 by Conn,[3] this condition has been described as a clinical syndrome characterized by hypertension, hypokalemia, and metabolic alkalosis resulting from autonomous production of aldosterone due to an adrenal adenoma.[3]

Currently, it has been estimated that unilateral adrenal adenoma accounts for 30% to 40% of PA cases, whereas the remaining 60% are caused by bilateral adrenal hyperplasia.[4] Recent data suggest molecular alterations (genetic variants in potassium channel genes) as causes of inappropriate aldosterone secretion.[5]

The prevalence of PA has been debated in recent years. This condition has been underestimated because the presence of hypokalemia was considered essential for the diagnosis. Recent data report that hypokalemia is present in only a small group of patients (9%–37%),[6] allowing extending biochemical screening for PA in patients with resistant hypertension and without hypokalemia. Consequently, if in the past PA was believed to account for less than 1% of hypertension, more recent studies reported a prevalence ranging up to 20%, especially in selected hypertensive patients (those with resistant hypertension, diabetes, and sleep apnea).[7]

In pregnancy, hyperaldosteronism is more rare: it has been extrapolated that PA can be diagnosed in 0.6% to 0.8% of pregnancies.[2] In the literature, approximately 50 cases of pregnant women with PA have been reported, but probably the incidence is significantly underestimated due to the difficult diagnosis.

Diagnosis of primary hyperaldosteronism in pregnancy

During pregnancy physiologic changes of the renin-angiotensin-aldosterone (RAA) system occur, making a diagnosis of PA more difficult. During pregnancy, the components of RAA system are stimulated,[8] in particular due to the role of extrarenal tissues.

The placenta represents one of the most important extrarenal RAA system.[9] Renin activity increases due to extrarenal synthesis by ovaries and maternal decidua.[10] It has been estimated that plasma renin activity (PRA) rises by approximately 4-fold in the first 8 weeks and by 7-fold in the third trimester.[11]

Estrogens stimulate the hepatic synthesis of angiotensinogen, leading to increased serum angiotensin II and aldosterone levels. Even if angiotensin II levels are increased during pregnancy, however, in normotensive conditions pregnant women are refractory to its vasopressor effects, probably due to the role of progesterone and prostacyclins, which can decrease the sensitivity to angiotensin II action.[9]

Aldosterone levels during pregnancy can reach concentrations 10-fold higher than baseline.[12] Its production remains sensitive to the physiologic regulation but less than in nonpregnant women. Furthermore, the physiologic effects of aldosterone are attenuated by progesterone, which represents a competitor of aldosterone in the distal convoluted tubule.[12] Therefore, despite the marked increase in blood volume, necessary to obtain an adequate placental perfusion, pregnant women are usually normotensive thank to the antagonizing effects of progesterone.

On the contrary, the reduction in sodium excretion during the standing position is higher during pregnancy.

Angiotensin-converting enzyme is the only component of RRA system that decreases during normotensive pregnancy,[13] even if can be increased in preeclamptic patients.[9]

On the basis of these physiopathologic changes, pregnancy is a condition of hyperreninemic hyperaldosteronism and the aldosterone-renin ratio during gestation can decrease, causing a false-negative result. An elevated aldosterone-renin ratio with suppressed PRA levels has been reported in approximately 60% of women with PA in pregnancy.[11] Malha and August propose[2] considering, for the diagnosis of PA in pregnancy, elevated plasma aldosterone together with PRA less than 4 ng/mL/h in the presence of hypertension and hypokalemia. Hypokalemia was reported in 25 of 37 pregnancies (68%) for which a value for serum potassium was available.[11]

Saline infusion or fludrocortisone suppression tests only rarely have been performed in pregnancy, considering the potential risk to increase the volume expansion occurring during gestation.[11] Magnetic resonance imaging (MRI) may be performed during the second or third trimester to determine the subtype of PA, whereas adrenal vein sampling is not performed because of the excess of radiation exposure.[11]

Management of primary hyperaldosteronism in pregnancy

Pregnancies in patients with PA thus have high risks of complications. No formal recommendations for the management of these patients have been proposed, however, even if several suggestions can be found in the literature. In particular, if the diagnosis is made before the conception:

- If aldosterone secretion is unilateral, adrenalectomy must be planned before the conception.
- If aldosterone secretion is due to bilateral adrenal hyperplasia, spironolactone or other drugs should be stopped approximately (at least) 1 month before conception. Pregnancy must be programmed and the PA adequately treated with the therapy usually recommended during pregnancy (α-methyldopa and β-blockers). Serum potassium must be periodically checked.

Spironolactone, which crosses the placenta, should be avoided during pregnancy because of its antiandrogenic effect and the risk of feminization of males.[12] The possible intrauterine growth retardation related to the natriuretic effect of the spironolactone also should be considered.[14] Studies on animal models suggest some caution in the use of spironolactone during the first weeks of pregnancy,[12] even if in humans data in about the effects on sexual development are conflicting. A case of sexual ambiguity in the female fetus of a woman treated with spironolactone until the fifth month of pregnancy has been reported, even if the relationship between sexual ambiguity and spironolactone has not been certainly proved.[12] Other studies report favorable outcomes of newborns exposed to spironolactone in utero.[12]

On the contrary, eplerenone has neither androgenic nor teratogenic effects. Few cases about the use of eplerenone during pregnancy have been described, with normal pregnancies and healthy offspring.[15] There are insufficient recommendations, however, about the use of eplerenone in pregnancy, due to lack of experience and marketing authorization for the treatment of PA.

Literature suggests the possible use of thiazides or amiloride both before and during pregnancy, on the basis of blood pressure and serum potassium.[12] The safety of amiloride during pregnancy, however, is still uncertain. A reasonable approach, both for diagnosis made before and during pregnancy, may be to use in the first instance drugs known to be safe during the first trimester. In cases of poor control of hypertension and/or hypokalemia, the use of thiazides, amiloride, or alternatively spironolactone should be considered during the second and third trimesters.[11]

Regarding unilateral aldosterone secreting adenoma detected during pregnancy, the benefit of adrenalectomy is unclear and the experience is based on case reports or case series. Adverse outcomes have been reported in 44% of pregnancies after laparoscopic adrenalectomy.[11] Despite the biochemical cure of inappropriate aldosterone secretion, significant fetal morbidity and mortality have been reported (intrauterine fetal death[16] as well as preterm deliveries associated with fetal distress[11]). It cannot be excluded, however, that intrauterine fetal death has been caused by reduced fetal blood flow (related to hypertension in mother) already present before surgery.[16] Other investigators report favorable outcomes,[17–19] concluding that laparoscopic adrenalectomy can be performed safety in pregnancy as long as preoperative adequate blood pressure control has been obtained. The more reasonable option is to perform adrenalectomy during the early second trimester, with open pneumoperitoneum creation and with less than 12 mm Hg pressure of pneumoperitoneum.[19] Fetal monitoring is mandatory during the procedure.

Pheochromocytoma/Paraganglioma

Epidemiology and clinical features of pheochromocytoma /paraganglioma in pregnancy

PCC in pregnancy is a rare condition, with a reported incidence of about 0.007%.[20,21] Correct diagnosis and a prompt treatment are mandatory to reduce fetal and maternal mortality which, if untreated, reaches approximately 40% to 50%.[22]

Diagnosis usually is made in prenatal period in 73% of cases, during the second trimester in 32%, and during the third trimester in 42%. Therefore, in 27% of cases the diagnosis was missed and the tumor is diagnosed as a result of an acute complication.[23]

The fetus is not exposed to maternal circulating levels of catecholamines due to the high placental expression of catechol O-methyltransferase and monoamine oxidase.[24] The placental exposure to maternal hypertension and to high catecholamines levels, however, can cause constriction of the maternal uterine circulation, inducing uteroplacental insufficiency. This may determinate spontaneous abortion, fetal growth restriction, fetal hypoxia, and intrauterine fetal death.[23] The fetal mortality rate related to maternal PCC dramatically decreased during the last decades from 55% (1969) to 7% if PCC is diagnosed antenatally.[25]

PCC in pregnancy is adrenal in 80% of cases and extra-adrenal in the remaining 20% of cases. Cases of concurrent bilateral PCC and extra-adrenal PG also have been reported.[23]

Pregnant woman with PCC sometimes can be asymptomatic.[25] In a majority of cases, however, symptoms of PCC in pregnant patients are similar to those detected in nonpregnant patients. The symptoms can progress because of several precipitating factors (increased intra-abdominal pressure due to the growing uterus, uterine contractions, fetal movements, labor and delivery, and finally anesthesia and surgery), which could stimulate the release of catecholamines.[23] Hypertension represents the most frequent symptom, reported in approximately 87% of cases. PCC-related hypotension is found in approximately 50% of the patients.[26] Furthermore, clinical presentation may include nonspecific signs and symptoms that usually are related to pregnancy or to other diseases in pregnancy (gestational hypertension, preeclampsia, eclampsia, gestational diabetes mellitus, and hyperemesis).

A rare but potential fatal complication of PCC is the development of a catecholamine-induced cardiomyopathy, manifesting as acute heart failure, cardiogenic shock, or acute coronary syndrome. This condition is seen more frequently during peripartum period[27,28] but it also can manifest as acute myocardial infarction during pregnancy.[29] In severe cases of multiple organ failure, intrauterine fetal death can occur.[30]

Diagnosis of pheochromocytoma in pregnancy

In the clinical suspicion of PCC, the differential diagnosis with preeclampsia is mandatory, because the diagnosis can be misleading (**Table 1**).[25]

The clinical suspicion of PCC must be confirmed by increased catecholamines or their metabolites levels. The most sensitive test currently available is represented by plasmatic and urinary metanephrines.[31] Catecholamine metabolism is unaltered during healthy pregnancy, and in patients with preeclampsia plasma catecholamine levels are only slightly increased.[32] Possible interferences must be considered if patients are using α-methyldopa or labetalol, which can determinate false-positive results.[33]

In cases of increased metanephrines levels, additional imaging studies are mandatory to confirm the diagnosis. As is well known, imaging based on ionizing radiation exposure is contraindicated in pregnancy for the possible negative effects on fetal outcome.[34] In pregnant women, ultrasound and MRI are the imaging techniques more used to localize a tumor. In the suspicion of PCC or abdominal PG, abdominal ultrasound can be useful (**Fig. 1**), even if it lacks sensitivity, particularly during the third trimester, when the enlarged uterus interferes with retroperitoneal examination. Neck ultrasound can be performed if a rare head-and-neck catecholamine-secreting tumor is suspected.[23]

Usually MRI is used for the diagnosis of PCC in pregnancy. This examination is considered accurate even if without gadolinium (**Fig. 2**), although gadolinium is not considered contraindicated during pregnancy.[35]

Meta-iodobenzylguanidine scintiscan is not considered safe for the fetus because of radioactive exposure.

After diagnosis and during follow-up, genetic consultation should be considered, because disease-related mutations can be found in approximately 30% of cases of PCC diagnosed during pregnancy, an incidence similar to that detected in nonpregnant population.[23]

The susceptibility genes that have been identified for PCC include *NF1*, *RET*, *Von Hippel Lindau (VHL)*, succinate dehydrogenase subunits (*SDHA*, *SDHB*, *SDHC*, and *SDHD*), cofactor for succinate dehydrogenase complex (*SDHAF2*), *TMEM127*, *MAX*, *EGLN1/PHD2*, *EGLN2/PHD1*, *KIF1β*, *IDH1*, *HIF2α*, *FH*, and *ATRX*.[23]

Treatment of pheochromocytoma in pregnancy

The mainstay of the management of PCC in pregnancy is the pretreatment with α-adrenergic receptor blockade to reduce the effects of the inappropriate catecholamines secretion and the surgical removal of the tumor. The recommendations for the treatment in pregnancy mainly derive by case reports, case series, and reviews reported in the literature.

Table 1
Differential diagnosis between pheochromocytoma and preeclampsia

	Pheochromocytoma	Preeclampsia
Hypertension	• Any gestational phase • Usually severe and paroxysmal • Orthostatic hypotension in up to 50% of cases	• Usually during second or third trimester • Usually moderate and sustained • Orthostatic hypotension is uncommon
Possible symptoms associated with hypertension	• Headache, sweating, tachycardia, pallor, visual abnormalities, nausea, chest pain, dyspnea	• Can be associated with headache, visual abnormalities, upper abdominal or epigastric pain, nausea, oliguria, chest pain, dyspnea, altered mental status
Ankle edema	Usually absent	Present
Proteinuria	Usually absent	Present ($\geq$300 mg in a 24-h urine specimen)
Weight gain	Usually absent (catecholamine-induced hypermetabolism)	Excess weight and increased weight gain during pregnancy predispose women to preeclampsia.
Plasma or 24-h urinary metanephrines	High levels	Normal levels
Plasma or 24-h urinary catecholamines	Normal or high levels	High levels have been rarely reported in severe cases of preeclampsia.
Other laboratory abnormalities	• Hyperglycemia • Glycosuria • Deranged liver function tests (rare) • Coagulation abnormalities (rare)	• High levels of serum uric acid • Serum creatinine >1.2 mg/dL (106 mmol/L) • Platelet count <100,000 cells/mm^3 • Microangiopathic hemolytic anemia ($\uparrow$ lactic acid dehydrogenase, $\uparrow$ bilirubin, $\downarrow$ serum haptoglobin levels, abnormal peripheral smear) • Elevated liver enzymes (twice the upper limit of normal)
Medical history	• Personal and/or familial history of PCC, PG, or genetic syndromes associated with catecholamine-secreting tumors (MEN2A, MEN2B, Neurofibromatosis type 1; VHL disease type 2; germline mutations of SDH subunits and cofactor genes; germline mutation of TMEM127 gene; germline mutation of MAX gene) • Multigravida women who have severe hypertension but no prior history of preeclampsia	• Personal and/or familial history of preeclampsia • Maternal age >40 y or <18 y • Nulliparity • Multifetal gestation • Black race • Preexisting medical conditions: body mass index $\geq$26.1; pregestational diabetes; chronic hypertension; chronic renal disease; antiphospholipid antibody syndrome or inherited thrombophilia; vascular or connective tissue disease

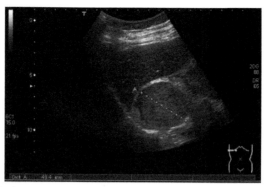

Fig. 1. Abdominal ultrasound performed in a 27-week pregnant patient with clinical and laboratory diagnosis of PCC. The examination reveals a 5-cm inhomogeneous, solid mass, isoechoic and characterized by peripheral vascularization (Salvatore M. Corsello, MD, personal communication, 2013).

Preoperative medical treatment Pretreatment with α-adrenergic receptor blockade results in a lower risk of perioperative and postoperative complications, because medical treatment assures a reduction in blood pressure and a reduced risk of paroxysmal blood pressure increase. There are not suggestions about the target of blood pressure in pregnant patients. In general, the target for chronic hypertension in pregnancy is less than 150/100 mm Hg (and diastolic blood pressure >80 mm Hg) in absence of signs of end-organ damage and less than

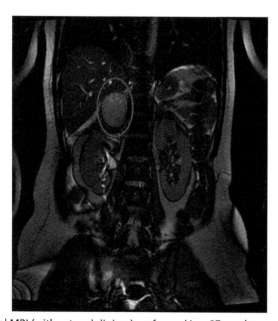

Fig. 2. Abdominal MRI (without gadolinium) performed in a 27-week pregnant patient with clinical and laboratory diagnosis of PCC. The MRI shows a 6-cm right adrenal mass (*red circle*), highly hyperintense in T2-weighted sequences. In this patient, the diagnosis has been confirmed by final histology (Salvatore M. Corsello, MD, personal communication, 2013).

140/90 mm Hg in presence of signs of end-organ damage.[32] In PCC pregnant patients, however, both an excess of catecholamines and a relative hypotension can compromise the uteroplacental circulation, which is directly affected by changes in maternal blood pressure. Therefore, the management of α-adrenergic receptor blockade is based on a delicate balance between the treatment of maternal hypertension and the maintenance of an adequate uteroplacental circulation.[32]

The treatment with α-adrenergic receptor blockade must be started for at least 10 days to 14 days before surgery. The most commonly used α-adrenergic receptor blockers are phenoxybenzamine (10–40 mg twice a day) and doxazosin (4–16 mg twice a day).[35]

Pregnant patients with normal blood pressure should be treated with low-dose α-adrenergic blockers as well to prevent paroxysmal peaks in blood pressure.

Phenoxybenzamine, which has been widely used for the favorable neonatal outcomes, is supposed to pass the placenta. As discussed previously, the fetus is not exposed to the effects of catecholamines for the activity of the catechol O-methyltransferase and of the monoamine oxidase in placental cells. Therefore, the fetus is exposed to a useless transplacental administration. Furthermore, phenoxybenzamine has been reported in association with neonatal hypotension and respiratory depression, and closely monitoring of the neonates born from mothers treated with phenoxybenzamine is recommended.[23] Doxazosin has been used more often during pregnancy, with good neonatal outcomes. Doxazosin is associated with lower incidence of reflex tachycardia and postoperative hypotension in mother. Furthermore, even if the drug crosses the placenta, neonatal hypotension and respiratory depression have not been reported.[26]

β-Adrenergic receptor blockers can be added to the treatment to contrast tachyarrhythmias and the possible α-adrenergic receptor blockade–associated reflex tachycardia.[23] This class is associated, however, with intrauterine growth restriction and their use is generally recommended only for a short period during pregnancy.[36]

If the hypertension is not adequately treated with α-adrenergic receptor blockade and there is not tachycardia, calcium channel blockers can be added to the treatment.[35]

Labetalol, which has a combined α-blocker and action β-blocker and often is suggested as single agent in the treatment of PCC, is not recommended in pregnancy, because of its relatively weak α-blockade activity, resulting in paroxysmal hypertension.[37] α-Methyldopa, the most frequently used drug to treat essential hypertension during pregnancy, is not recommended in pregnant patients with PCC because it can worsen hypertension.[23]

Finally, it is crucial to underline that several drugs commonly prescribed in pregnancy must be avoided in patients with PCC, because they can induce a PCC crisis. These drugs include corticosteroids, opioids (morphine), antiemetics (metoclopramide), anesthetics (thiopental, ketamine, and ephedrine), and muscle relaxants (mivacurium).[32]

Surgery Surgery represents the definitive treatment of PCC also in pregnancy. The time of surgery depends on gestational age, location of tumor, and maternal and fetal response to the medical treatment. The adrenalectomy should be planned at least 10 days to 14 days after starting medical treatment.[23]

When the diagnosis is made within the twenty-fourth week of gestation, it generally is recommended to remove the tumor in the second trimester (after the completion of the organogenesis). On the contrary, if the diagnosis is performed in the third trimester, it is recommended to plan the adrenalectomy after delivery, because the enlarged uterus could diminish the accessibility of the tumor.[32] For pregnant women with PCC in situ, there is no consensus about the preferred modality of delivery. Some cases reported higher mortality rate after vaginal delivery and cesarean was considered the preferred route of delivery.[32] Cesarean can cause, however, an excessive blood loss and can induce a catecholamine release due to the manipulation of the peritoneum. Furthermore, more recent literature describes successful vaginal delivery due to the current adequate obstetric and anesthesiologic management.[26] In particular, the epidural analgesia reduces pain and stress.

Cushing Syndrome in Pregnancy

Epidemiology and clinical features of cushing syndrome in pregnancy

CS in pregnancy is an extremely rare disorder in consideration of the influence of hypercortisolism on the hypothalamic-pituitary-gonadal axis, which causes impaired ovulation and reduces the fertility. A de novo diagnosis of CS during pregnancy is challenging for both diagnosis and treatment. The diagnosis can be difficult, considering the physiologic variations of hypothalamic-pituitary-adrenal axis during pregnancy and the factors that interfere with the biochemical cortisol evaluation. On the other hand, a correct diagnostic approach is mandatory, because untreated CS in pregnancy increases the risk of complications, both for mother and fetus. In the literature, fewer than 300 cases of CS in pregnancy have been reported.

A systematic review,[38] including 263 pregnancies with both active CS during pregnancy and treated and cured CS at the time of gestation, demonstrates that patients with active hypercortisolism had more problems in pregnancy and a worst fetal outcome. Women with active CS in pregnancy are at risk of developing gestational diabetes mellitus, gestational hypertension, and preeclampsia, compared with those with cured disease. Furthermore, fetal loss is higher in noncured CS in pregnancy and a diagnosis performed during pregnancy is predictor of increased risk of fetal mortality. Treatment of hypercortisolism (medical treatment or surgery) during pregnancy seemed protective in avoiding fetal loss.[38] Heart failure and psychiatric disorders also have been reported[39] Adrenal adenoma is the main cause of active CS during pregnancy (44.1%).[38]

Even if the fetus is partially protected from the hypercortisolemia by the activity of the placental 11β-hydroxysteroid dehydrogenase, which converts the 85% of maternal cortisol to biologically inactive cortisone,[40] neonatal complications are possible and include intrauterine deaths/spontaneous abortions, still births, premature delivery, intrauterine growth retardation, and neonatal adrenal insufficiency.[39]

A diagnosis of CS also can be performed in the postpartum period. A recent study reveals that more than one-quarter of women of reproductive age with CS had symptomatic disease within 1 year of childbirth.[41] Possible causal relationships are the stress of pregnancy and the pituitary corticotroph hyperactivity in the peripartum period.[41]

Diagnosis of cushing syndrome in pregnancy

On the basis of clinical features, patients can be divided in 3 groups:

1. Patients with known CS in pregnancy
2. Patients with de novo diagnosis of CS during pregnancy
3. Patients who develop clinical features and complications similar to CS during pregnancy (striae rubrae, arterial hypertension, and diabetes mellitus)

Pregnancy is a physiologic state of hypercortisolism related to the activation of the hypothalamic-pituitary-adrenal axis. Corticotropin-releasing hormone (CRH) plays an important role on maturation of the fetal adrenal gland and fetal-placental unit circulation. CRH production also occurs in thecal and stromal cells as well as in cells of the ovarian corpora luteum,[42] and CRH receptors are expressed by the epithelial cells of the endometrium. During pregnancy, CRH and corticotropin levels increase in the first trimester due to placental production. Under this stimulation, maternal adrenal glands gradually become hypertrophic, resulting in a small rise of cortisol levels, while the circadian rhythm is maintained.[43]

The high levels of estradiol in pregnancy cause an increase of corticosteroid-binding globulin (which is highest at the end of pregnancy) which in turn causes an overestimation of the serum total cortisol measured by commercial assays.[44] Serum free cortisol also increases (approximately 1.6-fold by the eleventh week of pregnancy) as a consequence of the pregnancy-induced hypothalamic-pituitary-adrenal activation. Therefore, urinary free cortisol increases up to 3-fold the normal range. Finally, the suppression of cortisol to low-dose dexamethasone suppression test is lower compared with the nonpregnant state[45] and the interference of estrogen-induced corticosteroid-binding globulin production also has to be considered in this test. Thus, the biochemical diagnosis of CS during pregnancy is more challenging than in the nonpregnant state.

The interpretation of biochemical test in pregnancy differs from that of nonpregnant patients. There are no pregnancy-specific guidelines about the biochemical diagnosis, but the combined use of urinary free cortisol and late-night salivary cortisol is recommended (**Tables 2** and **3**).[45,46]

An evaluation of circadian rhythm of cortisol secretion is suggested, because in normal pregnancy it is usually conserved despite higher serum and urinary cortisol levels.

Salivary cortisol represents an easy method to detect hypercortisolism. A recent study has determinate the reference values of night salivary cortisol in the 3 gestational trimesters (see **Table 3**).[47]

After the confirmation of hypercortisolism, corticotropin levels must be measured. In physiologic conditions, plasma corticotropin concentrations are lower during early pregnancy but gradually increase to slightly above normal, probably due to placental corticotropin and CRH secretion.[43] This is the reason why corticotropin may not be suppressed in patients with cortisol-secreting adrenal adenomas.[39] For the same reason, patients with CS diagnosed during pregnancy could have corticotropin levels in the upper normal range or even higher.[39]

Differential diagnosis for the corticotropin-dependent forms is the same than in nonpregnant patients: both high-dose dexamethasone suppression test and 100-μg CRH stimulation test correctly identified the cases of CS reported.[48] High-dose dexamethasone suppression test also can be helpful in identifying adrenal causes of CS (in which, as discussed previously, corticotropin can be not suppressed). Patients with adrenal etiology do not suppress,[49] whereas those with CS suppress serum cortisol.[39]

Table 2		
Biochemical test recommended for the diagnosis of Cushing syndrome in pregnancy		
Test	**Interpretation**	**Recommended Use**
Urinary free cortisol	More than 4 times the upper limit of normal	Yes
Salivary cortisol	Two to 3 times above the upper limit of normal	Yes
Low dose dexamethasone suppression test	Suppression of cortisol by dexamethasone is blunted, particularly in the second and third trimesters (risk of false-positive results)	NO

Table 3	
Reference values of night salivary cortisol in the 3 gestational trimesters	
Trimester	**Cutoff for Midnight Salivary Cortisol Value**[a]
First trimester	0.25 μg/dL
Second trimester	0.26 μg/dL
Third trimester	0.33 μg/dL

[a] In this study,[44] the upper reference value for nocturnal salivary cortisol of nonpregnant adults for this enzyme-linked immunosorbent assay method was 0.12 mg/dL.

The bilateral inferior petrosal sinus sampling should be performed only if strictly necessary, considering the radiation exposure and the thromboembolic events.[39]

About clinical imaging, performing abdominal ultrasound is suggested as the first step for the differential diagnosis, considering that adrenal adenoma is the most common cause of CS in pregnancy.[46] If necessary, abdominal MRI can be considered. In the suspicion of pituitary etiology, nongadolinium MRI may identify small microadenomas,[42] but it is mandatory to consider that the physiologic pituitary enlargement during pregnancy may mask a small tumor.

Management of cushing syndrome during pregnancy
Experience in treatment of CS in pregnancy derives from single small case series. The decision making is related to the severity of hypercortisolism: not all pregnant patients with active CS underwent treatment of hypercortisolism and the management can be conservative and based on the treatment of the metabolic comorbidities.

In general, however, in pregnancy, is considered the second line treatment after surgery.[50] Radiotherapy and mitotane are contraindicated for delayed results and potential teratogenic effects, respectively.[43]

Surgery should be evaluated on the basis of the severity of hypercortisolism and the timing of gestation.

Pituitary surgery can be performed between the end of first trimester and early second trimester with a lower rate of maternal and fetal complications.[43] Unilateral adrenalectomy, indicated for corticotropin-independent CS, can be performed at 16 weeks to 21 weeks of pregnancy.[46]

Medical therapy, usually starting in the second or third trimester, is considered the second line of treatment option after surgery. The most frequent option is based on steroidogenesis inhibitors use, in particular metyrapone.[51] Its most frequent side effects, related to the increase of precursors (11-deoxycorticosterone), are hypertension and risk for preeclampsia. It may become necessary to induce early delivery in presence of fetal complication related to eclampsia.[46]

Ketoconazole has been rarely used in pregnancy due to potential side effects (antiandrogenic effects and teratogenicity have been detected in animal studies, even if cases treated with ketoconazole in humans had good results).[43] Similarly, aminoglutethimide and mitotane can cause fetal masculinization and teratogenicity, respectively.[52] Pasireotide has not been used in pregnancy to date.

SUMMARY

The most important challenge in the management of hypertension in pregnancy is identifying the possible secondary causes and treating the potentially curable forms. This goal must be considered both during pregnancy and in women who would like to plan a pregnancy. No guidelines have been proposed for the diagnosis of the management of secondary hypertension in pregnancy, and operative suggestions derive from case reports, case series, and reviews.

The screening for secondary hypertension is mandatory in cases of suggestive clinical or biochemical features and the interpretation of biochemical test can be challenging, considering the physiologic changes occurring in pregnancy in the RRA system and the CRH-corticotropin-cortisol axis. Clinical management is very different on the basis on the underlying pathology.

In PA, the main goal is the medical treatment of hypertension, using as first choice drugs known to be safe in pregnancy and reserving the use of other drugs only for cases of uncontrolled blood pressure and hypokalemia. In CS, the choice of the treatment is related mainly to the severity of hypercortisolism. Normocortisolism can be achieved by pituitary or adrenal surgery preferably during the second trimester. In medical treatments, most experience has collected with metyrapone.

For PCC, surgery (after a careful preparation with medical therapy) represents the treatment of choice before the twenty-fourth week of gestation, although it can be postponed to the postpartum period if the pregnancy is more advanced. Thanks to the pretreatment of patients with α-blockade and technical progress in surgical and anesthesiologic techniques, over the last past decades, maternal and fetal prognosis improved extraordinarily.

REFERENCES

1. Barton JR, O'Brien JM, Bergauer NK, et al. Mild gestational hypertension remote from term: progression and outcome. Am J Obstet Gynecol 2001;184(5):979–83.
2. Malha L, August P. Secondary hypertension in pregnancy. Curr Hypertens Rep 2015;17(7):53.
3. Conn JW. The evolution of primary aldosteronism from 1954 to 1960. Acta Endocrinol Suppl (Copenh) 1960;34(Suppl 50):65–71.
4. Kaplan N. The current epidemic of primary aldosteronism: causes and consequences. J Hypertens 2004;22(5):863–9.
5. Xekouki P, Hatch MM, Lin L, et al. KCNJ5 mutations in the National Institutes of Health cohort of patients with primary hyperaldosteronism: an infrequent genetic cause of Conn's syndrome. Endocr Relat Cancer 2012;19(3):255–60.
6. Mulatero P, Stowasser M, Loh KC, et al. Increased diagnosis of primary aldosteronism, including surgically correctable forms, in centers from five continents. J Clin Endocrinol Metab 2004;89(3):1045–50.
7. Fagugli RM, Taglioni C. Changes in the perceived epidemiology of primary hyperaldosteronism. Int J Hypertens 2011;2011:162804.
8. Broughton Pipkin F. The renin-angiotensin system in pregnancy: why bother? Br J Obstet Gynaecol 1982;89(8):591–3.
9. Irani RA, Xia Y. The functional role of the renin-angiotensin system in pregnancy and preeclampsia. Placenta 2008;29(9):763–71.
10. Hsueh WA, Luetscher JA, Carlson EJ, et al. Changes in active and inactive renin throughout pregnancy. J Clin Endocrinol Metab 1982;54(5):1010–6.
11. Morton A. Primary aldosteronism and pregnancy. Pregnancy Hypertens 2015; 5(4):259–62.
12. Landau E, Amar L. Primary aldosteronism and pregnancy. Ann Endocrinol (Paris) 2016;77(2):148–60.
13. Merrill DC, Karoly M, Chen K, et al. Angiotensin-(1-7) in normal and preeclamptic pregnancy. Endocrine 2002;18(3):239–46.
14. Rigo J Jr, Glaz E, Papp Z. Low or high doses of spironolactone for treatment of maternal Bartter's syndrome. Am J Obstet Gynecol 1996;174(1 Pt 1):297.

15. Riester A, Reincke M. Progress in primary aldosteronism: mineralocorticoid receptor antagonists and management of primary aldosteronism in pregnancy. Eur J Endocrinol 2015;172(1):R23–30.
16. Kosaka K, Onoda N, Ishikawa T, et al. Laparoscopic adrenalectomy on a patient with primary aldosteronism during pregnancy. Endocr J 2006;53(4):461–6.
17. Baron F, Sprauve ME, Huddleston JF, et al. Diagnosis and surgical treatment of primary aldosteronism in pregnancy: a case report. Obstet Gynecol 1995;86(4 Pt 2):644–5.
18. Solomon CG, Thiet M, Moore F Jr, et al. Primary hyperaldosteronism in pregnancy. A case report. J Reprod Med 1996;41(4):255–8.
19. Shalhav AL, Landman J, Afane J, et al. Laparoscopic adrenalectomy for primary hyperaldosteronism during pregnancy. J Laparoendosc Adv Surg Tech A 2000; 10(3):169–71.
20. Harrington JL, Farley DR, van Heerden JA, et al. Adrenal tumors and pregnancy. World J Surg 1999;23(2):182–6.
21. Mannelli M, Bemporad D. Diagnosis and management of pheochromocytoma during pregnancy. J Endocrinol Invest 2002;25(6):567–71.
22. Schenker JG, Granat M. Phaeochromocytoma and pregnancy — an updated appraisal. Aust N Z J Obstet Gynaecol 1982;22(1):1–10.
23. Prete A, Paragliola RM, Salvatori R, et al. Management of catecholamine-secreting tumors in pregnancy: a review. Endocr Pract 2016;22(3):357–70.
24. Dahia PL, Hayashida CY, Strunz C, et al. Low cord blood levels of catecholamine from a newborn of a pheochromocytoma patient. Eur J Endocrinol 1994;130(3):217–9.
25. Iijima S. Impact of maternal pheochromocytoma on the fetus and neonate. Gynecol Endocrinol 2019;35(4):280–6.
26. Wing LA, Conaglen JV, Meyer-Rochow GY, et al. Paraganglioma in pregnancy: a case series and review of the literature. J Clin Endocrinol Metab 2015;100(8): 3202–9.
27. Cohen Y, Xing M, Mambo E, et al. BRAF mutation in papillary thyroid carcinoma. J Natl Cancer Inst 2003;95(8):625–7.
28. Rivkees SA, Mazzaferri EL, Verburg FA, et al. The treatment of differentiated thyroid cancer in children: emphasis on surgical approach and radioactive iodine therapy. Endocr Rev 2011;32(6):798–826.
29. Jessurun CR, Adam K, Moise KJ Jr, et al. Pheochromocytoma-induced myocardial infarction in pregnancy. A case report and literature review. Tex Heart Inst J 1993;20(2):120–2.
30. Cantwell-Dorris ER, O'Leary JJ, Sheils OM. BRAFV600E: implications for carcinogenesis and molecular therapy. Mol Cancer Ther 2011;10(3):385–94.
31. Boyle JG, Davidson DF, Perry CG, et al. Comparison of diagnostic accuracy of urinary free metanephrines, vanillyl mandelic Acid, and catecholamines and plasma catecholamines for diagnosis of pheochromocytoma. J Clin Endocrinol Metab 2007;92(12):4602–8.
32. van der Weerd K, van Noord C, Loeve M, et al. ENDOCRINOLOGY IN PREGNANCY: Pheochromocytoma in pregnancy: case series and review of literature. Eur J Endocrinol 2017;177(2):R49–58.
33. Kamoun M, Mnif MF, Charfi N, et al. Adrenal diseases during pregnancy: pathophysiology, diagnosis and management strategies. Am J Med Sci 2014;347(1): 64–73.
34. International Commission on Radiological Protection. Pregnancy and medical radiation. Ann ICRP 2000;30(1):1–43.

35. Lenders JW, Duh QY, Eisenhofer G, et al. Pheochromocytoma and paraganglioma: an endocrine society clinical practice guideline. J Clin Endocrinol Metab 2014;99(6):1915–42.
36. Butters L, Kennedy S, Rubin PC. Atenolol in essential hypertension during pregnancy. BMJ 1990;301(6752):587–9.
37. Lenders JW. Pheochromocytoma and pregnancy: a deceptive connection. Eur J Endocrinol 2012;166(2):143–50.
38. Caimari F, Valassi E, Garbayo P, et al. Cushing's syndrome and pregnancy outcomes: a systematic review of published cases. Endocrine 2017;55(2):555–63.
39. Lindsay JR, Jonklaas J, Oldfield EH, et al. Cushing's syndrome during pregnancy: personal experience and review of the literature. J Clin Endocrinol Metab 2005;90(5):3077–83.
40. Guilhaume B, Sanson ML, Billaud L, et al. Cushing's syndrome and pregnancy: aetiologies and prognosis in twenty-two patients. Eur J Med 1992;1(2):83–9.
41. Palejwala SK, Conger AR, Eisenberg AA, et al. Pregnancy-associated Cushing's disease? An exploratory retrospective study. Pituitary 2018;21(6):584–92.
42. Lindsay JR, Nieman LK. The hypothalamic-pituitary-adrenal axis in pregnancy: challenges in disease detection and treatment. Endocr Rev 2005;26(6):775–99.
43. Machado MC, Fragoso M, Bronstein MD. Pregnancy in Patients with Cushing's Syndrome. Endocrinol Metab Clin North Am 2018;47(2):441–9.
44. Nolten WE, Lindheimer MD, Rueckert PA, et al. Diurnal patterns and regulation of cortisol secretion in pregnancy. J Clin Endocrinol Metab 1980;51(3):466–72.
45. Odagiri E, Ishiwatari N, Abe Y, et al. Hypercortisolism and the resistance to dexamethasone suppression during gestation. Endocrinol Jpn 1988;35(5):685–90.
46. Nieman LK. Cushing's syndrome in pregnancy. Available at: https://www.uptodate.com/contents/cushings-syndrome-in-pregnancy. Accessed May 23, 2019.
47. Lopes LM, Francisco RP, Galletta MA, et al. Determination of nighttime salivary cortisol during pregnancy: comparison with values in non-pregnancy and Cushing's disease. Pituitary 2016;19(1):30–8.
48. Haugen BR, Sherman SI. Evolving approaches to patients with advanced differentiated thyroid cancer. Endocr Rev 2013;34(3):439–55.
49. Barasch E, Sztern M, Spinrad S, et al. Pregnancy and Cushing's syndrome: example of endocrine interaction. Isr J Med Sci 1988;24(2):101–4.
50. Vilar L, Freitas Mda C, Lima LH, et al. Cushing's syndrome in pregnancy: an overview. Arq Bras Endocrinol Metabol 2007;51(8):1293–302.
51. Lim WH, Torpy DJ, Jeffries WS. The medical management of Cushing's syndrome during pregnancy. Eur J Obstet Gynecol Reprod Biol 2013;168(1):1–6.
52. McClamrock HD, Adashi EY. Gestational hyperandrogenism. Fertil Steril 1992;57(2):257–74.

Adrenal Venous Sampling
Where Do We Stand?

Gian Paolo Rossi, MD[a],*, Giuseppe Maiolino, MD, PhD[b],
Teresa M. Seccia, MD, PhD[b]

KEYWORDS

• Aldosterone • Diagnosis • Hyperaldosteronism • Adrenal vein sampling

KEY POINTS

• The high diagnostic accuracy, minimal rate of complications, and better outcome with adrenal venous sampling-guided adrenalectomy support the guidelines recommendation that adrenal venous sampling should serve as the gold standard diagnostic test for the subtyping of primary aldosteronism.
• With some exceptions, adrenal venous sampling should be used systematically before referring a patient to the surgeon.
• As for all invasive diagnostic tests appropriate training of the interventionists, a tight collaboration with experienced endocrinologists and hypertensiologists is needed.
• Adherence to the suggestions that are herein summarized for the interpretation of the test will make the best clinical use of adrenal venous sampling for the doctor and for the patient.

INTRODUCTION

Primary aldosteronism (PA) is the most common endocrine form of hypertension and carries an increased risk of damage to the target organs of hypertension with ensuing cardiorenal complications.[1–3] Accordingly, early identification of affected patients followed by early institution of a specific treatment is a key step for prevention of cardiovascular events and reversal of damage.

Selection of the most appropriate treatment for patients with PA requires the distinction between bilateral and unilateral forms of PA. The former comprise adrenal hyperplasia (also known as idiopathic hyperaldosteronism), which requires a target

Disclosures: The authors have nothing to disclose.
Funding: This study was supported in part by research grants to GPR from FORICA (The FOundation for advanced Research In Hypertension and CArdiovascular diseases) and the Società Italiana dell'Ipertensione Arteriosa.
[a] Arterial Hypertension Unit, Clinica dell'Ipertensione Arteriosa, Department of Medicine, DIMED University Hospital, University of Padova, Via Giustiniani, 2, Padova 35126, Italy;
[b] Clinica dell'Ipertensione Arteriosa, Department of Medicine, DIMED, University of Padova, Via Giustiniani, 2, Padova 35126, Italy
* Corresponding author.
E-mail address: gianpaolo.rossi@unipd.it

Endocrinol Metab Clin N Am 48 (2019) 843–858
https://doi.org/10.1016/j.ecl.2019.08.012
0889-8529/19/© 2019 Elsevier Inc. All rights reserved.

medical therapy, whereas the latter, which are optimally treated with unilateral adrenalectomy, mainly entail aldosterone-producing adenoma (APA) and, less commonly, unilateral adrenal hyperplasia.[4]

To the aim of distinguishing unilateral from bilateral causes, all current clinical practice guidelines recommend adrenal vein sampling (AVS) to measure the plasma aldosterone concentration (PAC) and also a marker of selectivity, usually the plasma cortisol concentration (PCC), in adrenal vein blood.[5,6]

Unfortunately, AVS is not so widely available as it should be: for example, even in Europe there are entire countries where no center can offer AVS. Moreover, AVS is underused even at major referral centers as shown, by the Adrenal Vein sampling International Study (AVIS-1), a survey of AVS use worldwide.[7] The far from optimal clinical use of AVS translates into worse outcomes, as shown in the recently published AVIS-2 Study,[8] which provided evidence of a better outcome when adrenalectomy was AVS guided than when it was not.

Hence, the question, "Where do we stand now with AVS?" is timely and appropriate, and is addressed in this review.

WHY IS ADRENAL VEIN SAMPLING UNDERUSED?

AVS is a straightforward diagnostic test, but notwithstanding this, it is underused owing to a number of misconceptions, including the idea that AVS is technically challenging, invasive, risky, and, furthermore, that it is not always necessary, despite abundant evidence to the contrary.[7] Furthermore, a lack of accepted standards for the performance of AVS and of established criteria for interpretation of its results, contributes to prevent appropriate use of AVS in many patients with PA. The publication of a severely biased[9] randomized clinical trial[10] added further fuel to worsen this already worrying scenario. As a result of this study, far too many patients with PA are denied curative adrenalectomy, because lateralized aldosterone excess could not be convincingly demonstrated or, even worse, undergo adrenalectomy without such demonstration, which might translate into removal of the nonculprit adrenal gland.[11,12]

The largest registry of patients with PA submitted to AVS over 15 years in 19 referral centers showed that AVS was successful in 80.1% of all cases and allowed identification of unilateral PA in only 45.5%.[8] Moreover, adrenalectomy was performed in about 42% of all patients and cured arterial hypertension in roughly 20% of them, 2-fold more frequently in women than men ($P<.001$). When AVS-guided, surgery provided a higher rate of cure of hypertension than when not AVS-guided (40% vs. 30%; $P = .027$). Compared with surgical cases, patients treated medically needed more antihypertensive medications ($P<.001$) and exhibited a higher rate of persistent hypokalemia requiring potassium supplementation (4.9% vs. 2.3%; $P<.01$). Hence, the low rate of adrenalectomy and cure of hypertension indicates suboptimal AVS use in patients with PA seeking surgical cure. Although this suboptimal use is related to issues in patient selection, technical success, and AVS data interpretation, the better outcome of AVS-guided adrenalectomy calls for actions to improve the diagnostic use of this test.[8]

SELECTION OF THE PATIENTS FOR ADRENAL VEIN SAMPLING

Before considering AVS, it is mandatory to have reached an unequivocal biochemical diagnosis of PA, because this test aims at identifying the surgically curable cases of PA (**Fig. 1**).

An exception to this rule is patients with drug-resistant hypertension, who often have concealed PA. These patients are on multiple antihypertensive drugs, which renders very difficult, and sometimes even impossible, to reach a conclusive biochemical

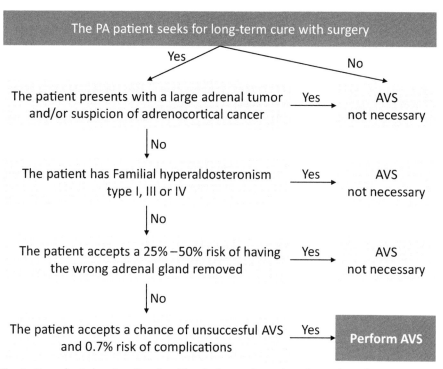

Fig. 1. Flow chart showing the algorithm to be used to select the patients for AVS.

diagnosis of PA. In these patients with very high cardiovascular risk, unilateral laparoscopic adrenalectomy often results in control of the high blood pressure values. If renin is not upregulated, AVS can be in performed in these patients, and demonstration of a lateralized aldosterone excess in the authors' experience is feasible.

Another exception entails the patients with germ-line mutations causing bilateral adrenal hyperplasia, for example, those with familial hyperaldosteronism (**Box 1**),[13] who should not undergo AVS, because they are unlikely to have a unilateral form of PA.

Finally, AVS is not indicated when either the patient prefers life-long medical treatment with a mineralocorticoid receptor (MR) antagonist, or the risks of surgery outweigh its benefits because of the patient's age or risk of general anesthesia and surgery itself, or when surgery is already mandated by the radiologic features, and/or size of the adrenal mass suspicious of adrenocortical carcinoma.

It has been contended that AVS might be skipped in young patients (eg, <35 years of age)[11] with a florid PA phenotype (as evidenced by spontaneous hypokalemia,

---

Box 1
Conditions for which AVS is not indicated in the patients with PA

1. Patients who are not candidate to general anesthesia and/or surgery;

2. Patients who prefer medical treatment;

3. Patients with familial hyperaldosteronism owing to germline mutations;

4. Patients with large adrenal tumors suggesting adrenocortical carcinoma.

undetectable renin, high plasma aldosterone concentration, and a clear-cut unilateral cortical adenoma with a contralateral normal adrenal on computed adrenal imaging),[14] because nonfunctioning adrenocortical adenomas ("incidentaloma") are infrequent in young people. However, the evidence supporting this proposition is weak and limited to only 6 patients, who fulfilled these criteria in a retrospective study.[11]

In summary, without AVS it is impossible to exclude (i) bilateral aldosterone secretion and (ii) unilateral aldosterone excess from a small adrenal computed tomography (CT)-invisible APA in the adrenal gland contralateral to a CT-detectable adrenal mass.

UNRELIABILITY OF IMAGING

It is intuitive, and also proved by overwhelming evidence, that imaging (with CT scans and MRI) cannot identify unilateral aldosteronism. Accordingly, all available evidences concur in demonstrating the poor accuracy of imaging in localizing the source of aldosterone excess. Furthermore, aldosterone-producing microadenoma and most cases of idiopathic hyperaldosteronism are, by definition, CT- and MR-undetectable. Therefore, in line with the global experience, to distinguish between unilateral and bilateral aldosterone excess, the US Endocrine Society and the Japan Endocrine Society guidelines recommend that AVS be offered to all patients with an unequivocal diagnosis of PA who want to pursue surgical cure.[5,6] For a more in-depth discussion of the reasons why AVS cannot be skipped the reader is referred to recent papers published elsewhere.[15,16]

OUTCOME OF ADRENAL VEIN SAMPLING-GUIDED ADRENALECTOMY

Nearly all patients who undergo AVS-guided adrenalectomy benefitted from surgery, as evidenced by correction of the hyperaldosteronism and improved blood pressure control; even if hypertension was not cured, drug treatment could be tapered and long-term regression of left ventricular hypertrophy occurred.[2] However, when proposing AVS the clinician should discuss with the patient realistic expectations of surgical outcomes.

Because surgical treatment is simply not feasible in the large proportion of the hypertensive patient population (6% to $\geq$11%) that has unilateral PA, a selection policy must be implemented in countries where health resources are limited. To this end, it is worth considering that some preoperative characteristics are associated with cure of hypertension after adrenalectomy, such as young age, shorter duration of hypertension (eg, <5 years), fewer antihypertensive medications (eg, $\leq$2), higher preoperative blood pressure and normal renal function, a body mass index of 25 kg/m^2 or less, female sex, lack of a family history of hypertension,[17–22] and no evidence of vascular remodeling.[17]

Therefore, in most public health care systems, priority should be given to (i) young patients, and particularly women as shown in the AVIS-2 Study,[8] who are the most likely to be cured and to gain the most in life-years off-treatment and (ii) patients with resistant hypertension (or antihypertensive drug intolerance), whose absolute risk of cardiovascular complications is the highest.

PREPARATION OF THE PATIENT FOR ADRENAL VEIN SAMPLING

The success of AVS requires an interdisciplinary team made of experienced hypertensiologists and/or endocrinologists and well-trained interventionists. Careful preparation of the patient for the procedure and standardization of the conditions for its performance are also essential steps. These recommendations are based on knowledge the factors that influence technical success and accuracy (**Box 2**).[18]

> **Box 2**
> **Summary of recommendations on how to perform AVS**
>
> 1. Prerequisites for performing AVS
>   - Prior correction of hypokalemia
>   - Prior adjustment of antihypertensive medications
>   - A multidisciplinary team in centers with extensive expertise
>   - One hour of supine rest
>   - Only if the success rate in achieving cannulation is low and the rapid cortisol assay is not available use cosyntropin stimulation
>
> 2. Preparation of the patient and preferred techniques for AVS
>   - Prevent and treat emotional and pain-related stress, because it can increase the SI, but lowers the LI
>   - The bilaterally simultaneous sampling should be the method of choice because it minimizes the time-related variability owing to the pulsatile pattern of secretion of cortisol and aldosterone, which can generate variability in hormone concentrations in the adrenal vein blood.
>
> 3. Pharmacologic stimulation
>   - Cosyntropin stimulation during AVS facilitates the assessment of selective adrenal vein catheterization; however, it confounds or even invert lateralization because it decreases the relative secretion index and there is no conclusive evidence that cosyntropin stimulation leads to a better outcome than unstimulated AVS
>   - Metoclopramide does not increase the SI or the LI. However, it helps in unmasking factitious contralateral suppression in non-APA cases

Hypokalemia, if present on the day of admission or during the previous days, should be corrected with oral or intravenous potassium supplements before AVS, because it decreases aldosterone secretion, thus potentially masking a unilateral aldosterone excess.[18]

Complete withdrawal of antihypertensive treatment is neither indicated nor necessary, but careful adjustment of the antihypertensive agents before and during AVS is important. Peripheral alpha1-adrenergic receptor blockers (eg, doxazosin mesylate) and/or the long-acting dihydropyridine or nondihydropyridine calcium-channel blockers (verapamil or diltiazem) are recommended, because these agents negligibly affect renin secretion. Even in stage 3, and/or drug-resistant hypertensive patients, who need multiple agents, including angiotensin I converting enzyme inhibitors, angiotensin receptor blockers, diuretics, and beta-adrenergic blockers, AVS can provide accurate diagnostic information, as long as renin is suppressed.[18] Nonsuppressed renin can stimulate aldosterone secretion from the unaffected side, thus minimizing the lateralization. As MR antagonists have the potential to increase renin, it is generally held that these drugs should be withdrawn for at least 6 weeks, and amiloride should be held for at least 2 weeks before AVS. The clinical risk of this withdrawal is probably small, even in patients with resistant hypertension,[19] but this is outweighed by the long-term benefits if a lateralized aldosterone excess is demonstrated. However, even though the issue of whether to withdraw MR antagonists and for how long has not been investigated prospectively, an anecdotal report,[20] and a retrospective study,[21] would suggest the possibility of using MRA as long as renin is not increased.

The use of plasma renin measurement to decide whether to perform AVS without withdrawing, or downtitrating, the MR antagonists is based on the premise that the finding of low renin is evidence for unlikely stimulation of the contralateral adrenal cortex at a level sufficient to confuse interpretation of lateralization. Nonetheless, in the presence of elevated renin (eg, a direct renin of >10 mIU/L) or hypokalemia, the results of AVS should be considered with caution because they are probably not valid.

TIME OF ADRENAL VEIN SAMPLING

To avoid false-negative results owing to diurnal fluctuation in adrenocorticotropic hormone having a more variable effect on many APAs than on the contralateral adrenal, AVS is best performed in the morning.

Some centers conduct AVS in outpatients, in which case time should be allowed for the patient to rest supine for 1 hour before AVS.[22,23] However, at the authors' institution we prefer to perform AVS during a 1-day hospital stay and to recommend 3 days of rest at home, because adrenal vein rupture (discussed elsewhere in this article) can occur suddenly, even after 24 hours, and is best managed in experienced hands in the hospital.

ASSESSMENT OF SUCCESSFUL CATHETERIZATION

In the early years of AVS when CT was not available, retrograde injection of contrast medium in the adrenal vein was used to confirm the success of catheterization with venography and to visualize the abnormal vascular tree of an APA.[24] This procedure carries an increased risk of adrenal vein rupture and contributed to create the fame of risky procedure for AVS.[7,22] Even though the injection of a small amount of dye with a gentle pressure is still commonly used to confirm the correct positioning of the catheter's tip inside the adrenal vein, with improved imaging techniques adrenal venography is no longer needed, and must be avoided.[25]

On the left side, the tip of the catheter should be placed distal to the orifice of the left inferior phrenic vein. On the right side, the right adrenal vein draining into the accessory hepatic vein should be identified beforehand on a CT scan and the location of the tip of the catheter in the right adrenal vein, instead of hepatic venous tributaries, should be confirmed by gentle injection of a very small amount of contrast just before blood sampling. The intraprocedural rapid cortisol assay during AVS,[26] (discussed elsewhere in this article) can be of help in this undertaking.

INTERPRETATION OF ADRENAL VEIN SAMPLING RESULTS

Selective catheterization of the left adrenal vein is achieved in almost 100% of the cases if the catheter's tip is positioned either at, or distal to, the orifice of the left inferior phrenic vein to avoid a dilution effect. Selective catherization is much more difficult on the right side because of the small size and short length of the right adrenal vein and because it drains directly into the inferior vena cava at various angles,[27] or directly into a small accessory hepatic vein.[22,28]

In about 10% of patients, the ascertainment of selectivity, and thus the success rate of AVS, can be affected by dilution from accessory vein blood flow.[29] Prior knowledge of the right adrenal vein anatomy can facilitate catheterization in difficult cases; hence, we recommend that a contrast-enhanced multidetector CT scan be performed before AVS to identify the right adrenal vein and delineate its anatomy, including its position in relationship to surrounding structures and the presence of an accessory hepatic vein.[18] This can improve the rate of success by guiding selective cannulation of the right adrenal vein instead of the common trunk composed of the accessory hepatic vein and the right adrenal vein, and also to locate the adrenal vein.[23] In case of anatomic variants, this recommendation is of paramount importance for success, as we recently reported.[30]

A particularly well-trained radiologist can also achieve subselective catheterization, which can allow the identification of the culprit nodule within the adrenal cortex, and thus guide the undertaking of spare adrenalectomy.[27] This approach is, however, confined to 1 center in Japan and remains to be validated in terms of improved outcomes.

INTRAPROCEDURAL RAPID CORTISOL ASSAY

Given that judgment of the achieved selectivity is possible only retrospectively when the hormonal data are available, a semiquantitative PCC measurement during AVS, which has the advantage of providing immediate feedback to the interventionist on whether selective blood sampling from each adrenal vein was accomplished or failed, has been proposed.[31] If selective catheterization failed, further attempts could be undertaken before removing the catheters, thus, avoiding the need for rescheduling the procedure.[31–33]

Thus far, this approach, which can improve the success rate during the interventionist's learning curve, was feasible only at centers where PCC could be measured rapidly, which implies a suitable logistic organization and a dedicated laboratory technician. However, the recent development of a quick cortisol assay, which needs neither a hardware nor an on-site technician, has made this strategy possible for the assessment of selectivity in a wider range of centers. Of note, a randomized study carried out in Japanese centers with a low level of experience in performing AVS showed an improved rate of success[26]; however, it remains to be determined if the same enhancement can be obtained in centers with a higher level of expertise in performing AVS. To answer this question, an international randomized prospective study, the Intra-Procedural cortisol Assay During Adrenal (I-Padua) vein sampling study, has been planned and is going.[34]

MINIMIZING STRESS DURING ADRENAL VEIN SAMPLING

Emotional and pain-related stress activates the hypothalamic pituitary adrenal axis, with ensuing adrenocorticotropic hormone-driven release of cortisol and aldosterone from both adrenals. The latter can be a major confounder of AVS results, particularly if bilaterally simultaneous blood sampling cannot be performed.[35] The latter technique was shown to provide better results in the AVIS-2 Study,[8] but owing to a number of misconceptions is not followed everywhere.

More cortisol than aldosterone is released during stress, which most patients experience when starting AVS; however, the cortisol can wane rapidly over about 15 minutes, and lateralization to the "culprit" adrenal can be obscured. A study that investigated the effect of stress on the selectivity index (SI) (**Table 1**) showed that a stress reaction increased the SI on both sides at the beginning of the procedure and influenced also the lateralization index (LI) values when using sequential AVS sampling.[35] Hence at the authors' institution, we systematically use the bilaterally simultaneous technique.

We also undertake precautions to minimize stress by explaining the procedure to the patient, providing reassurance by the doctor and nurses, administering benzodiazepines and local anesthesia before venipuncture and during AVS, and having the patient to rest quietly for at least 15 minutes before the blood sampling in a friendly environment with psychological assistance. Unfortunately, some of these measures were systematically used in only 5% of the centers participating in the AVIS Study.[7] Measures aimed at overriding stress effects by maximally stimulating cortisol release from both adrenals with cosyntropin are discussed elsewhere in this article.

In summary, the available evidence indicates that (i) a stress reaction can affect both the SI and LI, (ii) stress minimization measures should be taken when starting AVS (see **Box 2**), and (iii) a bilaterally simultaneous technique should be preferred.

Table 1 Indexes currently used for the interpretation of AVS results		
Index	**Formula**	**Interpretation**
Selectivity Index (SI)	$PCC_{side}/PCC_{IVC}{}^a$	Values above the cut-off confirm that the sample was obtained in the adrenal vein.
Relative secretion index (RASI)	$\dfrac{(PAC_{side}/PCC_{side})}{(PAC_{IVC}/PCC_{IVC})}$	Estimates aldosterone secretion of each adrenal gland relative to cortisol.
Contralateral suppression index (CLSI)	$\dfrac{(PAC_{non\ dominant}/PCC_{non\ dominant})}{(PAC_{IVC}/PCC_{IVC})}$	Values below the cut-off (generally 1.00) indicate suppression of aldosterone secretion in the non dominant gland.
Lateralization Index (LI)	$\dfrac{(PAC_{dominant}/PCC_{dominant})}{(PAC_{non\ dominant}/PCC_{non\ dominant})}$	Values above the cut-off indicate lateralized aldosterone excess.

At the author's institution androstenedione is also used for calculation of the SI and also for calculation of the other indexes, instead of PCC.

Abbreviations: Dominant, side with higher plasma aldosterone concentration; IVC, inferior vena cava; non dominant, contralateral side; PAC, plasma aldosterone concentration; PCC, plasma cortisol concentration.

[a] Peripheral venous blood can also be used.

BILATERAL SIMULTANEOUS CATHETERIZATION SHOULD BE THE PREFERRED METHOD

Owing to the pulsatile secretion of aldosterone, there are chances of creating artificial gradients between sides when the blood sampling is performed sequentially, that is, at different times, particularly if the interventionist is not proficient and fast enough. The untoward effect of the stress reaction occurring when starting AVS on assessment of lateralization can also worsen these problems. Undoubtedly, the time-dependent bias affecting AVS results can be avoided with bilaterally simultaneous AVS.[36]

These issues were clarified in a recent study where bilaterally simultaneous AVS was systematically used at time −15, that is, when starting the procedure, and again 15 minutes later and sequential AVS was then simulated by combining the samples obtained on each side at the different time points.[36] The simultaneously obtained samples at time 0 provided a more accurate identification of lateralization than those obtained sequentially; moreover, the chances of creating factitious lateralization to the last sampled side, regardless of its being right or left, were higher with the sequential technique, likely because of the waning of the aforementioned stress reaction.

Notwithstanding this factor, the AVIS study showed that only one-third of centers used the bilaterally simultaneous technique with no stimulation, whereas almost two-thirds still used the sequential technique with cosyntropin stimulation (discussed elsewhere in this article).[7] Similar results were obtained in the AVIS-2 Study.[8]

These findings could be anticipated, because (i) when cortisol secretion is maximally stimulated the time difference between blood sampling from one side and the other becomes less relevant, in the assessment of selectivity, and (ii) the bilateral simultaneity of blood sampling is crucial when AVS is performed without cosyntropin stimulation.

PHARMACOLOGIC STIMULATION DURING ADRENAL VEIN SAMPLING

Stimulation with a continuous cosyntropin infusion (50 µg/h started 30 min before sampling) or a bolus (250 µg) during AVS was introduced in 1979 and remains popular at many centers,[7,37] for 3 main reasons: (i) enhancing the PCC gradient between the adrenal vein and the inferior vena cava, thus increasing the SI values and physicians' confidence of successful sampling; (ii) decreasing stress-induced fluctuations in cortisol and aldosterone secretion during sequential AVS; (iii) and increasing aldosterone secretion from APA.

In 2012 the AVIS study showed that the major referral centers were almost equally split into those that used and those that did not use cosyntropin stimulation[7]; moreover, centers that systematically used cosyntropin reported use of higher SI cutoffs values than centers that used baseline (unstimulated) values.

A detailed discussion of the pros and cons for using cosyntropin was recently published elsewhere,[38] and is summarized here. In brief, there are no doubts that cosyntropin increased the rate of AVS studies judged to be selective, but this increase comes at the expense of decreased accuracy of the LI as repeatedly shown[39–41] and recently confirmed in the AVIS-2 Study,[8] and explained at the mechanistic level.[42]

In summary, in keeping with the theoretic premises, the bulk of the data indicate that cosyntropin increases the SI and, by doing so, facilitates the ascertainment of selective catheterization. To date, given the lack of conclusive evidence for the superiority of using pharmacologic stimulation with cosyntropin to determine lateralization of aldosterone excess, the recommendation needs to be limited to the following: (i) each center should use a consistent protocol, (ii) if cosyntropin stimulation is used, then higher SI and LI values are necessary, and (iii) if cosyntropin stimulation is not used, then bilateral simultaneous AVS should be performed.

As regards other stimuli, metoclopramide was used in only 2 studies[42,43] that reported that it did not increase the success of AVS or the LI to the culprit side. However, metoclopramide can be useful to unmask the factitious suppression of aldosterone production in the nondominant side in patients without APA.[44] A further study investigating the use of clarithromycin, which can blunt aldosterone secretion specifically from APA harboring the KCNJ5 mutation during AVS is ongoing.[45]

HOW TO INTERPRET ADRENAL VEIN SAMPLING RESULTS

A number of indexes have been developed for establishing whether catheterization was successful and for a proper interpretation of the results.[46] They easily can be calculated from the hormonal values measured in AVS-derived blood (see **Table 1**).

The SI (see **Table 1**) is the most popular technique to confirm the success of AVS,[43] based on the theoretic assumption that the hormone of interest is exclusively made in the adrenal cortex and, is not overproduced in the culprit adrenal. Therefore, the finding of a concentration gradient between a blood sample in a vein supposedly draining the adrenal cortex, and the inferior vena cava or a peripheral vein, indicates the correct placement of the catheter's tip into the adrenal vein. To this end, the most widely used hormone is cortisol, given its high rate of production, although attempts to use also chromogranin A,[47] epinephrine, metanephrine,[48] and other steroids have been made.

According to studies with liquid chromatography and tandem mass spectrometry that measured all steroids released by the human adrenal cortex, the step-up between the adrenal vein and the inferior vena cava or a peripheral vein blood would be greater for some steroids other than cortisol, suggesting that they can be better markers for selectivity.[49] A recent study that examined the performance of 17α hydroxyprogesterone and androstenedione in a number of AVS studies judged to be nonselective with cortisol-based SI, showed that this hypothesis was in fact correct[50]: 17α hydroxyprogesterone and androstenedione showed a 1.6-fold and 12-fold higher step-up than cortisol, respectively, thus allowing to rescue 43% and 72%, respectively, for diagnostic purposes. Hence, at the authors' institution we measure systematically androstenedione, besides cortisol, to confirm selectivity of AVS.

Although use of the SI is straightforward, the AVIS Study showed that even some major international referral centers continue to analyze their results using the absolute hormonal values without a prior assessment of the selectivity and correction for the degree of sample dilution, a practice that is not evidence-based and should be discouraged because the absolute hormonal values are markedly affected by the degree of proximity of the catheter's tip to the adrenal cortex. Of further concern, even in those centers that used the SI to assess selectivity, there was considerable variability in the SI cutoff values used.[7]

Some general considerations can, however, be made: the cutoffs are lower at centers that perform AVS with no pharmacologic stimulation than at those that use cosyntropin stimulation, an expected finding given that cosyntropin increases the cortisol release and therefore the gradient between adrenal vein and inferior vena cava blood.

Based on the experience gained and the results of the AVIS Study, the suggestion was made to use of a SI cutoff of 2.0 or greater for AVS performed under unstimulated conditions, and 3.0 or greater for AVS performed during cosyntropin stimulation (**Box 3**).[18] However, the choice of the SI cutoff is center-dependent and determined based on the accuracy of the laboratory in measuring these hormones.

To validate the findings and select the optimal cutoffs, it should be acknowledged that the only solid diagnosis that can be used as reference is that of APA. Studies that used the AVS results to validate the own AVS-based diagnosis and justify the choice of their cutoff values should be disregarded because they did not comply with the rules set by the Standards for Reporting of Diagnostic Accuracy committee.[51,52]

There is no doubt that (i) the higher the cutoff chosen to establish selectivity, the lower the proportion of AVS studies that could be defined as bilaterally selective and vice versa, as demonstrated conclusively in the AVIS-2 study[8]; (ii) too restrictive criteria lead to exclude a proportion of successful studies from diagnostic use; and (iii) conversely, too permissive SI cutoffs could limit the diagnostic accuracy of AVS.

Moreover, as the SI increases, so does the confidence of the interpretation. In some cases where unilateral aldosterone production is extremely high, a low SI can give the

---

Box 3
Interpretation of AVS

Assessment of selectivity
- Successful AVS should be determined by calculating the SI.
- AVS studies that are not bilaterally successful should not be used to establish lateralization.
- The cutoff value for the SI should be 2.0 or greater under unstimulated conditions and 3.0 or greater during cosyntropin stimulation.
- Where possible, the rapid intraprocedural cortisol measurement confers the advantage of drawing a repeat blood sample after catheter repositioning in case of unsuccessful initial catheterization.

Assessment of lateralization
- Lateralization of aldosterone secretion should be determined by the LI and not by absolute hormonal values.
- For assessing lateralization, there is no compelling evidence for the use of cosyntropin stimulation in terms of outcome.
- Most centers used LI between 2.0 and 4.0 under unstimulated conditions and between 2.6 and 4.0 during cosyntropin stimulation

correct interpretation, but, in cases when the overproduction is modest, wrong conclusions are possible.

A trade-off between too restrictive and too permissive cutoffs is needed, and it has also to be considered that the cutoffs depend on the accuracy (within-assay coefficient of variation) with which the hormone used to assess selectivity can be measured. For example, if this is greater than or around 10%, lower cutoffs such as 1.1 are not feasible, whereas if the assay coefficient of variation is less than 10%, an SI cutoff of 1.1 may be reasonable.[18,46]

A recent analysis of the large AVIS-2 database showed that use of less restrictive cutoffs for both the SI and the LI allowed to refer for surgery a much large proportion of the patients with PA, as discussed later. More important, more liberal cutoffs were not associated with a worse clinical outcome so that a greater number of patients could gain a clear-cut benefit.[53]

In summary, verification of bilateral selectivity is a prerequisite to the use of the data for diagnostic purposes, which implies that AVS studies that are not bilaterally successful must not be used to establish lateralization. Nonetheless, recognizing that many studies do not turn out to be bilaterally selective and/or can provide equivocal results, we refer the reader to what has been discussed in greater depth as regards how to make the diagnosis of unilateral PA in challenging cases.[54]

ASSESSMENT OF LATERALIZATION

The LI is the index to be used for assessment of lateralization of aldosterone excess (see **Table 1**). Because of the inevitable dilution of the samples by nonadrenal blood, PCC and/or androstenedione are used for correction of the adrenal aldosterone levels.

There are several caveats in assessing the accuracy of AVS criteria using outcome after adrenalectomy as a reference. Ideally, outcome should be defined using postoperative normalization of plasma aldosterone and renin to determine curative adrenalectomy.[2,55] In contrast, blood pressure normalizes in about 45% of biochemically cured patients, but it may not decrease if the patient has concomitant essential hypertension, chronic kidney disease, and/or vascular remodeling,[17,56] or it may decrease for reasons unrelated to biochemical cure of PA, such as the Hawthorne effect, lifestyle changes, and incident left ventricular systolic dysfunction, for example, owing to myocardial infarction.

In 2012 most of the referral centers performed AVS with sequential sampling and cosyntropin stimulation,[7] which is not the optimal way to perform it, for the reasons discussed elsewhere in this article.

Evidence for optimal diagnostic accuracy of LI cutoffs should come from prospective studies in patients undergoing unilateral adrenalectomy regardless of the AVS results, and in which the different LI are thereafter linked with postoperative biochemical cure of hyperaldosteronism rather than only high blood pressure, which is a composite phenotype. Unfortunately, the only such prospective randomized controlled studies available was underpowered to provide any conclusive information.[10]

In the AVIS study, referral centers used arbitrarily chosen LI cut-offs values that ranged between 2.0 and 4.0;[7] undoubtedly the choice of more restrictive (higher) cut-offs allows selection of a population with a higher chance of being cured with adrenalectomy, but precludes the chances of cure to several potentially curable patients.

The recent AVIS-2 study assessed the rate of patients deemed to have unilateral disease by LI cut-off definitions ranging from 2.0 to 5.0, in concert with SI cut-off definitions of 1.4, 2.0, and 3.0 for unstimulated measurements, and 5.0 for postcosyntropin values. It showed that, among bilaterally successful studies, the rate of lateralization dropped significantly with adoption of higher LI cut-off definitions and with each unit increase in LI cut-off definition. With commonly used biochemical definitions under unstimulated and cosyntropin-stimulated conditions, that is, an SI of 2.0 or greater with an LI of 3.0 or greater, and an SI of 5.0 or greater with an LI of 4.0 or greater, the proportion of patients deemed to have unilateral disease was about 40% and 37%, respectively (P = NS). It increased significantly to 56% ($P<.001$) with less stringent cutoff values of unstimulated SI and/or LI, that is, an SI of 1.4 or greater combined with a cut-off of 2.0 or greater for lateralization. Importantly, the rate of patients submitted to adrenalectomy was lower with application of more stringent definitions for unilateral disease, and decreased to a nadir of less than 25% with an SI of 3.0 or greater and an LI greater than 4.0. However, the proportion of patients referred for adrenalectomy among those with AVS evidence of unilateral disease was higher with more restrictive criteria for lateralization, suggesting that physicians' confidence in results that meet the stricter definitions was higher.[53]

SAFETY AND THE MANAGEMENT OF COMPLICATIONS

AVS should be performed in specialized referral centers with sufficient throughput and expertise. However, the limited number of such specialized centers may result in missed opportunities for optimal surgical management in many patients who have no access to AVS. Hence, appropriate training programs and certification of proficiency in performing AVS for radiologists should be implemented.

The only major complication of AVS is adrenal vein rupture with subsequent intraglandular and/or retroperitoneal hematoma.[18,57] Only occasionally these complications are curative if they occur in the adrenal gland harboring the APA. Clinically, adrenal vein rupture is characterized by acute onset of persistent lumbar pain during or after catheterization, which increases in intensity and requires analgesics over 24 to 48 hours. Under these circumstances a CT scan or MRI is necessary to confirm the diagnosis, and careful monitoring of vital signs should be undertaken. The complication usually resolves with conservative treatment in few days and does not carry sequelae, except that, if on the APA side, it can render subsequent laparoscopic adrenalectomy more difficult owing to extensive retroperitoneal adhesions.

Although early studies suggested a wide range of rates of adrenal vein rupture, in the AVIS Study the rate of this complication was only 0.6%,[7] with avoidance of routine adrenal venography and minimization of the injection volume for anatomic confirmation of the adrenal vein catheterization. Complications are more common at the right than left adrenal vein, because of the anatomic diversity and complexity; they do not depend on the methods of catheterization, that is, sequential, or bilaterally simultaneous, and the use of cosyntropin stimulation,[7] but they differ significantly, even among major referral centers, indicating that the expertise of the radiologist and the experience of each center are key issues inasmuch as adrenal vein rupture was inversely related to the number of AVS performed by each radiologist and the number of AVS performed per centers.

SUMMARY

The high diagnostic accuracy, minimal rate of complications, and better outcome with AVS-guided adrenalectomy support the guidelines recommendation that AVS should serve as the golden standard diagnostic test for the subtyping of PA. With some exceptions, AVS should be systematically used before referring a patient to the surgeon. As for all invasive diagnostic tests appropriate training of the interventionists, a tight collaboration with experienced endocrinologists and hypertensiologists, and adherence to the suggestions that are herein summarized for the interpretation of the test will make the best clinical use of AVS for the doctor and for the patient.

REFERENCES

1. Milliez P, Girerd X, Plouin PF, et al. Evidence for an increased rate of cardiovascular events in patients with primary aldosteronism. J Am Coll Cardiol 2005;45(8): 1243–8.
2. Rossi GP, Cesari M, Cuspidi C, et al. Long-term control of arterial hypertension and regression of left ventricular hypertrophy with treatment of primary aldosteronism. Hypertension 2013;62(1):62–9.
3. Reincke M, Fischer E, Gerum S, et al. Observational study mortality in treated primary aldosteronism: the German Conn's registry. Hypertension 2012;60(3): 618–24.
4. Rossi GP. Surgically correctable hypertension caused by primary aldosteronism. Best Pract Res Clin Endocrinol Metab 2006;20(3):385–400.
5. Funder JW, Carey RM, Mantero F, et al. The management of primary aldosteronism: case detection, diagnosis, and treatment: an Endocrine Society Clinical Practice Guideline. J Clin Endocrinol Metab 2016;101(5):1889–916.
6. Nishikawa T, Omura M, Satoh F, et al. Guidelines for the diagnosis and treatment of primary aldosteronism–the Japan Endocrine Society 2009. Endocr J 2011; 58(9):711–21.
7. Rossi GP, Barisa M, Allolio B, et al. The Adrenal Vein Sampling International Study (AVIS) for identifying the major subtypes of primary aldosteronism. J Clin Endocrinol Metab 2012;97(5):1606–14.
8. Rossi GP, Rossitto G, Amar L, et al. The clinical outcomes of 1625 patients with primary aldosteronism subtyped with adrenal vein sampling. Hypertension 2019.
9. Rossi GP, Funder JW. Adrenal venous sampling versus computed tomographic scan to determine treatment in primary aldosteronism (The SPARTACUS Trial): a critique. Hypertension 2017;69(3):396–7.
10. Dekkers T, Prejbisz A, Kool LJ, et al. Adrenal vein sampling versus CT scan to determine treatment in primary aldosteronism: an outcome-based randomised diagnostic trial. Lancet Diabetes Endocrinol 2016;4(9):739–46.
11. Lim V, Guo Q, Grant CS, et al. Accuracy of adrenal imaging and adrenal venous sampling in predicting surgical cure of primary aldosteronism. J Clin Endocrinol Metab 2014;99(8):2712–9.
12. Ladurner K, Hallfeldt J, Id O, et al. Accuracy of adrenal imaging and adrenal venous sampling in diagnosing unilateral primary aldosteronism. Eur J Clin Invest 2017;47(5):372–7.
13. Seccia TM, Caroccia B, Gomez-Sanchez EP, et al. The biology of normal zona glomerulosa and aldosterone-producing adenoma: pathological implications. Endocr Rev 2018;39(6):1029–56.
14. Funder JW, Carey RM, Fardella C, et al. Case detection, diagnosis, and treatment of patients with primary aldosteronism: an endocrine society clinical practice guideline. J Clin Endocrinol Metab 2008;93(9):3266–81.
15. Rossi GP, Mulatero P, Satoh F. 10 good reasons why adrenal vein sampling is the preferred method for referring primary aldosteronism patients for adrenalectomy. J Hypertens 2019;37(3):603–11.
16. Iacobone M, Mantero F, Basso SM, et al. Results and long-term follow-up after unilateral adrenalectomy for ACTH-independent hypercortisolism in a series of fifty patients. J Endocrinol Invest 2005;28(4):327–32.

17. Rossi GP, Bolognesi M, Rizzoni D, et al. Vascular remodeling and duration of hypertension predict outcome of adrenalectomy in primary aldosteronism patients. Hypertension 2008;51(5):1366–71.

18. Rossi GP, Auchus RJ, Brown M, et al. An expert consensus statement on use of adrenal vein sampling for the subtyping of primary aldosteronism. Hypertension 2014;63(1):151–60.

19. van der Wardt V, Harrison JK, Welsh T, et al. Withdrawal of antihypertensive medication. J Hypertens 2017;35(9):1742–9.

20. Haase M, Riester A, Kröpil P, et al. Outcome of adrenal vein sampling performed during concurrent mineralocorticoid receptor antagonist therapy. J Clin Endocrinol Metab 2014;99(12):4397–402.

21. Nanba AT, Wannachalee T, Shields JJ, et al. Adrenal vein sampling lateralization despite mineralocorticoid receptor antagonists exposure in primary aldosteronism. J Clin Endocrinol Metab 2019;104(2):487–92.

22. Daunt N. Adrenal vein sampling: how to make it quick, easy, and successful. Radiographics 2005;25(Suppl 1):S143–58.

23. Rossi GP. A comprehensive review of the clinical aspects of primary aldosteronism. Nat Rev Endocrinol 2011;7(8):485–95.

24. Davidson JK, Morley P, Hurley GD, et al. Adrenal venography and ultrasound in the investigation of the adrenal gland: an analysis of 58 cases. Br J Radiol 1975; 48(570):435–50.

25. Rossi GP. New concepts in adrenal vein sampling for aldosterone in the diagnosis of primary aldosteronism. Curr Hypertens Rep 2007;9(2):90–7.

26. Yoneda T, Karashima S, Kometani M, et al. Impact of new quick gold nanoparticle-based cortisol assay during adrenal vein sampling for primary aldosteronism. J Clin Endocrinol Metab 2016;101(6):2554–61.

27. Omura K, Ota H, Takahashi Y, et al. Anatomical variations of the right adrenal vein. Hypertension 2017;69(3):428–34.

28. Rossi GP. Diagnosis and treatment of primary aldosteronism. Endocrinol Metab Clin North Am 2011;12(1):313–32.

29. Miotto D, De Toni R, Pitter G, et al. Impact of accessory hepatic veins on adrenal vein sampling for identification of surgically curable primary aldosteronism. Hypertension 2009;54(4):885–9.

30. Rossi GP, Lerco S, Miotto D, et al. The key role of CT for success of adrenal venous sampling illustrated by a unique clinical case. High Blood Press Cardiovasc Prev 2019;26(2):139–41.

31. Rossi E, Regolisti G, Perazzoli F, et al. Intraprocedural cortisol measurement increases adrenal vein sampling success rate in primary aldosteronism. Am J Hypertens 2011;24(12):1280–5.

32. Mengozzi G, Rossato D, Bertello C, et al. Rapid cortisol assay during adrenal vein sampling in patients with primary aldosteronism. Clin Chem 2007;53(11): 1968–71.

33. Auchus RJ, Michaelis C, Jr FHW, et al. Rapid cortisol assays improve the success rate of adrenal vein sampling for primary aldosteronism. Ann Surg 2009;249(2): 318–21.

34. Cesari M, Ceolotto G, Rossitto G, et al. The Intra-procedural cortisol assay during adrenal vein sampling: rationale and design of a randomized study (I-Padua). High Blood Press Cardiovasc Prev 2017;24(2):167–70.

35. Seccia TM, Miotto D, Battistel M, et al. A stress reaction affects assessment of selectivity of adrenal venous sampling and of lateralization of aldosterone excess in primary aldosteronism. Eur J Endocrinol 2012;166(5):869–75.

36. Rossitto G, Battistel M, Barbiero G, et al. The subtyping of primary aldosteronism by adrenal vein sampling: sequential blood sampling causes factitious lateralization. J Hypertens 2018;36(2):335–43.
37. Weinberger MH, Grim CE, Hollifield JW, et al. Primary aldosteronism: diagnosis, localization, and treatment. Ann Intern Med 1979;90(3):386–95.
38. Deinum J, Groenewoud H, van der Wilt GJ, et al. Adrenal venous sampling: co-syntropin stimulation or not? Eur J Endocrinol 2019;181(3):D15–26.
39. Rossi GP, Pitter G, Bernante P, et al. Adrenal vein sampling for primary aldosteronism: the assessment of selectivity and lateralization of aldosterone excess baseline and after adrenocorticotropic hormone (ACTH) stimulation. J Hypertens 2008;26(5):989–97.
40. Seccia TM, Miotto D, De Toni R, et al. Adrenocorticotropic hormone stimulation during adrenal vein sampling for identifying surgically curable subtypes of primary aldosteronism: comparison of 3 different protocols. Hypertension 2009; 53(5):761–6.
41. Rossi GP, Ganzaroli C, Miotto D, et al. Dynamic testing with high-dose adrenocorticotrophic hormone does not improve lateralization of aldosterone oversecretion in primary aldosteronism patients. J Hypertens 2006;24(2):371–9.
42. Rossitto G, Maiolino G, Lenzini L, et al. Subtyping of primary aldosteronism with adrenal vein sampling: hormone- and side-specific effects of cosyntropin and metoclopramide. Surgery 2018;163(4):789–95.
43. Seccia TM, Miotto D, De Toni R, et al. Subtyping of primary aldosteronism by adrenal vein sampling: effect of acute D(2) receptor dopaminergic blockade on adrenal vein cortisol and chromogranin A levels. Eur J Endocrinol 2011;165(1): 85–90.
44. Rossitto G, Miotto D, Battistel M, et al. Metoclopramide unmasks potentially misleading contralateral suppression in patients undergoing adrenal vein sampling for primary aldosteronism. J Hypertens 2016;34(11):2258–65.
45. Maiolino G, Ceolotto G, Battistel M, et al. Macrolides for KCNJ5-mutated aldosterone-producing adenoma (MAPA): design of a study for personalized diagnosis of primary aldosteronism. Blood Press 2018;27(4):200–5.
46. Rossi GP, Sacchetto A, Chiesura-Corona M, et al. Identification of the etiology of primary aldosteronism with adrenal vein sampling in patients with equivocal computed tomography and magnetic resonance findings: results in 104 consecutive cases. J Clin Endocrinol Metab 2001;86(3):1083–90.
47. Seccia TM, Miotto D, De Toni R, et al. Chromogranin a measurement for assessing the selectivity of adrenal venous sampling in primary aldosteronism. J Clin Endocrinol Metab 2011;96(5):E825–9.
48. Dekkers T, Deinum J, Schultzekool LJ, et al. Plasma metanephrine for assessing the selectivity of adrenal venous sampling. Hypertension 2013;62(6):1152–7.
49. Eisenhofer G, Dekkers T, Peitzsch M, et al. Mass spectrometry – based adrenal and peripheral venous steroid profiling for subtyping primary aldosteronism. Clin Chem 2016;62(3):514–24.
50. Ceolotto G, Antonelli G, Maiolino G, et al. Androstenedione and 17-α-hydroxyprogesterone are better indicators of adrenal vein sampling selectivity than cortisol: novelty and significance. Hypertension 2017;70(2):342–6.
51. Rossi GP, Seccia TM, Pessina AC. A diagnostic algorithm–the holy grail of primary aldosteronism. Nat Rev 2011;7(12):697–9.
52. Bossuyt PM, Reitsma JB, Bruns DE, et al. The STARD statement for reporting studies of diagnostic accuracy: explanation and elaboration. Ann Intern Med 2003;49(1):7–18.

53. Rossitto G, Amar L, Azizi M, et al. Subtyping of primary aldosteronism in the AVIS-2 Study: assessment of selectivity and lateralisation. J Clin Endocrinol Metab, in press.

54. Rossi GP. Update in adrenal venous sampling for primary aldosteronism. Curr Opin Endocrinol Diabetes Obes 2018;25(3):160–71.

55. Quillo AR, Grant CS, Thompson GB, et al. Primary aldosteronism: results of adrenalectomy for nonsingle adenoma. J Am Coll Surg 2011;213(1):103–6.

56. Funder JW. Primary aldosteronism: clinical lateralization and costs. J Clin Endocrinol Metab 2012;97(10):3450–2.

57. Monticone S, Satoh F, Dietz AS, et al. Clinical management and outcomes of adrenal hemorrhage following adrenal vein sampling in primary aldosteronism. Hypertension 2015;67(1):146–52.

Drug-Induced Hypertension

Matthew C. Foy, MD[a,1], Joban Vaishnav, MD[b,1],
Christopher John Sperati, MD, MHS[c],*

KEYWORDS

- Drug-induced hypertension • Secondary hypertension • Polypharmacy

KEY POINTS

- Polypharmacy is common and may contribute to secondary causes of hypertension.
- Optimal management of drug-induced hypertension is discontinuation or minimization of the offending agent.
- For most causes of drug-induced hypertension, the optimal antihypertensive is unknown.
- Understanding mechanisms of drug-induced hypertension may allow for a more rational selection of antihypertensive therapy.

One must be in perfect health to withstand the blessings of modern medicine.
—General Creighton Abrams

From caffeine to state-of-the-art biological therapies, untoward side effects of pharmaceuticals can result in considerable morbidity and expense to the health care system. Although it is difficult to know the prevalence of drug-induced hypertension, as 15% of the United States population uses more than or equal to 5 prescription medications, there is likely a sizable fraction of the hypertensive population with disease induced or exacerbated by polypharmacy.[1] The elevation of blood pressure (BP) in drug-induced hypertension occurs through a variety of mechanisms, most notably, sodium and fluid retention, activation of the renin-angiotensin-aldosterone system (RAAS), alteration of vascular tone, or a combination of these pathways[2,3] (**Fig. 1**). Recognition of common medications causing drug-induced hypertension is important to effectively control BP (**Table 1**). The epidemiology, pathophysiology, and management of these agents are discussed.

Disclosures: None.
[a] Division of Nephrology, Louisiana State University Health Science Center, 5246 Brittany Dr, Baton Rouge, LA 70808, USA; [b] Division of Cardiology, Johns Hopkins University School of Medicine, 600 N Wolfe Street, Baltimore, MD 21287, USA; [c] Division of Nephrology, Johns Hopkins University School of Medicine, 1830 East Monument Street, Room 416, Baltimore, MD 21287, USA
[1] Drs Foy and Vaishnav contributed equally to the article and share first authorship.
* Corresponding author.
E-mail address: jsperati@jhmi.edu

Endocrinol Metab Clin N Am 48 (2019) 859–873
https://doi.org/10.1016/j.ecl.2019.08.013
0889-8529/19/© 2019 Elsevier Inc. All rights reserved.

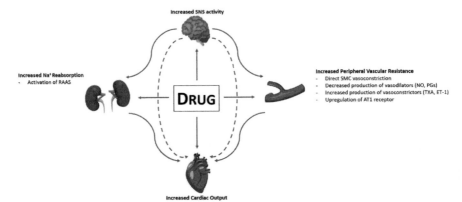

Fig. 1. Mechanisms contributing to drug-induced hypertension include (1) increased SNS activity; (2) alteration in peripheral vascular tone through decreased secretion of NO and PG, increased secretion of TXA and ET-1 from endothelial cells, upregulation of AT-1 receptor, and direct vasoconstriction; and (3) alteration in Na + homeostasis. AT1, angiotensin II receptor type 1; ET-1, endothelin 1; NO, nitric oxide; PGs, prostaglandins; RAAS, renin-angiotensin-aldosterone system; SMC, smooth muscle cell; SNS, sympathetic nervous system; TXA, thromboxane.

VASCULAR ENDOTHELIAL GROWTH FACTOR INHIBITORS
Epidemiology

Bevacizumab, a monoclonal antibody that binds circulating vascular endothelial growth factor (VEGF) A, was the first anti-VEGF chemotherapy to be approved for use in cancer treatment in 2004.[4] Subsequently, tyrosine kinase inhibitors (TKI), including sorafenib, sunitinib, pazopanib, lucitanib, and lenvatinib, have become major therapies for renal cell, thyroid, and other advanced solid tumors. The incidence of hypertension in older drugs ranges from 17% to 36%; in newer drugs, hypertension occurs in up to 70% to 90% of patients, likely due to increased potency.[5–9]

Pathophysiology

Antagonism of VEGFR-2, the major endothelial cell receptor in VEGF signaling, decreases nitric oxide (NO) production through numerous downstream pathways.[10] The resultant vasoconstriction may underlie much of the hypertension with VEGF inhibitors.[11] In mice, treatment with anti-VEGFR2 antibody decreases expression of renal endothelial NO synthases and rapidly increases BP by a mean of 10 mm Hg. Direct inhibition of NO generation reproduces the BP effect.[12] In humans, treatment with TKI leads to a decrease in plasma nitrate and nitrite levels that recover after cessation of therapy.[13,14]

An important consequence of NO downregulation is endothelial dysfunction and microvascular rarefaction—a reduced spatial density of microvascular networks.[11] After 6 months of bevacizumab therapy in patients with colon cancer, endothelial function as assessed by acetylcholine analogue administration and capillary density measurements were reduced.[15] Vasomotor tone is also enhanced through increases in endothelin (ET-1), a potent vasoconstrictor. In rats, sunitinib increased plasma and urinary levels of ET-1 with a concomitant increase in BP. In addition, with administration of the ET receptor antagonist macitentan, hypertension was prevented.[16] Altered vascular tone within the renal vasculature contributes to the maintenance of hypertension over time.[11]

Table 1
Estimated prevalence and mechanism of drug-induced hypertension by class

Drug	Prevalence of Hypertension	Proposed Mechanism
VEGF inhibitors	15%–90%[5–8]	VEGFR-2 antagonism with subsequent decreased NO production.
Calcineurin inhibitors	23%–60%[21,22]	Endothelin-1 overproduction with decreased NO production. Renal Na^+ retention through stimulation of thiazide-sensitive NaCl cotransporter via increased WNK kinase activity. Direct postsynaptic excitation via glutaminergic transmission with increased SNS activity.
NSAIDs[a]	14%–20%[45]	Reduced prostaglandin E2 with subsequent decrease in urine Na^+ excretion. Increased intrarenal aldosterone levels secondary to decreased hormone glucuronidation. Reduced prostaglandin I_2 with increased systemic vascular resistance.
Glucocorticoids	20%[50]	Renal Na^+ retention via stimulation of mineralocorticoid receptors. Upregulation of AT1 receptors on vascular smooth muscle with subsequent increased vascular tone.
Erythropoietin stimulating agents	20%–30%[57]	Increased thromboxane and reduced prostacyclin levels with blunted response to NO. Increased endothelin levels with resulting vasoconstriction.
Oral contraceptive pills	Unknown	Increased renin (estrogenic component) leading to RAAS activation and subsequent Na^+ and water retention.
Selective norepinephrine reuptake inhibitors	1%–5%[77]	Activation of the SNS with increased norepinephrine.
Drugs of abuse MDMA PCP Methamphetamine Cocaine	33%[80] 17%–46%[81]	Increased release and inhibited reuptake of monoamine neurotransmitters with subsequent SNS activation. Increased CNS catecholamine release with decreased neuronal uptake. Cocaine-induced increase in arterial wall stiffness and atherosclerosis.
Stimulants Modafinil Methylphenidate Amphetamines	~7%[99]	Block reuptake of norepinephrine or dopamine. Promote release of catecholamines.

Abbreviations: CNS, central nervous system; NO, nitric oxide; PNP, phencyclidine; SNS, sympathetic nervous system; VEGF, vascular endothelial growth factor; VEGFR, vascular endothelial growth factor receptor.
[a] Increase of baseline systolic BP of 20 mm Hg or more.

Management

The National Cancer Institute recommends monitoring BP weekly for the first cycle of therapy and then every 2 to 3 weeks for the duration of treatment.[17] If new-onset or worsening hypertension occurs, the necessity of ongoing therapy should be assessed. If therapy is essential, the lowest acceptable dose for the shortest duration of time should be used. The presence of albuminuria should be assessed. If present, angiotensin-converting enzyme inhibitors (ACEI) or angiotensin II receptor antagonists (ARB) are preferred therapies. Nondihydropyridine calcium channel blockers (non-DHP-CCBs) (eg, verapamil and diltiazem) should be avoided due to CYP3A4 inhibition in setting of TKI use.[18] Nifedipine may induce VEGF secretion, so DHP-CCBs such as amlodipine or felodipine are preferred.[19]

CALCINEURIN INHIBITORS
Epidemiology

Calcineurin inhibitors (CNIs), including cyclosporine and tacrolimus, are potent immunosuppressive drugs used to prevent posttransplant rejection and to treat autoimmune disease. A meta-analysis including 17 randomized controlled trials (RCTs) comparing cyclosporine with placebo demonstrated mean BP increase by 5 to 11 mm Hg with a dose-related effect.[20] The incidence of hypertension after initiation of cyclosporine therapy ranges from 65% to 100% in posttransplant patients, although this is confounded by the use of glucocorticoids and presence of pretransplant hypertension.[21] Tacrolimus is less likely to result in hypertension as compared with cyclosporine.[22,23]

Pathophysiology

The mechanisms of CNI-induced hypertension are multifactorial. Cyclosporine causes renal vasoconstriction through ET-1 production and decreased NO generation in preglomerular vessels. In rats, ET-A receptor antagonism largely prevents cyclosporine-induced hypertension.[24,25] Compared with cyclosporine, tacrolimus induces less vasoconstriction, in part through less extracellular calcium influx into the cytoplasm.[26]

Moreover, CNI-induced hypertension may be sodium dependent. Hypertension may be characterized by hyperkalemia and metabolic acidosis, thereby resembling familial hyperkalemic hypertension. Tacrolimus increases WNK kinase activity and, through phosphorylation of SPAK (STE20/SPS1-related proline/alanine-rich kinase) protein kinase, stimulates the thiazide-sensitive sodium chloride cotransporter (NCC) and inhibits renal outer medullary potassium channel activity. In NCC knockout mice, tacrolimus does not induce hypertension, compared with an exaggerated hypertensive response with overexpression of NCC.[27]

Increased sympathetic nervous system (SNS) activity also plays an important role in the vasoconstriction and alteration in sodium handling seen with CNIs. Cyclosporine increases SNS activity by direct postsynaptic excitation mediated by glutaminergic transmission or by increased renal afferent signaling through cyclosporine induced vasoconstriction.[27,28]

Management

DHP-CCBs are often first-line therapy because they reduce renal vascular resistance and increase renal blood flow. Superiority to other classes, however, has not been well established. In a meta-analysis of RCTs of antihypertensive treatment in kidney transplant recipients, CCBs reduced the risk of graft loss by approximately 25% and improved glomerular filtration rate (GFR) and creatinine.[29] In a crossover trial of renal transplant recipients receiving tacrolimus, both thiazide diuretics and amlodipine reduced systolic BP (SBP) by an average of 10 mm Hg. Thiazide diuretics may be especially effective in patients who have other renal tubular effects of CNIs including hyperkalemia and metabolic acidosis.[30] There are no high-quality data to support a benefit of ACEI/ARB relative to DHP-CCBs.[31–33] Thus, selection of antihypertensive drugs in the posttransplant patient should be individualized to their risk factor profile. In reality, many posttransplant patients require a multiple drug regimen for BP control in which case DHP-CCB, ACEI/ARB, and thiazide diuretics can all be considered.[34]

NONSTEROIDAL ANTIINFLAMMATORY DRUGS
Epidemiology

Nonselective nonsteroidal antiinflammatory drugs (NSAIDs) (eg, ibuprofen, naproxen, diclofenac, and indomethacin) inhibit cyclooxygenase (COX-1 and COX-2), whereas COX-2 inhibitors (eg, celecoxib and valdecoxib) were developed to decrease gastrointestinal toxicity. Cardiovascular effects, such as hypertension, are a major drawback to NSAID use. NSAID use has been shown to increase SBP by an average of 5 mm Hg and in those with established hypertension, by as much as 14 mm Hg.[35,36]

Pathophysiology

COXs regulate the synthesis of prostaglandins and are ubiquitously expressed. Inhibition of COX-2 is associated with a reduction in prostaglandin E2, which mediates natriuresis, leading to a 30% reduction in daily urine sodium excretion.[37,38] NSAIDs can also inhibit the glucuronidation of aldosterone, leading to elevated intrarenal concentrations.[39] Patients with chronic kidney disease are particularly susceptible to this sodium and fluid retention.[38,40] NSAIDs also reduce generation of vasodilatory prostaglandin I_2, a potent smooth muscle vasodilator, leading to an increase in systemic vascular resistance and mean arterial BP and reduced GFR.[40]

Data are mixed in regard to the magnitude of effect on BP of different NSAIDs.[41–44] In the PRECISION Trial, an RCT comparing cardiovascular safety of celecoxib, naproxen, and ibuprofen in patients with osteoarthritis and rheumatoid arthritis, ibuprofen demonstrated the greatest increase in SBP and a higher incidence of new-onset hypertension compared with celecoxib. In addition, the risk of hospitalization with hypertension was 69% higher in patients on ibuprofen compared with celecoxib.[45] Nevertheless, observational data suggest while intensification of antihypertensive treatment may be necessary when using NSAIDs, short-term safety issues may be infrequent even in high-risk patients.[46,47]

Management

Best management obviously centers on discontinuation of the NSAID. If therapy is essential, consider the use of an NSAID less likely to induce significant hypertension, such as nabumetone or celecoxib.[48]

GLUCOCORTICOIDS
Epidemiology

Excess glucocorticoids (GC), whether endogenous as in Cushing syndrome or from exogenous administration, induce hypertension. Hypertension occurs in approximately 20% of patients given GC.[49,50] Both dose and duration of steroid therapy contribute to risk of hypertension over time. In a retrospective analysis of patients with giant cell arteritis, there was a statistically significant increased risk of hypertension with each 1 g increase in cumulative GC use (hazard ratio 1.04 [1.01, 1.07], $P<.05$).[51] In a large US autoimmune patient cohort, both higher dosages and extended use (>60 days) of GC were associated with a significantly higher incidence of hypertension.[52]

Pathophysiology

Sodium and fluid retention through activation of mineralocorticoid receptors is an important mechanism for GC-related hypertension. Various studies, however, suggest this alone is insufficient. The GC receptor is present in both vascular smooth muscle and endothelium. Studies in smooth muscle cell culture demonstrate upregulation of AT1 receptors that mediate increased influx of Na^+ or Ca^+ into cells, thereby increasing vascular tone. In vitro experiments with endothelial cells suggest GC suppress production of vasodilators and alter vascular reactivity.[53] Beyond vascular tissue, the GC receptor is present in multiple tissues such as the kidney, adipose tissue, brain, and liver. Thus a combination of mechanisms contributes to hypertension with GC use.

Management

Given the multiple different pathways implicated in the development of GC-associated hypertension, the optimal antihypertensive regimen is unclear. If hypertension manifests early in GC use, DHP-CCBs can address the increased vascular tone. If hypertension persists, a diuretic or RAAS antagonist can be added to mitigate fluid retention.

ERYTHROPOIESIS-STIMULATING AGENTS
Epidemiology

Most commonly used in the treatment of anemia in patients with chronic kidney disease (CKD) or those receiving chemotherapy, erythropoiesis-stimulating agents (ESAs) have long been recognized for the capacity to increase BP.[54,55] A 2014 Cochrane analysis demonstrated increased odds of hypertension when compared with placebo (odds ratio ranging from 1.14, 95% confidence interval [CI] 0.99–1.32 for darbepoetin alfa to 4.10, 95% CI 2.16–7.76 for epoetin alfa).[56] Three randomized-controlled trials have raised concern about the cardiovascular safety of normalizing hemoglobin in this population, leading to a black-box label warning for serious adverse cardiovascular events.[57–59] Although the mechanism for adverse cardiovascular events is likely multifactorial, arterial hypertension may be a significant contributor. A 5 to 8 mm Hg increase in SBP and 4 to 6 mm Hg in diastolic BP (DBP) may occur in dialysis patients.[60]

Pathophysiology

ESA-induced hypertension occurs independently of red blood cell mass and viscosity.[61] With coadministration of erythropoietin-binding protein, there is preservation of the erythropoietic response and prevention of hypertension.[62] ESAs increase thromboxane and reduce prostacyclin levels, blunt response to NO-mediated vasodilation, and induce vasoconstriction through increased plasma endothelin levels. In a cross-sectional study of patients with end-stage renal disease, increased plasma levels of ET-1 directly correlated to increase in SBP.[63,64] Increased renal NO production can antagonize endothelin, serving as a counterregulatory mechanism against hypertension. This may in part explain why patients with chronic kidney disease (CKD) with reduced renal mass are more prone to hypertension from ESAs compared with normal subjects.[60,64]

Management

BP should be optimized before ESA initiation and then monitored regularly during treatment.[65] Therapeutic options for the management of ESA-associated hypertension include reduction or cessation of the ESA, optimization of volume status for patients on dialysis, or institution of antihypertensive medication. In patients with CKD who develop hypertension in association with ESA use, a potential future therapeutic alternative could be hypoxia-inducible factor prolyl hydroxylase inhibitors, as these agents may be associated with less elevation in BP.[66]

ORAL CONTRACEPTIVE PILLS
Epidemiology

In the United States, oral contraceptive pills (OCPs) are one of the most commonly prescribed birth control methods, used by approximately 10.6 million women.[67] Older literature reports new hypertension in approximately 5% of OCP users. However, there have been evolutions in OCP dose, formulation, and delivery method. Initial OCPs contained relatively high doses of estrogen and progestin, whereas contemporary OCPs contain approximately 20 to 35 mcg of ethinyl estradiol. A cohort study of 68,297 women that relied on self-reported BP measurements found an increased risk of hypertension that was highest among long-term users (risk ratio 1.8, 98% CI 1.5–2.3). After 2 years of use, there was a statistically significant, albeit small, difference in SBP and DBP compared with never users (0.9 mm Hg and 0.5 mm Hg, respectively). Twenty-four hour ambulatory BP also increased after 6 to 9 months of OCP use compared with women with an intrauterine device (BP increased from 120 ± 3/75 ± 2 to 128 ± 4/81 ± 2 mm Hg, $P<.04$).[68] A nonsignificant trend toward increased risk of hypertension with potency of progestin exists.[69]

Pathophysiology

It is likely that both exogenous estrogen and progesterone are responsible for the BP effect. The estrogenic component of OCPs increases renin and leads to stimulation of RAAS, thus mediating increased salt and water retention and vasoconstriction.[70,71] Natural progesterone produced by ovulating women counteracts this effect by aldosterone antagonism; however, synthetic progesterone lacks this ability. Although weight gain has been reported with OCP use, it has not been found to correlate to increases in BP.[68] Drospirenone, a newer progestogen derivative, has antialdosterone activity similar to natural progesterone. Clinical trials have demonstrated that drospirenone reduces BP in hypertensive postmenopausal women.[72] Importantly, drosperinone increases aldosterone concentration, thereby interfering with the diagnosis of primary hyperaldosteronism.[73] Thus, this drug should be withdrawn in women undergoing testing for secondary hypertension.

SEROTONIN NOREPINEPHRINE REUPTAKE INHIBITORS
Epidemiology

Patients with depression are more likely to suffer from cardiovascular disease. In addition, many classes of antidepressants have an adverse cardiovascular safety effect profile including QT interval prolongation, changes in BP, and sudden cardiac death.[74] Serotonin norepinephrine reuptake inhibitors (SNRIs), including venlafaxine and duloxetine, may have the greatest effect on BP. In a meta-analysis of 23 clinical trials, use of SNRIs resulted in modest SBP increases compared with selective serotonin reuptake inhibitors (mean difference 1.5 mm Hg, $P <.0001$).[75] This is consistent with 2 previously published meta-analyses evaluating the cardiovascular effects of venlafaxine. Thase[76] found a dose-dependent increase in BP when comparing venlafaxine with imipramine and placebo with a 9% increase in BP compared with placebo at doses greater than 300 mg/d. Feighner[77] similarly found a dose-related clinically significant increase in BP (defined as an increase in DBP greater than 15 mm Hg or to greater than 105 mm Hg) in 5.5% of patients on doses greater than 200 mg daily.

Pathophysiology

The likely mechanism of SNRI-induced hypertension is activation of the sympathetic nervous system secondary to increased levels of norepinephrine and potentiation of noradrenergic neurotransmission.

Management

Close monitoring of BP while using venlafaxine is reasonable. When selecting an anti-hypertensive agent, consideration of drug-drug interactions is important. A retrospective study compared venlafaxine and metabolites in patients receiving amlodipine compared with ramipril.[78] Venlafaxine metabolites were higher in patients on amlodipine, which could lead to an increase in noradrenergic affects, potentially exacerbating hypertension or negating antihypertensive effects of treatment.

DRUGS OF ABUSE
Epidemiology

MDMA (ecstasy), phencyclidine (PCP), methamphetamine, and cocaine are associated with acute hypertensive episodes. According to the 2017 National Survey on Drug Abuse and Health, lifetime use of these drugs for individuals 12 years of age or older living in the United States were estimated to be 7% for MDMA, 2.2% for PCP, 5.4% for methamphetamine, and 14.9% for cocaine.[79] In a pooled analysis of 166 healthy patients, MDMA led to SBP greater than 160 mm Hg in 33% of participants.[80] In a single-center emergency department case series of 184 patients with urine drug screens positive for PCP, hypertension was reported in 87 subjects, although in this study, criteria for hypertension was not defined, and a substantial number of patients also had coingestions that could have affected BP.[81] Of those patients who were only positive for PCP (N = 61), 32 had hypertension. Hypertension during acute methamphetamine intoxication has been described in numerous studies.[82]

Pathophysiology

MDMA, a derivative of methamphetamine, leads to an increase in the release of monoamine neurotransmitters or blockage of their reuptake.[83] PCP similarly blocks neuronal dopamine and norepinephrine reuptake.[84] Similar to MDMA and PCP, methamphetamine use leads to central nervous system (CNS) catecholamine release and also incompletely blocks neuronal reuptake.[85] Cocaine affects BP in several ways. In addition to blocking catecholamine reuptake in presynaptic neurons, the primary vasoactive metabolite of cocaine blocks sodium channels and enhances sympathetic activity.[86] In addition, chronic cocaine use is associated with arterial stiffness and atherosclerosis, potentially through impairment of NO release, increased levels of vascular cell adhesion molecules and intracellular adhesion molecules,[87] or increased generation of reactive oxygen species that further increase vascular wall stiffness.[88]

Management

Because these drugs result in CNS sympathetic excess, therapy for acute hypertension is sedation, typically with benzodiazepine therapy. CCBs and nitrates are also recommended for elevated BP that does not respond to sedation.[86,89,90] Although beta-blocker therapy has traditionally been avoided, particularly in cocaine intoxication out of concern for unopposed alpha receptor agonism, recent evidence calls this notion into question. Two meta-analyses of patients with cocaine ingestion did not demonstrate a significant difference in myocardial infarction or all-cause mortality when comparing patients who received beta-blocker therapy to those who did not.[91,92]

STIMULANTS
Epidemiology

Stimulants are most often used in the treatment of excessive daytime somnolence and narcolepsy, as well as attention deficit hyperactive disorder (ADHD). For caffeine, 200 to 300 mg can increase BP acutely an average of 8.1/5.7 mm Hg, without evidence of clear long-term effect.[93,94] Modafinil, a nonamphetamine CNS stimulant, blocks dopamine transporters and increases brain dopamine levels.[95] Although data suggest modafinil is associated with increased sympathetic activity[96] and increases in BP,[97] a more recent meta-analysis of modafinil use in pediatric patients did not show significant increase in SBP or DBP.[98] In a retrospective study of supratherapeutic modafinil exposures, hypertension was present in 6 (6.9%) patients.[99]

Stimulant medications, including methylphenidate and amphetamines, are commonly prescribed in the treatment of ADHD.[100,101] These medications either block reuptake of norepinephrine and dopamine into presynaptic neurons (methylphenidate and atomexatine) or promote the release of catecholamines (dextroamphetamine and lisdexamfetamine). In a South Korean cohort study of 1224 children designed to assess the association of methylphenidate with cardiovascular events, there was no difference in hypertension between exposed and unexposed patients.[102] In contrast, a meta-analysis of adults receiving CNS stimulant therapy for ADHD demonstrated a small elevation in SBP (2 mm Hg, CI 0.8–3.2, $P = .005$).[103]

Management

Current recommendations advise monitoring BP within the first 1 to 3 months of initiating therapy for ADHD and then every 6 to 12 months thereafter.[104] The use of beta-blockers and/or alpha-blockers can be considered.

SUMMARY

Thorough dietary and social history is important in assessing contributors to drug-induced hypertension. If a patient is to start therapy with a drug known to cause hypertension, adequate control of BP and cardiovascular risk factors beforehand is imperative. Once therapy is started, more frequent monitoring of BP is prudent. The optimal management of drug-induced hypertension is to discontinue the offending agent. If its use must continue, the selection of antihypertensive therapy should be guided by pathophysiologic and outcome data where available. In the absence of specific guidelines, management should follow current ACC/AHA guidelines.[105]

REFERENCES

1. Kantor ED, Rehm CD, Haas JS, et al. Trends in prescription drug use among adults in the United States From 1999-2012. JAMA 2015;314(17):1818–31.
2. Grossman E, Messerli FH. Drug-induced hypertension: an unappreciated cause of secondary hypertension. Am J Med 2012;125(1):14–22.
3. Lovell AR, Ernst ME. Drug-induced hypertension: focus on mechanisms and management. Curr Hypertens Rep 2017;19(5).

4. Hurwitz H, Fehrenbacher L, Novotny W, et al. Bevacizumab plus irinotecan, fluorouracil, and leucovorin for metastatic colorectal cancer. N Engl J Med 2004; 350(23):2335–42.

5. Maitland ML, Kasza KE, Karrison T, et al. Ambulatory monitoring detects sorafenib-induced blood pressure elevations on the first day of treatment. Clin Cancer Res 2009;15(19):6250–7.

6. Schlumberger M, Tahara M, Wirth LJ, et al. Lenvatinib versus placebo in radioiodine-refractory thyroid cancer. N Engl J Med 2015;372(7):621–30.

7. Soria JC, DeBraud F, Bahleda R, et al. Phase I/IIa study evaluating the safety, efficacy, pharmacokinetics, and pharmacodynamics of lucitanib in advanced solid tumors. Ann Oncol 2014;25(11):2244–51.

8. Zhu X, Wu S, Dahut WL, et al. Risks of proteinuria and hypertension with bevacizumab, an antibody against vascular endothelial growth factor: systematic review and meta-analysis. Am J Kidney Dis 2007;49(2):186–93.

9. Katsi V, Magkas N, Georgiopoulos G, et al. Arterial hypertension in patients under antineoplastic therapy: a systematic review. J Hypertens 2019;37(5): 884–901.

10. Robinson ES, Khankin EV, Karumanchi SA, et al. Hypertension induced by vascular endothelial growth factor signaling pathway inhibition: mechanisms and potential use as a biomarker. Semin Nephrol 2010;30(6):591–601.

11. Pandey AK, Singhi EK, Arroyo JP, et al. Mechanisms of VEGF (Vascular Endothelial Growth Factor) Inhibitor–Associated Hypertension and Vascular Disease. Hypertension 2018;71(2):e1–8.

12. Facemire CS, Nixon AB, Griffiths R, et al. vascular endothelial growth factor receptor 2 controls blood pressure by regulating nitric oxide synthase expression. Hypertension 2009;54(3):652–8.

13. de Jesus-Gonzalez N, Robinson E, Penchev R, et al. Regorafenib induces rapid and reversible changes in plasma nitric oxide and endothelin-1. Am J Hypertens 2012;25(10):1118–23.

14. Robinson ES, Khankin EV, Choueiri TK, et al. Suppression of the nitric oxide pathway in metastatic renal cell carcinoma patients receiving vascular endothelial growth factor–signaling inhibitors. Hypertension 2010;56(6):1131–6.

15. Mourad JJ, des Guetz G, Debbabi H, et al. Blood pressure rise following angiogenesis inhibition by bevacizumab. A crucial role for microcirculation. Ann Oncol 2008;19(5):927–34.

16. Veronese ML, Mosenkis A, Flaherty KT, et al. Mechanisms of hypertension associated with BAY 43-9006. J Clin Oncol 2006;24(9):1363–9.

17. Maitland ML, Bakris GL, Black HR, et al. Initial assessment, surveillance, and management of blood pressure in patients receiving vascular endothelial growth factor signaling pathway inhibitors. J Natl Cancer Inst 2010;102(9):596–604.

18. Hayman SR, Leung N, Grande JP, et al. VEGF inhibition, hypertension, and renal toxicity. Curr Oncol Rep 2012;14(4):285–94.

19. Miura S, Fujino M, Matsuo Y, et al. Nifedipine-induced vascular endothelial growth factor secretion from coronary smooth muscle cells promotes endothelial tube formation via the kinase insert domain-containing receptor/fetal liver kinase-1/NO pathway. Hypertens Res 2005;28(2):147–53.

20. Robert N, Wong GWK, Wright JM. Effect of cyclosporine on blood pressure. Cochrane Database Syst Rev 2010;(1):CD007893.

21. Cifkova R, Hallen H. Cyclosporin-induced hypertension. J Hypertens 2001; 19(12):2283–5.

22. Gojowy D, Adamczak M, Dudzicz S, et al. high frequency of arterial hypertension in patients after liver transplantation. Transplant Proc 2016;48(5):1721–4.

23. Vincenti F, Jensik SC, Filo RS, et al. A long-term comparison of tacrolimus (FK506) and cyclosporine in kidney transplantation: evidence for improved allograft survival at five years1. Transplantation 2002;73(5):775–82.

24. Cavarape A, Endlich K, Feletto F, et al. Contribution of endothelin receptors in renal microvessels in acute cyclosporine-mediated vasoconstriction in rats. Kidney Int 1998;53(4):963–9.

25. Takeda Y, Miyamori I, Wu P, et al. Effects of an endothelin receptor antagonist in rats with cyclosporine-induced hypertension. Hypertension 1995;26(6 Pt 1): 932–6.

26. Grześk E, Malinowski B, Wiciński M, et al. Cyclosporine-A, but not tacrolimus significantly increases reactivity of vascular smooth muscle cells. Pharmacol Rep 2016;68(1):201–5.

27. Hoorn EJ, Walsh SB, McCormick JA, et al. The calcineurin inhibitor tacrolimus activates the renal sodium chloride cotransporter to cause hypertension. Nat Med 2011;17(10):1304–9.

28. Schlaich MP, Grassi G. Sympathoexcitation in calcineurin inhibitor-induced hypertension: villain or innocent bystander? J Hypertens 2010;28(9):1809–10.

29. Cross NB, Webster AC, Masson P, et al. Antihypertensives for kidney transplant recipients: systematic review and meta-analysis of randomized controlled trials. Transplantation 2009;88(1):7–18.

30. Moes AD, Hesselink DA, van den Meiracker AH, et al. Chlorthalidone versus amlodipine for hypertension in kidney transplant recipients treated with tacrolimus: a randomized crossover trial. Am J Kidney Dis 2017;69(6):796–804.

31. Hiremath S, Fergusson DA, Fergusson N, et al. Renin-angiotensin system blockade and long-term clinical outcomes in kidney transplant recipients: a meta-analysis of randomized controlled trials. Am J Kidney Dis 2017;69(1): 78–86.

32. Zakrzewska A, Tylicki L, Debska-Slizien A. Cardiovascular and renal outcomes of renin-angiotensin system blockade in renal transplant recipients. Transplant Proc 2018;50(6):1834–7.

33. Lenihan CR, O'Kelly P, Mohan P, et al. MDRD-estimated GFR at one year post-renal transplant is a predictor of long-term graft function. Ren Fail 2008;30(4): 345–52.

34. Mangray M, Vella JP. Hypertension after kidney transplant. Am J Kidney Dis 2011;57(2):331–41.

35. Johnson AG. NSAIDs and increased blood pressure: what is the clinical significance? Drug Saf 1997;17(5):277–89.

36. Wehling M. Non-steroidal anti-inflammatory drug use in chronic pain conditions with special emphasis on the elderly and patients with relevant comorbidities: management and mitigation of risks and adverse effects. Eur J Clin Pharmacol 2014;70(10):1159–72.

37. Whelton A, Schulman G, Wallemark C, et al. Effects of celecoxib and naproxen on renal function in the elderly. Arch Intern Med 2000;160(10):1465.

38. White WB. Cardiovascular effects of the cyclooxygenase inhibitors. Hypertension 2007;49(3):408–18.

39. Knights KM, Winner LK, Elliot DJ, et al. Aldosterone glucuronidation by human liver and kidney microsomes and recombinant UDP-glucuronosyltransferases: Inhibition by NSAIDs. Br J Clin Pharmacol 2009;68(3):402–12.

40. Snowden S, Nelson R. The effects of nonsteroidal anti-inflammatory drugs on blood pressure in hypertensive patients. Cardiol Rev 2011;19(4):184–91.
41. Aw T-J, Haas SJ, Liew D, et al. Meta-analysis of cyclooxygenase-2 inhibitors and their effects on blood pressure. Arch Intern Med 2005;165:7.
42. Farkouh ME, Kirshner H, Harrington RA, et al. Comparison of lumiracoxib with naproxen and ibuprofen in the Therapeutic Arthritis Research and Gastrointestinal Event Trial (TARGET), cardiovascular outcomes: randomised controlled trial. Lancet 2004;364(9435):675–84.
43. MacDonald TM, Reginster J-Y, Littlejohn TW, et al. Effect on blood pressure of lumiracoxib versus ibuprofen in patients with osteoarthritis and controlled hypertension: a randomized trial. J Hypertens 2008;26(8):1695–702.
44. Schwartz JI, Thach C, Lasseter KC, et al. Effects of etoricoxib and comparator nonsteroidal anti-inflammatory drugs on urinary sodium excretion, blood pressure, and other renal function indicators in elderly subjects consuming a controlled sodium diet. J Clin Pharmacol 2007;47(12):1521–31.
45. Ruschitzka F, Borer JS, Krum H, et al. Differential blood pressure effects of ibuprofen, naproxen, and celecoxib in patients with arthritis: the PRECISION-ABPM (Prospective Randomized Evaluation of Celecoxib Integrated Safety Versus Ibuprofen or Naproxen Ambulatory Blood Pressure Measurement) Trial. Eur Heart J 2017;38(44):3282–92.
46. Bouck Z, Mecredy GC, Ivers NM, et al. frequency and associations of prescription nonsteroidal anti-inflammatory drug use among patients with a musculoskeletal disorder and hypertension, heart failure, or chronic kidney disease. JAMA Intern Med 2018;178(11):1516–25.
47. Fournier JP, Sommet A, Bourrel R, et al. Non-steroidal anti-inflammatory drugs (NSAIDs) and hypertension treatment intensification: a population-based cohort study. Eur J Clin Pharmacol 2012;68(11):1533–40.
48. Palmer R, Weiss R, Zusman RM, et al. Effects of nabumetone, celecoxib, and ibuprofen on blood pressure control in hypertensive patients on angiotensin converting enzyme inhibitors. Am J Hypertens 2003;16(2):135–9.
49. Goodwin JE, Geller DS. Glucocorticoid-induced hypertension. Pediatr Nephrol 2012;27(7):1059–66.
50. Mantero F, Boscaro M. Glucocorticoid-dependent hypertension. J Steroid Biochem Mol Biol 1992;43(5):409–13.
51. Gale S, Wilson JC, Chia J, et al. Risk associated with cumulative oral glucocorticoid use in patients with giant cell arteritis in real-world databases from the USA and UK. Rheumatol Ther 2018;5(2):327–40.
52. Rice JB, White AG, Johnson M, et al. Quantitative characterization of the relationship between levels of extended corticosteroid use and related adverse events in a US population. Curr Med Res Opin 2018;34(8):1519–27.
53. Hand MF, Haynes WG, Johnstone HA, et al. Erythropoietin enhances vascular responsiveness to norepinephrine in renal failure. Kidney Int 1995;48(3):806–13.
54. Berglund B, Ekblom B. Effect of recombinant human erythropoietin treatment on blood pressure and some haematological parameters in healthy men. J Intern Med 1991;229(2):125–30.
55. Lebel M, Kingma I, Grose JH, et al. Hemodynamic and hormonal changes during erythropoietin therapy in hemodialysis patients. J Am Soc Nephrol 1998; 9(1):97–104.
56. Palmer SC, Saglimbene V, Mavridis D, et al. Erythropoiesis-stimulating agents for anaemia in adults with chronic kidney disease: a network meta-analysis. Cochrane Database Syst Rev 2014;(12):CD010590.

57. Drüeke TB, Locatelli F, Clyne N, et al. normalization of hemoglobin level in patients with chronic kidney disease and anemia. N Engl J Med 2006;355(20): 2071–84.
58. Pfeffer MA, Burdmann EA, Chen C-Y, et al. A trial of darbepoetin alfa in type 2 diabetes and chronic kidney disease. N Engl J Med 2009;361(21):2019–32.
59. Singh AK, Barnhart H, Reddan D. Correction of anemia with epoetin alfa in chronic kidney disease. N Engl J Med 2006;355(20):2085–98.
60. Krapf R, Hulter HN. Arterial hypertension induced by erythropoietin and erythropoiesis-stimulating agents (ESA). Clin J Am Soc Nephrol 2009;4(2): 470–80.
61. Agarwal R. Mechanisms and mediators of hypertension induced by erythropoietin and related molecules. Nephrol Dial Transplant 2018;33(10):1690–8.
62. Lee MS, Lee JS, Lee JY. Prevention of erythropoietin-associated hypertension. Hypertension 2007;50(2):439–45.
63. Lebel M, Moreau V, Grose JH, et al. Plasma and peritoneal endothelin levels and blood pressure in CAPD patients with or without erythropoietin replacement therapy. Clin Nephrol 1998;49(5):313–8.
64. Vaziri ND. Mechanism of erythropoietin-induced hypertension. Am J Kidney Dis 1999;33(5):821–8.
65. Fishbane S, Spinowitz B. Update on anemia in ESRD and earlier stages of CKD: core curriculum 2018. Am J Kidney Dis 2018;71(3):423–35.
66. Gupta N, Wish JB. hypoxia-inducible factor prolyl hydroxylase inhibitors: a potential new treatment for anemia in patients with CKD. Am J Kidney Dis 2017; 69(6):815–26.
67. Jones J, Mosher W, Daniels K. Current contraceptive use in the united states, 2006–2010, and changes in patterns of use since 1995. Natl Health Stat Report 2012;(60):1–25.
68. Cardoso F, Polónia J, Santos A, et al. Low-dose oral contraceptives and 24-hour ambulatory blood pressure. Int J Gynaecol Obstet 1997;59(3):237–43.
69. Chasan-Taber L, Willett WC, Manson JE, et al. Prospective study of oral contraceptives and hypertension among women in the United States. Circulation 1996; 94(3):483–9.
70. Boldo A, White WB. Blood pressure effects of the oral contraceptive and postmenopausal hormone therapies. Endocrinol Metab Clin North Am 2011;40(2): 419–32, ix.
71. Ribstein J, Halimi JM, du Cailar G, et al. Renal characteristics and effect of angiotensin suppression in oral contraceptive users. Hypertension 1999; 33(1):90–5.
72. White WB, Pitt B, Preston RA, et al. Antihypertensive effects of drospirenone with 17beta-estradiol, a novel hormone treatment in postmenopausal women with stage 1 hypertension. Circulation 2005;112(13):1979–84.
73. Ahmed AH, Gordon RD, Taylor PJ, et al. Effect of contraceptives on aldosterone/ renin ratio may vary according to the components of contraceptive, renin assay method, and possibly route of administration. J Clin Endocrinol Metab 2011; 96(6):1797–804.
74. Dhar AK, Barton DA. Depression and the link with cardiovascular disease. Front Psychiatry 2016;7:33.
75. Zhong Z, Wang L, Wen X, et al. A meta-analysis of effects of selective serotonin reuptake inhibitors on blood pressure in depression treatment: outcomes from placebo and serotonin and noradrenaline reuptake inhibitor controlled trials. Neuropsychiatr Dis Treat 2017;13:2781–96.

76. Thase ME. Effects of venlafaxine on blood pressure: a meta-analysis of original data from 3744 depressed patients. J Clin Psychiatry 1998;59:502–8.
77. Feighner JP. Cardiovascular safety in depressed patients: focus on venlafaxine. J Clin Psychiatry 1995;56(12):574–9.
78. Augustin M, Schoretsanitis G, Grunder G, et al. How to treat hypertension in venlafaxine-medicated patients-pharmacokinetic considerations in prescribing amlodipine and ramipril. J Clin Psychopharmacol 2018;38(5):498–501.
79. 2017 National Survey on Drug Use and Health. Available at: https://www.samhsa.gov/data/sites/default/files/cbhsq-reports/NSDUHDetailedTabs2017/NSDUHDetailedTabs2017.htm#tab1-1B. Accessed April 24, 2019.
80. Vizeli P, Liechti ME. Safety pharmacology of acute MDMA administration in healthy subjects. J Psychopharmacol 2017;31(5):576–88.
81. Dominici P, Kopec K, Manur R, et al. Phencyclidine intoxication case series study. J Med Toxicol 2015;11(3):321–5.
82. Cruickshank CC, Dyer KR. A review of the clinical pharmacology of methamphetamine. Addiction 2009;104(7):1085–99.
83. Kalant H. The pharmacology and toxicology of "ecstasy" (MDMA) and related drugs. CMAJ 2001;165(7):917–28.
84. Akunne HC, Reid AA, Thurkauf A, et al. [3H]1-[2-(2-thienyl)cyclohexyl]piperidine labels two high-affinity binding sites in human cortex: further evidence for phencyclidine binding sites associated with the biogenic amine reuptake complex. Synapse 1991;8(4):289–300.
85. Courtney KE, Ray LA. Methamphetamine: an update on epidemiology, pharmacology, clinical phenomenology, and treatment literature. Drug Alcohol Depend 2014;143:11–21.
86. Bachi K, Mani V, Jeyachandran D, et al. Vascular disease in cocaine addiction. Atherosclerosis 2017;262:154–62.
87. Kim ST, Park T. Acute and chronic effects of cocaine on cardiovascular health. Int J Mol Sci 2019;20(3).
88. Zhu W, Wang H, Wei J, et al. Cocaine exposure increases blood pressure and aortic stiffness via the mir-30c-5p-malic enzyme 1-reactive oxygen species pathway. Hypertension 2018;71(4):752–60.
89. Paratz ED, Cunningham NJ, MacIsaac AI. The cardiac complications of methamphetamines. Heart Lung Circ 2016;25(4):325–32.
90. Richards JR, Garber D, Laurin EG, et al. Treatment of cocaine cardiovascular toxicity: a systematic review. Clin Toxicol (Phila) 2016;54(5):345–64.
91. Shin D, Lee ES, Bohra C, et al. In-hospital and long-term outcomes of betablocker treatment in cocaine users: a systematic review and meta-analysis. Cardiol Res 2019;10(1):40–7.
92. Pham D, Addison D, Kayani W, et al. Outcomes of beta blocker use in cocaineassociated chest pain: a meta-analysis. Emerg Med J 2018;35(9):559–63.
93. Mesas AE, Leon-Munoz LM, Rodriguez-Artalejo F, et al. The effect of coffee on blood pressure and cardiovascular disease in hypertensive individuals: a systematic review and meta-analysis. Am J Clin Nutr 2011;94(4):1113–26.
94. Steffen M, Kuhle C, Hensrud D, et al. The effect of coffee consumption on blood pressure and the development of hypertension: a systematic review and meta-analysis. J Hypertens 2012;30(12):2245–54.
95. Volkow ND, Fowler JS, Logan J, et al. Effects of modafinil on dopamine and dopamine transporters in the male human brain: clinical implications. JAMA 2009;301(11):1148–54.

96. Hou RH, Langley RW, Szabadi E, et al. Comparison of diphenhydramine and modafinil on arousal and autonomic functions in healthy volunteers. J Psychopharmacol 2007;21(6):567–78.

97. Taneja I, Diedrich A, Black BK, et al. Modafinil elicits sympathomedullary activation. Hypertension 2005;45(4):612–8.

98. Wang SM, Han C, Lee SJ, et al. Modafinil for the treatment of attention-deficit/hyperactivity disorder: a meta-analysis. J Psychiatr Res 2017;84:292–300.

99. Carstairs SD, Urquhart A, Hoffman J, et al. A retrospective review of supratherapeutic modafinil exposures. J Med Toxicol 2010;6(3):307–10.

100. Cooper WO, Habel LA, Sox CM, et al. ADHD drugs and serious cardiovascular events in children and young adults. N Engl J Med 2011;365(20):1896–904.

101. Volkow ND, Swanson JM. Clinical practice: adult attention deficit-hyperactivity disorder. N Engl J Med 2013;369(20):1935–44.

102. Shin JY, Roughead EE, Park BJ, et al. Cardiovascular safety of methylphenidate among children and young people with attention-deficit/hyperactivity disorder (ADHD): nationwide self controlled case series study. BMJ 2016;353:i2550.

103. Mick E, McManus DD, Goldberg RJ. Meta-analysis of increased heart rate and blood pressure associated with CNS stimulant treatment of ADHD in adults. Eur Neuropsychopharmacol 2013;23(6):534–41.

104. Fay TB, Alpert MA. Cardiovascular effects of drugs used to treat attention deficit/hyperactivity disorder part 2: impact on cardiovascular events and recommendations for evaluation and monitoring. Cardiol Rev 2019;27(4):173–8.

105. Whelton PK, Carey RM, Aronow WS, et al. 2017 ACC/AHA/AAPA/ABC/ACPM/AGS/APhA/ASH/ASPC/NMA/PCNA guideline for the prevention, detection, evaluation, and management of high blood pressure in adults. J Am Coll Cardiol 2018;71(19):e127–248.

Surgical Approach to Endocrine Hypertension in Patients with Adrenal Disorders

Jessica Shank, MD, Jason D. Prescott, MD, PhD, Aarti Mathur, MD*

KEYWORDS

- Endocrine hypertension • Secondary hypertension • Hyperaldosteronism
- Hypercortisolism • Cushing syndrome • Pheochromocytoma • Adrenalectomy

KEY POINTS

- Primary hyperaldosteronism, pheochromocytoma, and Cushing syndrome are examples of surgically treatable endocrine hypertension arising from the adrenal gland.
- Management of secondary hypertension owing to adrenal abnormalities includes treatment with specific antihypertensive agents and surgery, which can be performed by various surgical approaches.
- A lower number of antihypertensive agents, female sex, shorter duration of hypertension, and lower body mass index are among the factors that have a favorable effect on blood pressure outcome after surgery for primary aldosteronism. Surgical intervention is more cost-effective than mineralocorticoid antagonist therapy in the treatment of unilateral disease in patients with primary aldosteronism.
- In patients with Cushing syndrome and bilateral adrenal disease, adrenal venous sampling may be used to guide surgery.
- Hormone-specific preoperative and postoperative considerations are critical for optimal outcomes.

SURGICAL APPROACH IN PATIENTS WITH ENDOCRINE HYPERTENSION

Introduction

Hypertension affects approximately 31% of Americans, of which 15% of cases are attributable to secondary causes, including endocrine and nonendocrine origins.[1] Endocrine hypertension owing to adrenal gland pathologic condition can result from diagnoses of primary hyperaldosteronism, Cushing syndrome, or pheochromocytoma. Secondary hypertension owing to adrenal abnormalities can be targeted by specific antihypertensive agents or even cured by surgical intervention. This article

Disclosure Statement: The authors have nothing to disclose.
Department of Surgery, Johns Hopkins University School of Medicine, 600 North Wolfe Street, Blalock 606, Baltimore, MD 21287, USA
* Corresponding author.
E-mail address: amathu10@jhmi.edu

Endocrinol Metab Clin N Am 48 (2019) 875–885
https://doi.org/10.1016/j.ecl.2019.08.014
0889-8529/19/© 2019 Elsevier Inc. All rights reserved.
endo.theclinics.com

focuses on patient selection and perioperative considerations of each type of endocrine hypertension followed by various surgical approaches.

Hyperaldosteronism

Primary aldosteronism (PA), owing to autonomous aldosterone production by either one or both adrenal glands, is the most common cause of secondary hypertension affecting around 10% of hypertensive patients.[2] Only 40% of cases of PA occur secondary to unilateral adrenal gland hypersecretion owing to unilateral aldosterone-producing adenomas (APAs), unilateral adrenal hyperplasia, or aldosterone-producing carcinomas.[2] The remaining cases of PA occur secondary to bilateral adrenal hyperplasia.[2] Patients with unilateral disease can be cured by unilateral adrenalectomy compared with patients with bilateral adrenal hyperplasia, best treated with medical optimization. Surgical intervention is more cost-effective than mineralocorticoid antagonist therapy in the treatment of unilateral disease with an estimated cost savings of $6870 for surgical treatment compared with medical therapy for APAs in patients projected to have 41 remaining life-years.[3,4]

Preoperative considerations

Once a biochemical diagnosis of PA is confirmed, bilateral adrenal venous sampling (AVS) is pivotal in discerning unilateral versus bilateral aldosterone hypersecretion in patients who are deemed surgical candidates.[2] Although the Endocrine Society Practice guidelines recommend that younger patients (age <35) with spontaneous hypokalemia, marked aldosterone excess, and unilateral adrenal lesions with radiologic features consistent with a cortical adenoma may not need AVS, many other single-institution studies have demonstrated that up to 50% of patients would have been inappropriately managed based on imaging alone.[5–7] For this reason, the investigators obtain AVS with corticotropin (ACTH) stimulation on all patients with PA planned for surgical intervention regardless of age (**Fig. 1**). Before surgical intervention, patients require medical optimization with mineralocorticoid antagonist therapy and potassium replacement.[8]

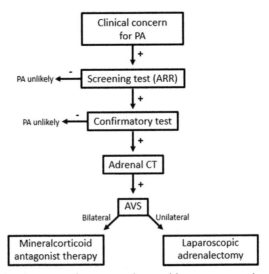

Fig. 1. Algorithm for diagnosis of PA. ARR, plasma aldosterone to renin ratio.

Postoperative considerations

Postoperatively, the remaining adrenal gland may not initially produce adequate levels of aldosterone to compensate, thereby leading to transient hypoaldosteronism and increased risk of hyperkalemia. A retrospective analysis of 192 patients after unilateral adrenalectomy for APA found 6.3% developed hyperkalemia.[9] Although this is an uncommon complication with undefined risk factors, caution must be taken to prevent hyperkalemia by instituting a low-potassium diet with increased fluid and salt intake as well as avoidance of renal aggravating medications.[10] In select patients, a short dose of fludrocortisone may be considered. In addition, serum potassium levels should be evaluated on postoperative days 1 and 14 with subsequent laboratory evaluation at 2-week intervals thereafter until normalization.[10]

After adrenalectomy, nearly all patients have reduction in antihypertensive regimen, and up to 60% of patients are cured of hypertension, likely depending on duration of hypertension before surgery.[1,2,11,12] Zarnegar and colleagues[13] established a model to predict resolution of hypertension after adrenalectomy in patients with PA, which assigns a point value to the following preoperative factors: fewer than 2 antihypertensive agents, female sex, hypertensive duration equivalent to or less than 6 years, and body mass index less than or equal to 25 kg/m^2. Likelihood of complete resolution of hypertension increases proportionally with the score.[13] Regardless of cause and treatment, hyperaldosteronism-induced cardiovascular morbidity is reduced once appropriate therapy is administered.[2]

Adrenocorticotropic-Independent Cushing Syndrome

Up to 80% of patients diagnosed with endogenous hypercortisolism are from an ACTH-dependent secreting pituitary adenoma, termed Cushing disease. ACTH-independent hypercortisolism, however, constitutes 20% of endogenous hypercortisolism cases.[14] Adrenal hypercortisolism can arise from a unilateral adenoma, unilateral hyperplasia, adrenocortical carcinoma (ACC), and rarely, primary bilateral macronodular adrenal hyperplasia (PBMAH) and primary pigmented nodular adrenocortical disease.[14-16] Subclinical Cushing syndrome results in hypercortisolism in the absence of overt signs the syndrome but is also associated with increased cardiovascular risk and mortality.[17] Subclinical Cushing may be due to unilateral hypersecretion, bilateral micronodular disease, or PBMAH.[17]

Preoperative considerations

Once a biochemical diagnosis of ACTH-independent Cushing syndrome is confirmed, cross-sectional imaging delineates anatomy and evaluates for risk of malignancy.[14,15] Patients with clinical or subclinical Cushing syndrome from an adrenal adenoma or unilateral hyperplasia are cured by unilateral adrenalectomy.[14,17] Patients with Cushing syndrome from PBMAH are cured with bilateral adrenalectomy, which results in lifelong adrenal insufficiency. However, given life-long steroid dependence and annual risk of adrenal insufficiency crisis, unilateral adrenalectomy with close follow-up has been proposed as a treatment alternative.[16] In contrast, patients with subclinical disease and bilateral adrenal abnormalities present a therapeutic conundrum.[7] AVS has been suggested in case reports to distinguish between unilateral and bilateral disease processes to guide therapy decision making.[17] However, studies thus far have been retrospective in nature with small sample sizes and inconsistent protocols to determine lateralization.[17] Some have used aldosterone to establish successful catheterization, whereas others have used epinephrine or metanephrine after administration of dexamethasone to eliminate endogenous ACTH interference.[17,18] ACC occurs in approximately 0.7 to 2 cases per million population with 40% presenting with elevated cortisol.[19] Surgery remains the only opportunity for cure, and an open incision is used to adequately obtain negative margins and decrease rates of recurrence.[19]

For patients undergoing adrenalectomy, administration of 100 mg hydrocortisone upon anesthesia induction is recommended.[20] Even patients with subclinical disease have an associated risk of inadequate cortisol surge during a stress response.[20] Subcutaneous heparin should also be administered before induction because these patients are at increased risk of development of deep venous thromboses.[21]

Postoperative considerations

Surgery results in cure of biochemical hypercortisolism along with improvement in symptoms of obesity, glucose metabolism, and hypertension.[22] Most prototypical physical characteristics of Cushing syndrome also resolve on average 7 to 9 months after surgery.[23] Immediately postoperatively, adrenal insufficiency occurs in 99.7% of frank Cushing syndrome owing to atrophy of the contralateral gland as a result of ACTH suppression from chronic cortisol excess.[24,25] Therefore, it is critical to administer postoperative stress dose steroids with an appropriate taper followed by maintenance therapy.[13] Glucocorticoids may be weaned over months to allow the hypothalamic-pituitary-axis to reestablish normal cortisol secretion from the remaining gland.[25]

Another important postoperative consideration in patients with Cushing syndrome is an increased, up to 10-fold, risk of development of venous thromboembolism owing to a hypercoagulable state.[26] An American College of Surgeons National Surgical Quality Improvement Program database retrospective study of 4217 patients who underwent adrenalectomy discovered higher rates of postoperative thromboembolism events in patients diagnosed with Cushing syndrome (2.6%) compared with patients with alternative diagnoses (1%).[27] Rates of thrombosis postoperatively rival those of major orthopedic operations, and thus, prophylaxis should be administered and maintained.[26] However, optimal duration and dose have yet to be determined.[26]

Pheochromocytoma/Paraganglioma

Pheochromocytomas originate from neural crest-derived chromaffin cells, and most (95%) arise from the adrenal medulla.[28] Of those found within the adrenal gland, 10% are malignant, and approximately one-quarter are hereditary with more than 20 germline and somatic mutations identified thus far.[1,29] Familial syndromes and genetic mutations need to be considered based on family history and presentation, including von Hippel-Lindau (VHL), RET mutation in multiple endocrine neoplasia-2 and -3 (MEN-2, MEN-3), neurofibromatosis type 1 and succinate dehydrogenase mutations.[28] Patients diagnosed with sporadic pheochromocytoma should undergo genetic testing to evaluate for one of these mutations.

Preoperative considerations

Catecholamine excess results in hypertension in 70% to 80% of patients, with paroxysmal hypertension constituting 37% of those, and normotension in the remainder.[28,30] A small portion, 30% to 40%, of patients present with the classic triad of episodic palpitations, headache, and diaphoresis.[30] Once a diagnosis is biochemically confirmed, tumor localization with imaging is crucial for surgical planning, especially in the case of extraadrenal or bilateral pheochromocytomas.[28] Adrenal protocol computed tomography (CT) imaging provides a localization sensitivity of 88% to 100%.[28] Imaging characteristics include Hounsfield units greater than 10 on noncontrast imaging, hyperenhancement after contrast administration, and delayed washout.[28,31] On MRI, pheochromocytomas appear hyperintense on T2-weighted images.[28] Functional imaging, such as a metaiodobenzylguanidine (MIBG) scan, may also be obtained to evaluate for extraadrenal lesions, bilateral disease, or metastases with an associated sensitivity of 70% to 100%.[30] Compared with MIBG and traditional PET with fludeoxyglucose/CT, 68Ga-Dotatate PET/CT better identifies primary tumors as well as extraadrenal activity.[32]

In the era before alpha- and beta-blockade agent availability, resection of pheochromocytomas resulted in unacceptably high mortalities of 13% to 45% secondary to cerebrovascular accidents and myocardial infarctions.[33] Therefore, the principal goal of preoperative management is to prevent an intraoperative hypertensive crisis. A multidisciplinary approach is recommended because these tumors are challenging, and any procedure, including those to remove the offending gland, can lead to hypertensive crises.

Initiation of antihypertensive therapy with alpha-adrenergic receptor blockers (phenoxybenzamine or doxazosin) to oppose catecholamine-induced vasoconstriction is recommended for even normotensive patients because hemodynamic instability can occur with induction or maintenance of anesthesia.[34] Alpha-blockade is titrated to nasal stuffiness or orthostatic hypotension 7 to 14 days before the operation.[28] After adequate titration of an alpha-blocker, beta-blockade may then be initiated for control of tachycardia or arrhythmias. Beta-blockade should never be the first-line agent owing to complications of unopposed alpha-receptor stimulation.[28] Calcium channel blockers may also be used in addition, if necessary. Because catecholamine excess leads to volume contraction, patients are encouraged to consume liberal fluid and salt intake perioperatively.[28] Catecholamine excess leads to suppression of insulin as well as increased glycogenolysis, which can result in hyperglycemia in pheochromocytoma patients.[34] Insulin therapy is initiated as appropriate.[34]

Anesthesia and cardiovascular evaluation, including an electrocardiogram and echocardiogram, is necessary to determine baseline cardiac function, which can be compromised secondary to coronary artery vasoconstriction and arrhythmias.[34]

Intraoperative/postoperative considerations

Laparoscopic adrenalectomy is the mainstay of therapy with bilateral cortical-sparing adrenalectomy reserved for patients with bilateral pheochromocytomas.[1,28] Intraoperative invasive blood pressure monitoring is essential to assess real-time hemodynamic changes that may occur.[34] Intraoperative hypertension is most appropriately managed with short-acting vasodilators, such as sodium nitroprusside and esmolol.[34] Excision of the gland and catecholamine source can result in profound vasodilation requiring vasoactive substances, fluid resuscitation, and blood products, which may necessitate placement of a central venous catheter.[34]

Postoperatively, these patients require intensive care monitoring because catecholamine withdrawal can lead to hemodynamic instability requiring vasopressor support. In addition, close glucose monitoring is required for potential hypoglycemia as well as neurologic sequela that may occur in approximately 4.2% patients.[35] This phenomenon is likely due to the catecholamine-initiated increase in glycogenolysis with insulin suppression and resistance resulting in hypoglycemia once the catecholamine source has been removed.[35] Retrospective studies reveal that development of hypoglycemia is associated with longer operations, larger tumor size, and extreme elevations of 24-hour urine metanephrines.[35]

Currently, the only definitive determinate of a malignant pheochromocytoma is recurrence and metastasis.[34] Therefore, long-term follow-up with plasma metanephrine level evaluations 2 to 6 weeks postoperatively and annually thereafter with imaging is required for these patients.[34]

SURGICAL TECHNIQUE FOR ADRENALECTOMY
Approach

Surgical techniques include open, laparoscopic, and robotic with various approaches, including transperitoneal or retroperitoneal. Since its first introduction in 1992, laparoscopic adrenalectomy has become widely adopted for benign tumors of the adrenal glands.[33] The laparoscopic approach has proven superior to the open approach with regards to decreased blood loss, reduction in postoperative analgesia requirements, and decreased hospital stay.[33] In retrospective comparisons, laparoscopic adrenalectomy had significantly decreased operative time and rates of ileus development, which defined the approach as more cost-effective.[36] Robot-assisted laparoscopic adrenalectomy has been shown to have similar conversion rates to the laparoscopic procedure with equivalent hospital stays and relatively similar costs.[37,38] Therefore, the laparoscopic versus robotic approach is dependent on surgeon preference, because neither has shown superiority in direct comparisons. Regardless of surgical approach, a limited touch technique should be adhered to in order to avoid transient hypertension in pheochromocytomas and to avoid capsular disruption.[33]

Although rare with an incidence of 0.5% to 1% of cases per million per year, suspicion of ACC based on imaging requires an open approach to decrease the risk of capsular rupture and seeding.[1,38,39] Adequate visualization of surrounding and potentially involved nearby structures allow for an appropriate R0 resection to reduce chances of local recurrence.[1,38,39] However, various retrospective studies have demonstrated the ability to safely remove ACC laparoscopically.[40] In one of the largest series to date of 201 cases of ACC all less than 10 cm in size, there was no difference in morbidity, mortality, margin status, 5-year disease-free survival, or overall survival rates of those resected with a minimally invasive approach compared with open approach.[40] However, prospective studies are necessary, particularly to avoid selection bias. The Society of American Gastrointestinal and Endoscopic Surgeons guidelines recommend an open resection when malignancy is likely.[40] Malignancy risk increases with imaging findings of tumors greater than 4 to 6 cm in size, Hounsfield unit values greater than 10, irregular margins, or internal heterogeneity.[39]

Right Transperitoneal Laparoscopic Adrenalectomy

Regardless of approach, the principles of adrenalectomy remain similar. Because of familiarity and authors' preference, the transperitoneal laparoscopic technique is described in detail in this text. The patient is positioned in the lateral decubitus after placement of a urinary catheter and orogastric or nasogastric tube (**Fig. 2**). Prophylactic antibiotic administration is indicated to reduce surgical site infections, and 5000

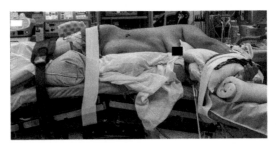

Fig. 2. Positioning for a transperitoneal laparoscopic adrenalectomy in lateral decubitus with a break in the operating room table, which allows for optimal distance between the iliac crest and costal margin.

units of subcutaneous heparin before induction decreases rates of deep venous thromboses. Three to 5 ports are placed below the costal margin, and the procedure commences with lateral mobilization of the liver (**Fig. 3**). Upward retraction of the liver with a soft paddle exposes peritoneal attachments, which when incised reveal the superior portion of the gland.[41] The kidney is identified, bringing the adrenal gland into view and delineating its inferior border.[41] Medial dissection is accomplished by incising the peritoneal attachments below the liver, separating it from the inferior vena cava.[41] In this space, the right adrenal vein is isolated, clipped, and divided. The remaining attachments are divided, and the gland is placed into an Endo Catch bag for removal (**Fig. 4**).

Left Transperitoneal Laparoscopic Adrenalectomy

After similar preparation and trocar insertion under the left costal margin, a left adrenalectomy necessitates splenic flexure mobilization that continues with lateral peritoneal attachment dissection up to the diaphragm, taking care to avoid injury to the stomach and spleen. The spleen and pancreas subsequently fall medially, allowing for adrenal gland and kidney visualization. Gerota fascia is incised on the anterior surface, which is continued laterally toward the retroperitoneal muscle. That maneuver creates separation between Gerota fascia overlying the kidney and a superior fat pad encasing the adrenal gland, which avoids inadvertent injury to the pancreas. Identification of the phrenic vein often verifies that the dissection is occurring in the correct plane. Once the adrenal gland is isolated, the left adrenal vein can be found on the medial aspect, allowing for clip placement and vein ligation.

Retroperitoneoscopic Adrenalectomy

A retroperitoneal approach is advantageous in avoidance of the intraabdominal space and, therefore, the potential sequelae of abdominal surgery, including adhesions from previous operations and a more direct route to access the adrenal glands.[42] The primary disadvantage is the size limitation because this approach offers only a small working space and is recommended for glands less than 6 cm in dimension.[42,43] Patients require prone positioning with the operating room table in the prone jack-knife configuration.[42] Port placement is triangulated around the tip of the 12th rib, the largest of which is the camera port at the apex.[42] Following entry into the retroperitoneal space, the fat is retracted inferiorly, which creates the operative field with medial vertebral muscle, lateral intraabdominal organs with spleen on the left and liver on the

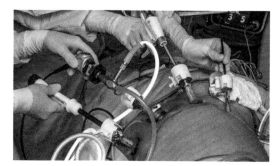

Fig. 3. Ideal port placement is along the costal margin for a transperitoneal laparoscopic adrenalectomy. The function of the working ports in order from medial to lateral are as follows: port for liver retraction, camera port, working port with harmonic scalpel, and port for inferior kidney retraction.

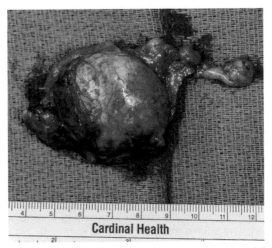

Fig. 4. An excised adrenal gland with a hyperfunctioning cortical nodule.

right, and the diaphragm cranially.[42] Dissection commences with exposure of the upper aspect of the kidney, which is retracted caudally with the fat.[42] Blunt dissection is continued until the vein is identified, clipped, and ligated.

Comparisons between retroperitoneoscopic and transabdominal laparoscopic approaches have been equivocal, and no definitive recommendations have been made.[43,44] Thus, surgeon preference continues to guide operative-approach decision making.

Cortical-Sparing Adrenalectomy

Bilateral pheochromocytomas occur in cases of familial syndromes, particularly MEN-2 and VHL. Treatment with bilateral adrenalectomy results in risk of adrenal insufficiency and obligate lifelong steroid therapy. Therefore, these patients can be treated more optimally with bilateral cortical-sparing adrenalectomy foregoing the aforementioned potential complications.[45] The surgical concepts are similar to complete adrenalectomy, but also include mindful preservation of a portion of vascularized cortex.[45] The transabdominal laparoscopic technique requires repositioning after partial gland excision in order to operate on the contralateral side, whereas the retroperitoneoscopic approach requires no repositioning. Regardless of technique, a cortical rim is identified separately from the medullary tumor with circumferential dissection of the specimen and double ligation with laparoscopic clips of the main adrenal vein.[46] A laparoscopic stapler can then be taken across the remaining cortex, which preserves the superior/medial aspect of the cortex to remain in situ.[46]

Complications

Recent studies suggest that patients who undergo adrenalectomy have few complications with an average hospital length of stay around 3 days and a zero 30-day mortality.[47] Bleeding requiring transfusion remains the most common complication at 2.6% followed by local infection at 1.2%, and laceration of viscus at 0.8%.[47] Complications tend to be more common among patients younger than the age of 60, female patients, obese patients, and patients of lower socioeconomic status.[48] Overall adrenalectomy is a well-tolerated procedure with potential for significant benefits and improvement in symptoms.

SUMMARY

Adrenal hormonal hypersecretion of aldosterone, cortisol, and catecholamines causes secondary hypertension. Endocrine hypertension potentially results in higher cardiovascular and cerebrovascular complication rates compared with essential hypertension counterparts. Select patients may undergo surgical resection for potential cure. Surgical interventions range from laparoscopic adrenalectomy, robot-assisted laparoscopic adrenalectomy, to open procedures. Perioperative management is unique to each pathologic adrenal entity and remains essential for optimal outcomes. Surgical intervention can be curative and can reverse the risk of cardiovascular events once hypertension is controlled.

ACKNOWLEDGMENTS

The corresponding author would like to acknowledge grant K23 AG053429.

REFERENCES

1. Koch CA, Chrousos GP. Overview of endocrine hypertension. In: Feingold KR, Anawalt B, Boyce A, et al, editors. Endotext [Internet]. South Dartmouth (MA): MDText.com, Inc; 2016. p. 1–25. Available at: https://www.ncbi.nlm.nih.gov/books/NBK278980/.
2. Vilela LAP, Almeida MQ. Diagnosis and management of primary aldosteronism. Arch Endocrinol Metab 2017;61:305–12.
3. Sywak M, Pasieka JL. Long-term follow-up and cost benefit of adrenalectomy in patients with primary hyperaldosteronism. Br J Surg 2002;89:1587–93.
4. Reimel B, Zanocco K, Russo MJ, et al. The management of aldosterone-producing adrenal adenomas—does adrenalectomy increase costs? Surgery 2010;148(6):1178–85.
5. Funder JW, Carey RM, Mantero F, et al. The management of primary aldosteronism: case detection, diagnosis, and treatment: an Endocrine Society clinical practice guideline. J Clin Endocrinol Metab 2016;101:1889–916.
6. Wachtel H, Zaheer S, Shah PK, et al. Role of adrenal vein sampling in primary aldosteronism: impact of imaging, localization, and age. J Surg Oncol 2016; 113(5):532–7.
7. Mathur A, Kemp CD, Dutta U, et al. Consequences of adrenal venous sampling in primary hyperaldosteronism and predictors of unilateral adrenal disease. J Am Coll Surg 2010;211:384–90.
8. Chen ZW, Hung CS, Wu VC, et al. Primary aldosteronism and cerebrovascular diseases. Endocrinol Meab (Seoul) 2018;33(4):429–34.
9. Shariq OA, Banco I, Cronin PA, et al. Contralateral suppression of aldosterone at adrenal venous sampling predicts hyperkalemia following adrenalectomy for primary aldosteronism. Surgery 2018;163(1):183–90.
10. Tahir A, McLaughlin K, Kline G. Severe hyperkalemia following adrenalectomy for aldosteronoma: prediction, pathogenesis and approach to clinical management-a case series. BMC Endocr Disord 2016;16(1):43.
11. Vorselaars WMCM, Nell S, Postma EL, et al. Clinical outcomes after unilateral adrenalectomy for primary aldosteronism. JAMA Surg 2019;154(4):e185842.
12. Miller BS, Turcu AF, Nanba AT, et al. Refining the definitions of biochemical and clinical cure for primary aldosteronism using the primary aldosteronism surgical outcomes (PASO) classification system. World J Surg 2018;42(2):453–63.

13. Zarnegar R, Young WF, Lee J, et al. The aldosteronoma resolution score: predicting complete resolution of hypertension after adrenalectomy for aldosteronoma. Ann Surg 2008;247:511–8.

14. Chaudhry HS, Singh G. Cushing syndrome. StatPearls [Internet]. Treasure Island (FL): StatPearls Publishing; 2018. Available at: https://www.ncbi.nlm.nih.gov/books/NBK470218/.

15. Hirsch D, Shimon I, Manisterski Y, et al. Cushing's syndrome: comparison between Cushing's disease and adrenal Cushing's. Endocrine 2018;62:712.

16. De Venanzi A, Alencar GA, Bourdeau I, et al. Primary bilateral macronodular adrenal hyperplasia. Curr Opin Endocrinol Diabetes Obes 2014;21(3):177–84.

17. Maghrabi A, Yaqub M, Denning KL, et al. Challenges in the diagnostic work-up and management of patients with subclinical Cushing's syndrome and bilateral adrenal masses. Endocr Pract 2013;19(3):515–21. Available at: https://search-proquest-com.proxy1.library.jhu.edu/docview/1518679894?accountid=11752.

18. Ueland GÅ, Methlie P, Jøssang DE, et al. Adrenal venous sampling for assessment of autonomous cortisol secretion. J Clin Endocrinol Metab 2018;103(12):4553–60.

19. Puglisis S, Perotti P, Pia A, et al. Adrenocortical carcinoma with hypercortisolism. Endocrinol Metab Clin North Am 2018;47(2):395–407.

20. Tsinberg M, Liu C, Duh QY. Subclinical Cushing's syndrome. J Surg Oncol 2012; 106(5):572–4.

21. Weatherill D, Spence AA. Anesthesia and disorders of the adrenal cortex. Br J Anaesth 1984;56(7):741–9.

22. Iacobone M, Citton M, Scarpa M, et al. Systematic review of surgical treatment of subclinical Cushing's syndrome. Br J Surg 2015;102(4):318–30.

23. Sippel RS, Elaraj DM, Kebebew E, et al. Waiting for change: symptom resolution after adrenalectomy for Cushing's syndrome. Surgery 2008;144(6):1060–1.

24. Di Dalmazi G, Berr CM, Fassnacht M, et al. Adrenal function after adrenalectomy for subclinical hypercortisolism and Cushing's syndrome: a systematic review of the literature. J Clin Endocrinol Metab 2014;99(8):2637–45.

25. Raff H, Carroll T. Cushing's syndrome: from physiological principles to diagnosis and clinical care. J Physiol 2015;593:493–506.

26. Van der Pas R, Leebeek FWG, Hofland LJ, et al. Hypercoagulability in Cushing's syndrome: prevalence, pathogenesis and treatment. Clin Endocrinol 2013;78: 481–8.

27. Babic B, De Roulet A, Volpe A, et al. Is VTE prophylaxis necessary on discharge for patients undergoing adrenalectomy for cushing syndrome? J Endocr Soc 2019;3(2):304–13.

28. Gunawardane PK, Grossman A. Phaeochromocytoma and paraganglioma. In: Islam MS, editor. Hypertension: from basic research to clinical practice. Advances in experimental medicine and biology, vol. 956. Cham (Switzerland): Springer; 2016. p. 239–59.

29. Fishbein L, Leshchiner I, Walter V, et al. Comprehensive molecular characterization of pheochromocytoma and paraganglioma. Cancer Cell 2017;31(2):181–93.

30. Davison AS, Jones DM, Ruthven S, et al. Clinical evaluation and treatment of phaeochromocytoma. Ann Clin Biochem 2018;55(1):34–48.

31. Northcutt BG, Trakhtenbroit MA, Gomez EN, et al. Adrenal adenoma and pheochromocytoma: comparison of multidetector CT venous enhancement levels and washout characteristics. J Comput Assisted Tomogr 2016;40(2):194–200.

32. Moreau A, Giraudet AL, Kryza D, et al. Quantitative analysis of normal and pathologic adrenal glands with 18F-FDOPA PET/CT: focus on pheochromocytomas. Nucl Med Commun 2017;38(9):771–9.
33. Aggeli C, Nixon AM, Parianos C, et al. Surgery for pheochromocytoma: a 20-year experience of a single institution. Hormones (Athens) 2017;16(4):388–95.
34. Naranjo J, Dodd S, Martin YN. Perioperative management of pheochromocytoma. J Cardiothorac Vasc Anesth 2017;31(4):1427–39.
35. Chen Y, Hodin RA, Pandolfi C, et al. Hypoglycemia after resection of pheochromocytoma. Surgery 2014;156:1404–9.
36. Soares RL Jr, Monchik J, Migliori SJ, et al. Laparoscopic adrenalectomy for benign adrenal neoplasms. Surg Endosc 1999;13(1):40–2.
37. Probst KA, Ohlmann CH, Saar M, et al. Robot-assisted vs open adrenalectomy: evaluation of cost-effectiveness and peri-operative outcome. BJU Int 2016; 118(6):952–7.
38. Paduraru DN, Nica A, Carsote M, et al. Adrenalectomy for Cushing's syndrome: do's and don'ts. J Med Life 2016;9(4):334–41.
39. Sgourakis G, Lanitis S, Kouloura A, et al. Laparoscopic versus open adrenalectomy for stage I/II adrenocortical carcinoma: meta-analysis of outcomes. J Invest Surg 2015;28(3):145–52.
40. Jing H, Li F, Wang L, et al. Comparison of the 68Ga-DOTATATA PET/CT, FDG PET/CT, and MIBG SPECT/CT in the evaluation of suspected primary pheochromocytomas and paragangliomas. Clin Nucl Med 2017;42(7):525–9.
41. Giulea MA, Nădrăgea M, Enciu O. Laparoscopic partial adrenalectomy. Chirurgia (Bucur) 2017;112(1):77–81.
42. De Crea C, Raffaelli M, D'Amato G, et al. Retroperitoneoscopic adrenalectomy: tips and tricks. Updates Surg 2017;69(2):267–70.
43. Lombardi CP, Raffaelli M, De Crea C, et al. Endoscopic adrenalectomy: is there an optimal operative approach? Results of a single-center case-control study. Surgery 2008;144(6):1008–14.
44. Constantinides VA, Christakis I, Touska P, et al. Systematic review and meta-analysis of retroperitoneoscopic versus laparoscopic adrenalectomy. Br J Surg 2012;99(12):1639–48.
45. Biteman BR, Randall JA, Brody F. Laparoscopic bilateral cortical-sparing adrenalectomy for pheochromocytoma. Surg Endosc 2016;30(12):5622–3.
46. Sackett WR, Bambach CP. Bilateral subtotal laparoscopic adrenalectomy for phaeochromocytoma. ANZ J Surg 2003;73(8):664–6.
47. Thompson LH, Nordenström E, Almquist M, et al. Risk factors for complications after adrenalectomy: results from a comprehensive national database. Langenbecks Arch Surg 2016;402(2):315–22.
48. Hauch A, Al-Qurayshi Z, Kandil E. Factors associated with higher risk of complications after adrenal surgery. Ann Surg Oncol 2015;22(1):103–10.

Printed and bound by CPI Group (UK) Ltd, Croydon, CR0 4YY

08/05/2025

01864746-0003